OXFORD MEDICAL PUBLICATION

An Introduction to Health Planning in Developing Countries

An Introduction to Health Planning in Developing Countries

SECOND EDITION

ANDREW GREEN

Senior Lecturer and Head of the International Division,
Nuffield Institute for Health, University of Leeds, Leeds

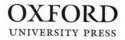

OXFORD
UNIVERSITY PRESS

OXFORD
UNIVERSITY PRESS

Great Clarendon Street, Oxford OX2 6DP

Oxford University Press is a department of the University of Oxford.
It furthers the University's objective of excellence in research, scholarship,
and education by publishing worldwide in

Oxford New York

Athens Auckland Bangkok Bogotá Buenos Aires Calcutta
Cape Town Chennai Dar es Salaam Delhi Florence Hong Kong Istanbul
Karachi Kuala Lumpur Madrid Melbourne Mexico City Mumbai
Nairobi Paris São Paulo Singapore Taipei Tokyo Toronto Warsaw

with associated companies in Berlin Ibadan

Oxford is a registered trade mark of Oxford University Press
in the UK and in certain other countries

Published in the United States
by Oxford University Press Inc., New York

First published 1992
First published as paperback 1994
Reprinted 1995, 1996, 1997, 1998
Second edition published 1999

British Library Cataloguing in Publication Data
Data available

Library of Congress Cataloging in Publication Data
Green, Andrew, 1952–
An introduction to health planning in developing countries/
Andrew Green. – 2nd ed.
Includes bibliographical references and index.
ISBN 0 19 262985 9 (Hbk.). ISBN 0 19 262984 0 (Pbk.)
1. Health planning–Developing countries.   2. Medicine, State–Developing countries.
I. Title.
RA395.D44G74 1999   362.1'09172'4–dc21   99–27071

1 3 5 7 9 10 8 6 4 2

ISBN 0 19 262984 0 (Pbk)

Typeset in Berkeley
by J&L Composition Ltd, Filey, North Yorkshire
Printed in Great Britain
on acid-free paper by
Biddles Ltd, Guildford & King's Lynn

Preface to second edition

The first edition of this book was written in 1991 and published a year later. In the period since, there have been a number of changes in the international context which have implications for health planning and which it is hoped this new edition will reflect and address. Of particular significance are the political changes in central and eastern Europe, the economic crisis that has hit parts of the world, and in particular south-east Asia, and the emergence of Health Sector Reform (HSR) as the policy agenda of the decade.

Although the basic dilemma that planning attempts to deal with (a shortage of resources compared to health needs) is shared by all the health systems of the world and thus the principles of planning are the same, the particular characteristics of individual health systems and socio-economic and political contexts suggest that the specific application of these principles may need to be different. I have always felt uncomfortable with the term 'developing countries', which has a number of negative connotations particularly when put alongside the term 'developed countries'. However, I originally chose it for the title, in the absence of a better and accepted term, to indicate a target group of countries sharing a particular set of constraints. In particular the primary focus was on the health sectors in countries in Africa, the Middle East, and parts of Asia and South America. The changes in central and eastern Europe have left many of these countries trying to develop new, more flexible and decentralized approaches to health-care under clear resource constraints and facing similar concerns to those of the original target audience and it is hoped that planners and policy-makers in these countries may also find something of use in this book. Furthermore, a number of countries in south-east Asia, which five years ago were seen as economic growth success stories, are now facing considerable difficulties with significant implications for their health sectors and it is hoped that there may be something of interest in this edition for them. Lastly, it is my belief that health systems even in higher income, industrialized countries can learn from the approaches and experiences of developing countries and that this book may assist this learning process.

The previous edition was founded on the principles of Primary Health Care (PHC) which, for many countries, was the major policy paradigm of the 1980s. I believe strongly that these principles still should form the bedrock of health systems, though recognize that this is seen in some quarters as an old-fashioned view. The main policy thrust of the 1990s has been HSR which, for some policy-makers, has replaced PHC as the focus of attention. At one level, reform of the health sector is, of course, an inevitable, dynamic and important process that should be continuously occurring in response to the changing environment that all health systems face. There can be no single and simple solution to how the health sector is configured. Indeed, PHC policies themselves clearly suggest the need for reform of health sector structures in most if not all countries, and planners should be in the forefront of such changes. However, the reform agenda of the early 1990s encouraged particular health system models based on principles of competition. This reflected the neo-liberal ideology underpinning parts of the 'reform' movement which were not confined to developing countries and indeed were often manifest in market oriented reforms such as those of the UK. Such models are less obviously consistent with the principles of PHC and in particular that of equity. At the time of writing this, there appears to be some signs that the early evangelism for the market is being replaced by a recognition that there are no universal solutions, and indeed that reform can provide no easy panacea to the underlying resource constraints. However the reforms have focused critical attention on not just the current practice of the public sector but also the role of the State including in the area of strategic planning, the focus of this book. The first edition made no pretence at suggesting that all was well with the practice of health planning and indeed was founded on a belief that significant changes were needed. HSR policies may in themselves force planners to reconsider their roles and capacities and this is to be welcomed. However, this book continues to be based on a belief that the State does have a key strategic role in the health sector and that planning is an important mechanism for carrying out this role.

This is reflected in the changes to the content of the book. The basic chapter structure remains the same, but Chapter 3 is significantly expanded to include discussion of HSR policies. Elsewhere in the book, changes have also been made to reflect the implications of HSR on health planning. The limitation of being able to make only a limited number of changes in updating to a second edition has, however, provided a practical constraint and prioritizing decisions (familiar to all planners!) on where to make changes.

In addition, the production of a second edition has allowed me the opportunity to correct a number of minor errors that existed in the first edition. I have been alerted to some of these by students and colleagues to whom I am grateful. One embarrassing example was Figure 2.4, in which I used the analogy of political 'winds' affecting the speed and direction of the implementation of plans. It was pointed out to me, shortly after publication of the first edition, that the way I had drawn the winds would lead to no movement at all, and possible capsize, demonstrating my ignorance of matters nautical! I have also ironically had to remove references to Health For All by the Year 2000, as we move into the next century. It is hoped, however, that the new millennium may prove to be the beginning of the restrengthening of strategic planning, and that this new edition will play some small part in this.

Leeds   A. G.
May 1999

Acknowledgements to the second edition

A number of people have contributed in different ways to this second edition. Colleagues at the Nuffield Institute have been helpful in a number of different ways; in particular Michelle Abbott, Charles Collins, Deborah Hale, Steve Harrison, Maureen Hastie, David Hunter, Marianne Lubben, Ann Matthias, James Newell, Maye Omar, Nicola Ruck, Jane Shaw, and Terry Nicholson. Colleagues in the Information Resource Centre at the Institute have also, as always, been helpful with references; in particular Lorraine Bate, Jackie Gerrard, Liz Lodge, and Susan Mottram. Students and former students, both at the Nuffield Institute and elsewhere, have provided inputs both knowingly and unknowingly. The interest shown in planning in classes and the feedback given, particularly when illustrated with examples from the experience of participants, has provided an important learning source for me. Some have gone beyond this and made specific textual suggestions and I would wish to acknowledge their input; in particular Lia Van Antwerpen, Mike Curtis, Allan Johnson, Margaret Kaseje, Sidney Ndeki, Mohammad Rana, Jondi Flavier and Gotfried Mubyazi. I have also learnt greatly from the experience of projects with which I have been involved over the last eight years. In particular I would draw attention to discussions with Barkat Ali, Abdul Naeem, Duncan Ross and Colin Thunhurst in Pakistan, and Andres Rannamae in Estonia which have all helped me to understand, better, strategic planning.

Lastly, as in the first edition, I would wish to acknowledge the support from my family and in particular Mary over both the period since the first edition and during the process of revising, which has at times felt like a new book.

Preface to the first edition

The origins of this book are straightforward, and twofold. The first dates back to 1976, when I was employed by the Swaziland government with the specific remit to set up a national planning unit in the Ministry of Health. I was a development economist with exposure to the health sector from previous work as an economist in West Africa. My experience of national health planning was, however, very limited and second-hand. I expected to be supported in this new position by books from practising health planners, academics, WHO — anyone! To my dismay there were very few readily available publications which dealt with the real and practical issues with which I was concerned — health planning from the perspective of the public sector in developing countries.

A number of years later I joined the Nuffield Institute for Health Services Studies as the member of teaching staff responsible for courses in health planning. My students were experienced health professionals from a variety of developing countries who had risen to positions in planning and management. In the period since I had started in a similar position, there had been various publications; but still none seemed to deal with the real issues which I had confronted. The closest was a short book by Oscar Gish, who had worked in a similar capacity in Tanzania earlier. However, its brevity left one wishing for more! In order to satisfy the needs of my students I had to develop my own teaching materials.

This book stems directly from this lack of material on planning the health sector. Since that time, the situation has improved. As the introductory readings at the end of the first two chapters show, there are now a number of texts on health planning. However, though all are useful in their own fields, none quite hit the spot that I was looking for. My own experience of planning both from my days in Southern Africa and on numerous consultancy visits since have taught me that the successful planner (if such a rare breed exists!) is a combination of a technician and a politician. Texts on planning tend to deal with one or other of these aspects. Some texts provide excellent introductions to the technical aspects of planning; others concentrate on the political aspects. Few combine these in a way that I feel is essential. This book tries to complement these other, more specialist books. Whether it succeeds or not, I leave to you to judge.

The objective of this book, then, is to introduce prospective practitioners to the wonders and mysteries of the art of planning. By practitioners, I do not mean just those who will work in offices with the title 'Health Planner' outside the door. One theme of this book is that, if the art of health planning is to succeed, it must be owned by as wide a constituency as possible. This book is aimed therefore not just at 'health planners', but at the health service professionals who recognize the need to engage in the planning process. I also use the words 'art of planning' carefully. Planning is not a science; and there are no correct answers to the multitudinous dilemmas that face planners. Attempts to reduce planning to a series of techniques are doomed to failure by their lack of recognition of the politics of planning. If there is one theme that does run through this book it is this. Planning is about change — and change inevitably has its losers, and hence opponents. Planning is as much concerned with analysing who are the losers and winners of situations, and deciding how to handle them, as it is with technical analysis. The book therefore aims to introduce readers to the technical aspects of planning *within* the context of the wider political arena. It is not intended as a comprehensive planning manual, but rather as a taster of some of the issues and techniques.

A number of further points need to be made about the scope of the book. Firstly, this book has a public sector emphasis. Though many of the issues and techniques are the same for NGOs and others outside the public health sector, and indeed it is hoped that people working in such organizations will find it of use and interest, its perspective is that of the public sector planning system. Thus, though it recognizes very clearly the importance of other sectors in health-care provision and related health matters, it looks at these from the viewpoint of the public sector. Early in the book we explore the different roles that the state can, in theory, play in health-care delivery. In this book I make the broad assumption that the state *is* a major player in the health-care arena. Such a role is well understood in many African, Asian, and to a lesser degree South American countries.

Secondly, the book is aimed primarily at developing countries. Many of the issues and themes of the book are of course, common to *all* health care systems. For example, the relationship between techniques and political analysis is common to all systems, and the broad characteristics of a planning system based in primary health care should be universal. Indeed the health planning systems of many 'more developed' countries have much to learn from the health planning systems of developing countries, and it is hoped that readers with a primary interest in industrialized health systems may also find the book of interest. However the book is written from the context of developing countries. No attempt is made, in the book, to define what I mean by 'developing', and I am well aware of the difficulties of using such a broad and inaccurate term. However, it is used here to denote countries whose health systems are grappling with major health problems in the face of severe resource shortages and embryonic infrastructures. In the course of writing the book, there have been major changes in the political structures of Eastern Europe; and these dual elements of severe resource constraints and organizational change face planners in those countries very starkly. It is hoped that, in addition to planners in the countries more conventionally described as developing, there may be some parts of this book that such Eastern European planners may find of use.

Thirdly, the book does not try to provide a blueprint for planning. Such an arrogant attitude would run counter to the very spirit of primary health care and of this book. In addition, the very varied socio-political and economic contexts of different countries make such an approach not only unwise but impossible. However it is easy to use such arguments as an excuse for dealing only in generalities; but for many readers practical examples are needed as pegs on which to hang the underlying concepts. As such, at various stages in the book, examples are given of how a planning system might approach particular issues. The most comprehensive of these is provided in the last chapter in the book, where the various elements of planning are brought together in the form of a case study of an overall health planning system. They must however be treated in the spirit in which they are provided — as exemplars and not as prescriptions.

Lastly, while health planning and policy are closely connected, this book does not attempt to discuss alternative policy options. This is for two reasons. Firstly, in contrast to the area of health planning, there are numerous other books around which deal with specific aspects of policy. A number of these are referenced at the end of Chapter 3. Secondly, however, of more importance here is the recognition that health policy cannot be formed in isolation. The development of health policy should result from the planning process itself, and should be specific to each context. This book is concerned therefore with the *process* of forming and implementing policy, rather than with the specific policies resulting from that process. Having said that, however, there is one major policy assumption that underlies the whole book, and that is an acceptance of the principles and philosophy of primary health care. This policy foundation has major implications for the type of planning process developed.

The structure of the book is straightforward. The first half looks at a number of background issues to health planning. Chapter 1 provides a general introduction to the rationale for planning as a means of making decisions about the future. As part of this rationale it examines the arguments as to why planning, rather a market mechanism for allocating health care, is appropriate within a primary health care context. This is followed in Chapter 2 by a description of different approaches to, and theories of, planning. The importance of recognizing the dual nature of planning as technical and a political process is introduced, and the different emphases given to techniques and political analysis within different approaches to planning are examined. Chapter 3 looks at the origins of primary health care and at the implications of this philosophy, as set out in the Alma-Ata Declaration, for planning. One major aspect of this philosophy is the need to recognize the inputs both of other health agencies and of health-related agencies. Chapter 4 examines how a framework for this wider view can be developed. There has been little recognition in many countries of the current roles of non-governmental organizations, and this chapter looks in particular at how government can use the planning process to consider policies towards this sector. Finally in this first half of the book, different approaches to the financing of health care are discussed. Planning is concerned with managing the inevitable disparities between needs and available resources. One planning strategy concerns attempting to increase the available resources; and Chapter 5 looks at the potential for, and the problems of, such strategies.

The second half of the book then takes each of the different conceptual stages of the planning spiral introduced in Chapter 2 and examines them in more detail. Information is essential in the planning process; and Chapter 6 looks at the needs for information and at the planning information systems that will help to provide appropriate information. Chapter 7 builds on this by examining the first step of any planning process, the analysis of the current situation.

Possibly the most difficult part of the planning process is that of setting priorities. Indeed, it is this activity that most graphically demonstrates the interaction between techniques and value judgements which underlies all planning activity. Chapter 8 sets out the issues involved in the setting of priorities, relating these back to the principles of primary health care.

Underlying all planning decisions is the concept of opportunity cost: the fact that every time a decision is made to carry out an action, this automatically implies that some other action cannot be undertaken — an opportunity is lost. Costing, as a technique, is important both as a component of the option appraisal process and as part of budgeting. Chapter 9 looks at cost concepts and different techniques of costing. Chapter 10 introduces approaches to option appraisal and evaluation. It initially looks at economic techniques as a commonly used framework, and then widens this to incorporate a number of other perspectives which economic appraisal alone would ignore. Evaluation asks many similar questions to appraisal; and the second half of Chapter 10 looks more specifically at issues in evaluation.

Plans are only possible to achieve if the resources are allocated in a manner consistent with the priorities set. However, for many health systems the resource-allocation process is divorced from the planning process. This is discussed in Chapter 11, and various ways in which resources can be allocated and budgets can be set are outlined.

One of the commonest and severest criticisms of planning is that it is full of good intentions that never materialize into action. Chapter 12 looks at the common causes of poor implementation, and how they can be improved. Many of the difficulties in implementation can in fact be traced back to poor planning at an earlier stage of the process. However there are also a number of techniques at the implementation stage itself which can be useful, and these are introduced. The penultimate chapter is concerned with the most important resource available in the health sector — human resources. Planning human resources (or manpower planning, as it is often called) is a strangely neglected part of planning. Yet personnel account for the greater part of health sector expenditure; and without an appropriate supply of staff, plans cannot be implemented. Chapter 13 sets out different approaches to human-resource planning.

The final chapter brings together the various elements of the planning spiral. It develops criteria for a health planning system which is relevant to the needs of primary health care and provides a framework for the different elements of planning.

Each chapter follows a similar format. At the beginning of the chapter is an introduction to the topics covered, and at the end a short summary. Within the chapters, boxes, figures, and tables are used to illustrate the text. Figures and tables are conventionally used. Boxes are reserved for self-standing examples or concepts. For each chapter there is also a list of references, including suggested introductory readings. At the end of most chapters there is also a short exercise, which is intended to help readers to develop their own thoughts on the subject, or to try out simple techniques introduced in the chapter. Many of these can be done alone; but some are more appropriate to group work.

Underlying all health planning is a belief that the low and unacceptable health status faced by many communities and individuals in developing countries *can* be improved, and that the process of planning is an important means to that end. Planning is concerned with creating the future from the constraints of the present. It is, however, not an easy process — and indeed it can be a very lonely one for planners. The type of radical changes needed to improve health status are not popular with many groups within the health sector, and such changes will continue to meet with resistance. The development of a planning culture and planning system is a slow, a continuous, and indeed a never-ending process. This book has been written as a contribution to that process.

Leeds   A. G.
1992

Acknowledgements to the first edition

Thanks are due to a number of people for their input into the production of this book. Firstly to previous students who have pointed out the lack of such a text and encouraged me to fill the gap. Colleagues within the International Division and elsewhere within the Institute have also been very supportive and positively critical. Staff at the specialist Information Resource Centre at the Institute have been tireless in their assistance in tracking down references. I also owe a great debt of thanks to Hilary Sharp, whose skills have been greatly stretched in trying to make sense of my own crude attempts at word processing. She has persevered and succeeded where many others would have failed.

Lastly, the major debt of thanks is due to my family, who have supported me in this task. My parents, Tom and Mab Green, have tried to remind me of the basic rules of the English language. Remaining split infinitives are entirely my responsibility! I hope that the associations between books and late nights and weekend working do not have a permanent negative effect on my children, Laura, Christopher, and Martin, who have been extremely tolerant with me during this last year. Above all, my greatest thanks are reserved for Mary for her patience and support.

Contents

Abbreviations   xx

1   What is planning, and why plan?   1

Development of formalized planning   1
Health planning   2
Rationale for health planning   2
What is allocative planning?   3
Scarcity and choice — the basis for planning   3
What is meant by the term 'health'?   7
Different perspectives on health and health-care   8
The market as a means of determining allocations   9
The state's responsibilities in the health sector   11
State attitudes to different types of health-care   14
Attitudes to health planning   15
Planning as an open transparent process   18
Planning as a technocratic or as a political activity   18
Summary   19
Introductory reading   20
Exercise 1   20
References and further reading   20

2   Approaches to planning   24

Planning models   24
Realistic rational planning   31
Planning as a political process   33
Private and public sector planning   34
Levels of planning   36
Planning, management, and policy   37
Planning activities and terms   37
Summary   40
Introductory reading   40
Exercise 2   40
References and further reading   41

3 The policy context: Primary Health Care and
   Health Sector Reform   43
   Origins of Primary Health Care   43
   The Alma-Ata declaration   49
   Equity   50
   Community participation   55
   A multisectoral approach to health   57
   Appropriate technology and service mix   58
   A health-promotive and preventive approach   59
   Decentralization   59
   Multiagency collaboration   61
   Obstacles to the implementation of a PHC approach   61
   Health sector reform   63
   HSR, PHC, and planning   66
   Summary   68
   Introductory reading   68
   Exercise 3   69
   References and further reading   69

4 Planning for health   74
   Planning for the health-care sector   75
   Development of government policies and plans towards
   non-State organizations   81
   Planning for health promotion   88
   Planning for health   91
   Summary   93
   Introductory reading   93
   Exercise 4   93
   References and further reading   94

5 Financing health-care   95
   The context   95
   Alternative strategies to increase effective resource levels 98
   Criteria for choosing a financing system   100
   Alternative approaches to financing health-care   103
   Planning and financing   110
   Summary   111
   Introductory reading   111
   Exercise 5   113
   References and further reading   113

6 Information for planning   116
   What is information and why do we need it?   116
   Paralysis by analysis   118

Accuracy of information 118
Spatial and time considerations 121
Level of aggregation of information 122
Type of information 123
Information systems 127
Summary 133
Introductory reading 133
Exercise 6 134
References and further reading 134

7 **Situational analysis** **137**
Population characteristics 138
Area characteristics and infrastructure 139
Policy and political environment 141
Health needs 141
The non-health sector: plans and services provided 143
Health services 143
Resources 144
Efficiency, effectiveness, equity, and quality of current services 147
Analysis of the situation 147
Who should carry out the situational analysis? 148
Summary 149
Introductory reading 149
Exercise 7 149
References and further reading 149

8 **Setting priorities** **151**
Health and need 151
Need as perceived by the community and by
    the health professions 153
Underlying perceptions of health 154
Who should set priorities? 159
Establishing priorities within a planning framework 161
Priority-setting and PHC 165
Summary 166
Introductory reading 167
Exercise 8 167
References and further reading 168

9 **Costs and costing** **170**
What is meant by costs? 170
Whose costs? 171
Real or market prices? 174
Costing methods 176

Levels of accuracy and sources of information   180
Unit costs   181
Recurrent cost coefficients   182
Costs relationships   182
Apportionment of joint costs   184
Cash-flow analysis   186
Summary   187
Introductory reading   187
Exercise 9: Marginal and average cost example   187
References and further reading   188

10 Option appraisal and evaluation   **190**
Economic appraisal techniques   191
Option appraisal and economic appraisal   203
Forms and checklists   206
Option appraisal and programming   206
Appraisal and evaluation   207
Evaluation   207
Evaluation questions   208
Evaluations and situational analysis   211
Summary   211
Introductory reading   212
Exercise 10   212
References and further reading   213

11 Resource allocation and budgeting   **215**
Different forms of budget   215
Budgeting and resource allocation approaches   219
The budgeting process   226
Financial management and accounting   229
Summary   234
Introductory reading   235
Exercise 11   235
References and further reading   235

12 Programmes, projects, implementation, and monitoring   **237**
Programmes and projects   237
Implementation   239
Causes of poor implementation   240
Improving the record on implementation   243
Monitoring   255
Location of projects and programmes   256
Implementation of services provided by other agencies   257
Summary   257

Introductory reading   257
Exercise 12   258
References and further reading   258

13 Planning human resources   260

What is human resource planning?   260
The record on human resource planning   261
Why is the record on human resource planning so poor?   262
Human resource planning — an approach   263
Assess demand   265
Assess supply   268
Determine mismatches between the estimated demand and supply over
   time and location   273
Determine appropriate action to minimize mismatches   273
Regularly review and update plan   274
Human resource planning implementation   274
Relationship to the planning process   275
Human resource planning and Health Sector Reform   276
Summary   277
Introductory reading   277
Exercise 13   278
References and further reading   279

14 The state of planning and planning for the State   280

Assessment criteria   281
An illustrative case study of a planning system   293
A planning culture   300
The future of State planning   301
Introductory reading   302
Exercise 14   302
References and further reading   302

Index   305

Abbreviations

BCR	benefit to cost ratio
BoD	Burden of Disease
CBA	cost–benefit analysis
CBD	community based distribution
CEA	cost–effectiveness analysis
CUA	cost–utility analysis
DALY	Disability Adjusted Life Year
DOTS	Directly Observed Treatment, Short Course
EPI	expanded program of immunization
FP	family planning
GNP	gross national product
HMO	Health Maintenance Organization
HSR	Health Sector Reform
ILO	International Labour Organization
IMF	International Monetary Fund
IRR	internal rate of return
IT	information technology
MCH	mother-and-child health
MIS	management information systems
MOV	means of verification
MPNHD	Managerial Process for National Health Development
NGO	non-governmental organization
NHS	National Health Service (UK)
NPV	net present value
OVI	objectively verifiable indicators
PHC	Primary Health Care
PPBS	Planning Programme Budgeting Systems
PQLI	Physical Quality of Life Indicator
QALY	Quality-Adjusted Life Year
TFR	total fertility rate

1

What is planning, and why plan?

For many health-care professionals, the term 'planning' may be confusing, as it is used by different people in very different ways. The activity itself may be seen as mysterious, complex, and possibly irrelevant to their daily lives either at work or at home. This introductory chapter explains the rationale for planning and its development, and discusses possible reasons for negative attitudes towards it in some quarters.

There are a number of different styles and approaches to planning. Later in the chapter a more precise definition of planning will be introduced. At this point, however, it is sufficient to recognize that all planning approaches share one common element — a concern about making decisions relating to the future.

When reduced to this fundamental, planning is of course neither new nor confined to organizations. At a personal level most of us plan to some degree or other. We are constantly making decisions about our futures — ranging from what we will do tomorrow, through holiday plans, to our careers. Indeed, we may be very scornful of those who fail to plan!

As a formalized, specialist discipline, however, planning is relatively new. Although this book makes no pretence to being a history of planning, it is worth spending a moment tracing some of the influences over this century which have led to the rise of planning.

DEVELOPMENT OF FORMALIZED PLANNING

Firstly, planning, as a separate identifiable activity in organizations, has been partly the result of the growth, during this century, of businesses from small family concerns to large organizations, including multi-billion dollar multinationals. The size and complexity of such organizations has resulted in the need for decisions about the future to be taken in both a more considered and a more explicit manner. This has led to a rise in business planning techniques, which include such specialist skills as market forecasting.

By contrast, the second influence came from the rise of State economic planning, initially in the former USSR following the Russian revolution. The attempt to build an economy based on nationally determined economic plans resulted in a major development of formalized State planning (and indeed of the planning bureaucracy). This rise in State planning was not confined to the non-capitalist economies of Eastern Europe, but can be seen in the period before the Second World War in the increasing State intervention in the UK during the depression of the 1930s and in the New Deal activities of Roosevelt in the USA.

The third influence came during the Second World War, when the shortages caused by a wartime economy, together with the specific military needs of a country at war, led to centralized controls in countries such as the UK.

In the period following the Second World War three major trends can be discerned which had further implications for the rise in planning:

- The reconstruction of Europe after the war inevitably involved major State intervention in the economies of the European countries.

- In some countries — notably the UK — shifts in political power and ideology led to an acceptance of government responsibility for the provision of certain social welfare services, including health and education, on a scale that required long-term decisions to be taken. These did not necessarily result immediately in explicit planning structures, however. In the UK, for example, which set up its National Health Service 50 years ago, a formalized health planning system was set up only in the 1970s.

- The drive for the independence of colonies during the 1950s and 1960s gave impetus to the need to develop clear strategies for economic development. Few countries, following independence, failed to develop national economic (and later social) planning structures. In India, for example, the first 5 year plan dates back to 1951.

HEALTH PLANNING

This book is concerned primarily with the role of the State in health planning. For many developing countries, the birth of State health planning can be traced to the 1970s, and to a shift in development thinking (discussed further in Chapter 3) away from pure economic growth to broader social (including health) goals. There are, however, notable exceptions: some, such as India and some Latin American countries, whose health planning activities can be traced back to a much earlier date, and others for whom planning is still in its gestation.

Given this long history in planning at an individual level, within business, and by the State, one might expect its rationale to be clearly understood and accepted. However, partly as a result of its relative newness to the health sector, its basis and role in the health field is often not well understood. It is important, therefore, to be clear why we need to plan for health and health-care.

RATIONALE FOR HEALTH PLANNING

Later in this chapter different forms of planning will be looked at in more detail. Essentially, however, the health planning that this book is concerned with can be viewed as falling into two broad types — activity planning and allocative planning.

- *Activity planning* relates to the setting of monitorable timetables and schedules for the implementation of pre-set activities. As good management practice, such planning is straightforward, provided it does not become too rigid. Chapter 12 deals particularly with this aspect of planning.

- The more complex and contentious side of planning, with which this book is primarily concerned, is *allocative planning* — the making of decisions on how resources should be spent.

WHAT IS ALLOCATIVE PLANNING?

Definitions of planning abound, although most carry with them the same essentials. The following tries to capture this essence, but makes no pretence to being a more useful definition than many others:

Planning is a systematic method of trying to attain explicit objectives for the future through the efficient and appropriate use of resources, available now and in the future.

The important components of this and other similar definitions are concepts of:

- where are we going (*objectives*)

- with what (*resources*)

- how (*efficient and appropriate implementation*)

- when? (*future*)

- degree of formalization (*explicitness*, *systematic* and *method*) about the process.

As such, planning involves a system of making decisions about how an organization will use its resources in and for the future. Note, however, that the above definition does not restrict planning to effecting change solely with the organization's own resources. An organization can stimulate change by direct changes in the services provided by itself, or by inducing change in other organizations. This will be discussed later, with particular reference to the dual role of the State in planning any services it provides directly, and in regulating the services and standards of other organizations, including the private sector.

    Plans, the result of such planning decisions, are therefore statements of intent concerning how resources will be used to achieve the organization's objectives.

SCARCITY AND CHOICE — THE BASIS FOR PLANNING

The need for such decisions is based on the recognition that resources are limited. At the individual level it is not difficult to recognize that most of us have wants that outstrip our available income, and that we have to make choices between these — decisions which are often difficult. Choices are also needed in organizations. For example, manufacturing organizations need to make decisions as to whether their current mix of products is appropriate for the future. They also need to decide whether to grow, contract, or consolidate. Such organizations have limited funds at their disposal to invest in new activities, and must make choices. Organizations providing services — such as the health sector — need to consider whether the current mix of services provided should change to meet future requirements, and whether the location and means of provision of services are appropriate. It will not be possible to meet all requirements, and decisions on which are the most important are also needed. Such prioritizing decisions again stem from the limited resources referred to above.

As economists would say, resources are scarce in comparison to the uses to which a society or an organization wishes to put them. Within the health sector, the resources available are insufficient to meet all the health-care needs or demands that society would ideally like satisfied. This scarcity is not confined to developing countries; the concept is equally applicable to the wealthier countries of the world. In the UK, for example, over £800 is currently spent on health-care for each citizen each year; yet significant health needs remain unmet — as evidenced, for example, by waiting lists for operations — and health professionals argue strongly for more funds. Despite the much higher levels of resources available to the health service in the UK compared with a country such as Bangladesh, or even a middle-income country such as Estonia, decisions are still necessary as to which needs will be met and — as significantly — which will therefore be left unmet. Although this gap exists within a well-resourced country such as the UK, it is far more severe in resource-poor countries, as illustrated in Table 1.1.

Table 1.1   Indicators of health-care resource and needs: selected countries and regions

Countries	Health expenditure per capita ($)	Health expenditure (% of GDP)	Child mortality rate (deaths per 1000 under 5 years)	Life expectancy at birth (years)
Sub-Saharan Africa	24	4.5	175	52
India	21	6.0	127	58
China	11	3.5	43	69
Other Asia and islands	61	4.5	97	62
Latin America and Caribbean	105	4.0	60	70
Middle Eastern crescent	77	4.1	111	61
Formerly socialist economies of Europe	142	3.6	22	72
Established market economies	1860	9.6	11	76
World	323	8.0	96	65

Source: Compiled from World Bank *World Development Report* (OUP 1993), using various tables; data generally refers to 1990.

Though this may be a politically unpalatable fact, it is increasingly recognized that no health-care system can meet all the health-care needs of its citizens and therefore that prioritizing decisions and a consequent rationing of resources have to be made. This is the hardest and most challenging aspect of health planning, but also potentially the most satisfying when resources are successfully channelled away from low priority uses to high priority ones. Figure 1.1 gives some examples of the sort of choices that the health sector needs to make at different levels.

Planning, then, is an activity that all organizations carry out with greater or lesser degrees of explicitness. Furthermore, as we have seen, planning is not an activity

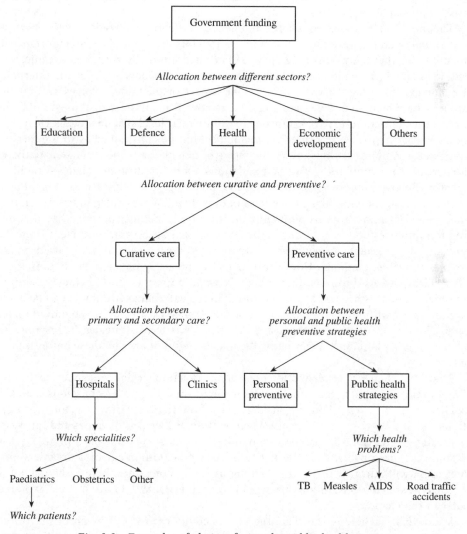

Fig. 1.1 Examples of choices facing the public health sector

confined to the public sector. Within the private sector, private hospitals need to plan — whether to expand or not and in what areas, where staff are to come from, what charges to levy, and so on. Most individuals also make comparable micro-level decisions, for example, about whether to build or extend a home, and whether or when to send their children to school. The degree to which we would normally refer to such decisions as 'planning' largely revolves around the degree to which the decision was open and explicit, and we explore this aspect later in the chapter.

Planning involves the making of choices — and so requires the possibility of *real* alternatives. Where such choices are *not* available, allocative planning has no function. People living in conditions of absolute poverty may have no alternative to their basic survival strategy, and hence may be in no position to plan, in the sense that the term has been used above.

The range of alternatives available, and hence the degrees of freedom with which an individual or an organization can operate, is therefore crucial to the real importance of planning for that body. This range may be curtailed internally within an organization (by, for example, its constitutional structure, or by professional attitudes) or externally (by, for example, legislative controls). One aspect of planning revolves around the amount by which such constraints can be removed or minimized, thus shifting the boundaries of planning. An example at the individual level may make this clearer. A house-owner may wish to extend her/his house, but be constrained as to the form of the extension by regulations, or by the views of neighbours. One strategy may therefore require attempting to get these regulations altered or attitudes changed to allow greater effective choice. Some definitions of planning stress this aspect. Planning is seen as a means of minimizing the effects of outside influences on an organization that may cause deviation from its optimal path. It is also sometimes portrayed as attempting to minimize the levels of uncertainty or risk that an organization faces from the outside environment. Sometimes a situation of great uncertainty is used as an argument against planning. However, it is in fact precisely under such circumstances that a clear view as the direction in which we want to travel is most obviously required in order that necessary responses to changes in the external environment can be made appropriately without losing sight of the sectoral aims. Clearly, what is required under such circumstances is a willingness to change short-term strategies in response to change, and a planning system that is flexible enough not only to allow but indeed to ensure this.

Decisions, then, are needed in the present about actions which will affect the future. For an individual such decisions may be made to some degree subconsciously, and as such may involve less explicit consideration of alternatives. However, for organizations which involve groups of people, each with their own sets of values and interests, a greater degree of transparency is required about such decisions. In this sense planning is inescapable. Real alternative courses of action do exist for organizations, and these will affect their futures. As long as such choices are there to be made (or created), explicit decision-making would seem inevitable. This is further explored later in the chapter.

We have so far referred to planning as an activity carried out by an organization, whether private or public. The aims of such organizations will of course differ, and this may affect the manner in which decisions are made. Strategic decisions as to the direction to be followed are, however, required by all organizations.

This book is primarily concerned with the role of the State in health planning. Inasmuch as the State may provide health-care, the importance and role of planning in the provision of such services is similar to that in other organizations — though its aims and methods may differ. In addition, however, the State is different from other organizations in that it has wider responsibilities in the promotion of the health of its citizens. These responsibilities suggest a particular form of health planning for the State, which is broader and qualitatively different from that undertaken by other organizations. Different countries have different views of these responsibilities, depending on a number of factors — in particular the ideology of the ruling group and historical factors. These influence what is meant by 'health' and how it is viewed, and are now examined.

WHAT IS MEANT BY THE TERM 'HEALTH'?

'Health' is a word widely used in everyday conversation, with little apparent ambiguity. However, closer examination reveals various different interpretations — each with different implications for the role of the State. It is important to recognize, first, the difference between 'health' and 'health-care'; terms which are frequently (and inaccurately) interchanged. This point is discussed in more detail later, but some preliminary remarks are necessary here. The term 'health' refers to a state either of an individual or of a community. This state of health may be influenced by a number of factors, including health-care. However, other factors affecting health range from poverty, education levels, food intake, employment, access to clean water, and sanitation and housing conditions through to personal practices such as sexual behaviour or smoking.

The narrowest concept of health sees it as a measure of the state of the physical bodily organs. An individual is unhealthy if there is a malfunctioning of a part of the body, for example the lungs or kidney. A broader, but related, definition sees health not just in terms of the mechanics of the different bodily organs, but in the ability of the body as a whole to function. In contrast, the WHO definition of health as 'a state of physical, mental and social well-being and not merely the absence of disease or infirmity', indicates a clear shift away from earlier narrow organic or functionally based definitions of health to a more holistic view. It sees the health of an individual or community as being concerned not only with physical (and mental) status, but also with social and economic relationships.

How one views health will affect the type of intervention and planning possible. The narrowest definitions are closely associated with a medical model of health, in which the role of health services is seen as paramount in restoring the functioning of the unhealthy body. Wider Primary Health Care (PHC) concepts (see Chapter 3) suggest that much broader interventions, including individual and community empowerment and anti-poverty measures, are necessary to promote health.

We turn now to differing perspectives on the importance of health, and hence on possible roles of the State in promoting it. Four main perspectives can be distinguished.

DIFFERENT PERSPECTIVES ON HEALTH AND HEALTH-CARE

Health as a right

Health is viewed by some as a right, analogous to justice or political freedom. Indeed the WHO constitution states that '. . . the enjoyment of the highest attainable standard of health is one of the fundamental rights of every human being without distinction of race, religion, political belief, economic or social condition' (WHO Constitution, quoted in Corrigan (1979), p. 7). Few would, however, believe that equal health status is attainable in the same way that equal political freedom may be. However, health is seen as so fundamental that constraints to its full attainment must be minimized. Part of this involves ensuring access to health-care, which is the second possible perspective. Logically it would also require a commitment to removing all the other constraints to full health, as health-care is only one of the factors affecting an individual's health.

Health-care as a right

A second position views access to health-care, rather than the unattainable equality of health, as the appropriate right. The State is seen as having a responsibility to ensure this, comparable with its role in ensuring equal justice. Under such a view a government will be particularly concerned with issues of equity in health-care. Access to health-care may be viewed as similar to access to a minimal level of food and shelter. Indeed, a frequent version of this attitude is that there is a right to *basic* health-care rather than *all* levels of health-care.

Health as a consumption good

For others health is seen as an important individual objective, which is not comparable with 'justice', but rather with material aspects of life. Such a view may refer to health or health-care as a consumption good. The State here has no special responsibilities in the promotion of health, but leaves decisions as to its comparative importance to an individual. The State role under such a view might be limited to ensuring that the health-care provided is of an adequate quality (such as ensuring professional standards are maintained), in the same way that it would monitor the quality of any goods or services, such as food.

Health as an investment

A final view of health is that it is important, but largely because it affects the productive ability of the workforce. Illness may affect overall production, either through absenteeism or by lowering productivity through its debilitating effects. The development strategies for many countries (both colonial and post-colonial) during the 1950s and 1960s saw the prime factor in, and indicator of, development as growth in Gross National Product (GNP). These strategies were reflected in the emphasis placed by the State on the productive sectors — industry, agriculture and mineral extraction. To compete for attention (and funding) the apparent effects of ill health on productivity were often stressed by advocates of the health sector (albeit with little clear evidence of the links).

Such a view of health-care as primarily an investment good or a means to an end, rather than as an end in itself, persists in some quarters, although its influence has been reduced by a variety of factors:

- the recognition that growth in GNP does not by itself lead to the form of develop-ment many would wish to see, but often instead to a widening of inequalities in society, with little alleviation of the condition of the poorest

- the recognition that changes in the health status of an individual, particularly within an agricultural economy affected by seasonal variations, with periods of underemployment and family-based labour systems, may not have the expected effect on production levels

- the fact that, if taken to its logical conclusion, the effects of such a strategy on provision for health-care for non-productive groups, such as the elderly, would be unacceptable.

The above contrasting views of health and health-care have been portrayed as existing in isolation. In practice no government or society is likely to subscribe to a simplistic view consisting of any one of these on its own. Furthermore, attitudes may differ between different types of health-care: life-saving interventions are likely to be viewed differently to cosmetic surgery, and preventive care for children, such as measles immunizations, may be viewed differently to hip replacements for the elderly. These attitudes can be seen as components of a more complex attitude to health. They demonstrate that governments with different views of health (linked to their ideologies) are likely to view their responsibilities to the health sector in very different ways. New Right governments are likely to see health as an individual responsibility with a minimal State role, whereas socialist governments may see access to health-care as a right with the State thus having a major role to play in promoting this.

Before examining these potential State roles in the health sector, a short diversion is needed to introduce the economic concept of 'the market'.

THE MARKET AS A MEANS OF DETERMINING ALLOCATIONS

Until now, the view of planning with which we have been concerned has concentrated on its role in assisting an organization to make decisions about how it will use its resources. The economic context within which these organizations operate has not been mentioned, and must now be introduced.

The simplest form of economic relationship is that of the private market, in which a number of providers of services or goods sell these to individuals wishing to buy them. Under nineteenth-century classical economic theory, this 'market' was regarded as the most efficient way of operating an economy, particularly when there were a large number of buyers and sellers competing with each other. Perfect competition was seen as a means of ensuring that prices were kept down and the demands of consumers were met, hence maximizing the welfare of the country. This theory forms the basis of the economic policy of capitalist states. Under such policies, decisions on the allocation of resources to different services and goods and the utilization of these services and consumption of goods are left to 'the market' to sort out, using the mechanism of supply and demand. An increase in the demand for one service results, in the medium term, in a concomitant increase in the supply of that service to meet the demand. In the short run, the price for that good may rise to 'choke off' the increased demand, until increased supplies (responding to the price increases) are available. Within the health-care field such a pure model would involve individuals paying for health-care purchased from independent practitioners and hospitals operating for the purpose of maximizing profits. Individuals unable to pay would fail to receive care. Hospitals and specialties that were popular would be able to increase their fee levels, whereas less popular practices would have to reduce fee levels or even go out of business as a result of the lack of demand. Resources would flow (be allocated) to the former away from the latter.

The overall theory of perfect competition can be fundamentally criticized, notably by Marxist economic theory, as being ultimately unstable and not welfare-promoting. In addition, there are particular reasons, advanced by welfare economists from the neo-classical school of economics, as to why the use of the private market as a means of allocating resources is likely to fail in the health-care field.

Firstly, the particular nature of health-care implies that the conditions which classical theory set out as being prerequisites for the functioning of the market are likely to break down in the area of health-care. Classical theory requires that there is perfect knowledge by the purchaser of the goods or services, and that buyers and suppliers operate independently. However, it is often the case that 'consumers' of health-care may not themselves have adequate knowledge to make decisions as to their precise needs, but look to a health professional to assist them in doing this. The provider of the service (the doctor) is then also determining the need or demand for the health-care, undermining the principle of independent action.

Classical theory also requires that the effect of a purchase by one individual does not affect a decision by another. In the area of health-care, however, there are many decisions which are not in this way 'private' to the individual. Two examples may clarify this. Firstly, some public health services (such as environmental protection leading to clean air) can only be provided to communities and cannot be provided solely to individuals. Secondly, knowledge that others are being immunized may lead an individual to decide not to be vaccinated, on the basis that s/he will be protected by the immunity of the others. (Of course, if everyone thought in this way, sufficient levels of immunity within the community to protect it — known as herd immunity — would not be reached.) Both of these are examples where market provision would not maximize welfare.

There is a second major reason why health-care is regarded by many as inappropriate for provision through the 'market'. As we have seen, access to health-care is regarded by many as a right, and so as something which should not be affected by an individual's ability to pay. Yet this is precisely what a market does: it discriminates according to ability to pay.

There are other reasons why the operation of the market is regarded by many as inappropriate for at least some, if not all, forms of health-care. This book is not an economics textbook, and the reader who wishes to pursue these arguments is advised to consult such a text (suggestions for further reading are given at the end of the chapter). Suffice it to say at this point that there is a wide consensus on the fact that at least some, if not all, forms of health-care are inappropriate for allocation through the market.

In the absence of a market to send messages as to how resources should be allocated, a different mechanism is required. Needs-based health planning — under which the State makes or influences these decisions on behalf of the citizens — is such an alternative. Such an approach occurs to some degree in every country in the world; there is no country in which a completely private health-care market exists. However, the exact role and degree of involvement of the State in this aspect of planning, the broad allocation of resources, varies — a variation we shall now examine.

THE STATE'S RESPONSIBILITIES IN THE HEALTH SECTOR

There are four main categories of activities that are needed for the functioning of a health system — policy formation, financing, service provision, and regulation. The State may have different types and levels of roles within these in different countries.

The State and health policy formation

The first potential role for government is that of setting health and health-care policy. A government that viewed health or access to health-care as a right could be expected to take a lead role in setting policy for the sector as a whole. Elements of such policy might range from broad statements concerning the relative roles in the health sector of different health-care organizations such as private hospitals, to setting requirements for health providers on such matters as location of health facilities and technical medical matters (for example, immunization schedules, professional standards and training, and pharmaceuticals). A government that viewed health-care as a consumption good with no special characteristics might still set policy concerning the operation of the medical market, for example ensuring that pricing mechanisms operated smoothly and enforcing regulations concerning health professional recognition. The links between policy formation and planning are very close and will be discussed further in Chapters 3 and 4.

The State and financing of health-care

Finance for health-care can be provided in a number of ways (discussed in Chapter 5). Ultimately, whichever system is used, it is the citizens of a country who pay for its health-care. However, the means and distribution of responsibility for payment have important implications. Individuals can pay directly at the time of consumption of health-care (through user charges or fees for service) in a number of ways, or can insure themselves against such bills through some form of prepayment. Alternatively, the State can take responsibility for financing health-care through some central funding mechanism, such as taxation or social insurance, which has no relationship to the level or type of personal service provided. (More complex variations of these approaches are discussed further in Chapter 5.)

Under a private market approach the State has a minimal role in the actual generation of funds for health-care, although it may have a regulatory role in ensuring that charges for health-care are set and administered fairly. Under a more collective financing mechanism, the State takes a more proactive role in collecting the finance for health-care (through taxes or insurance contributions) and distributing it to the service providers. Under such a system there is opportunity for the equitable collection and disbursement of funds as the State contracts with health-care agencies public (and/or private) to provide health-care under conditions it sets.

The State as a service provider

We referred above to the State's role in financing health-care. The next potential responsibility involves the actual provision of health-care. The governments of many developing countries, particularly in Africa and Asia and the transitional economies of central and eastern Europe, currently have a major role in directly providing health-care, in owning facilities, and in employing health staff. In some countries this is a legacy from the colonial period, when the health ministry may have been responsible directly for the health-care of certain groups of people (such as civil servants, colonial officers, and the army). In central and eastern Europe this is a legacy of former communist policy. In some countries it is the result of a deliberate current policy decision, based on a belief that State control of health-care is desirable. In particular, it may be viewed as the most efficient (through economies of scale, whereby large-scale integrated provision is seen as reducing unit costs) or the most equitable method.

Elsewhere the State may see a role for itself in organizing the financing of health-care, but considers that the job of providing health services is best done by non-State organizations (the private or voluntary sector). Under such a scenario it is still possible for the State as the financer (and therefore ultimately as the purchaser) of the health-care to exert a major control over the nature and the direction of the health providers.

The State as a regulator

Lastly, the State may have a role as a regulator of the type and quality of health-care provision. The regulatory function is, to a large degree, the converse of the policy function. It is the mechanism that ensures that the policies set are carried out. As such regulations could be set concerning any aspect of health-care, and the breadth and depth of such a role will again depend on the view the State has of health and hence its role within it. Thus regulation could be set in areas as diverse as health-care charges, standards for health-care provision, location of health facilities, the type and size of health facilities allowed, and professional standards. The ability of the government to carry out such regulatory functions will depend both on the resources it is able to devote to the function, often under-resourced in the past, and its political power.

Figure 1.2 sets out a matrix showing how different combinations of the role of the State are possible in two of these roles, financing and provision. As a means of illustrating the potential diversity, the following set out a number of caricatures of governments combining the above possible roles.

- An extreme libertarian capitalist government may see its role as a regulator of health-care (to minimize distortions to the market mechanisms), but have no interest in funding or providing services. In such a situation the actual provision and management of health-care is left to the private sector — a market solution to the dilemma of scarcity and choice. This may (more usually) be tempered by a recognition that extreme inequities result from such a market solution, and the government may provide some form of safety net to deal with those cases who might otherwise be an embarrassment to them through the failure of the market. Medicare and Medicaid in the USA are examples of safety nets under such a system,

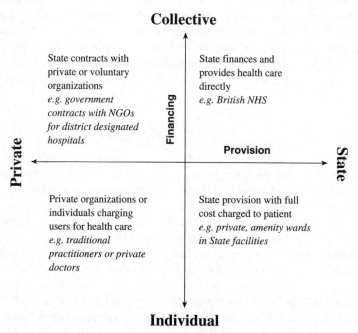

Fig. 1.2 Combinations of financing and provision of health-care

through which certain groups, including elderly and poor people, may be protected from the consequences of the failure of pure market provision.

- Further along the spectrum, the State may wish to control or influence the provision of health-care (including when it views it as a potential investment good) without necessarily directly providing it. In such situations there may be some central funding of health-care, but the provision of services is left to other agencies, whether private or closely related to the government. Some Latin American and central and east European countries fall into this category, with social security institutions playing a role in financing and often in service provision. Here the government is likely to exert a degree of control over the type of health-care provided (although not necessarily through the health ministry, which may well be politically weak).

- The next point on the spectrum involves the financing and provision of health-care facilities by the State directly. Such a situation may exist either for historical reasons (it can be argued for example that the Conservative governments of the UK in the 1980s and 1990s had little ideological sympathy with the National Health Service, but found it politically difficult to discard), or through a belief that direct State provision is either more efficient or more equitable, or both. Such State provision may be one of only a few services so provided, as a result of a particular regard for health-care; or,as in centrally planned states, it may take its place alongside a variety of others.

We have been using the term 'State' to refer to organizations under the direct control of government, although it has to be recognized that the boundaries are not always well defined. Some institutions, such as the health ministry, clearly fall within the definition, but for others such as social security institutions or hospital trusts which have a greater degree of autonomy, the situation less clear. In this book 'State' is used to refer to organizations for which the government has the ultimate power to control strategic direction.

STATE ATTITUDES TO DIFFERENT TYPES OF HEALTH-CARE

Up to now the term 'health-care' has been used to denote a wide variety of activities, ranging from public health services (such as environmental sanitation), through personal preventive services (such as immunization), to personal curative services. The above scenarios may thus vary, in that the attitudes and responsibilities of the State to each of these may differ. Governments that do not regard provision of individual curative care as a proper activity for the State may well regard the provision of public health services as their responsibility (because of their collective nature).

This book is set within the context in which many countries (particularly in Africa, Asia, the Caribbean, and central and eastern Europe) find themselves, with the State historically having had a major role in the provision of all types of health-care.

Although in some countries there may in addition be a significant private or voluntary sector, it is here assumed that the State plays the leading role.

This is still the case despite policies by agencies such as the World Bank which promote the role of the private sector in health-care. Such policies have been fuelled in part by the global recession, which has hit many developing countries hard, and affected the ability of the public sector to maintain levels of health-care expenditure. This, together with policies of Structural Adjustment imposed by the International Monetary Fund (IMF), has forced expenditure restrictions on their public health sectors. There appears, however, to be a broad recognition that the socio-economic condition of these countries is such that the private sector cannot totally supplant the State health sector. Furthermore, needs-focused policies are, we shall argue, inconsistent with reliance on the private sector. Chapter 4 deals specifically with the relations between these sectors.

This book assumes, then, that, in addition to its financing role, the State has roles in policy-making, regulation, and service provision. These require planning functions and skills; however, it is important that, conceptually at least, they are kept apart. In many countries planning within the health ministry has concentrated on plans for its own services. This has led to a failure to consider adequately the wider issues of co-ordinating planning for the sector as a whole. In addition, the very size of the public sector, coupled with a shortage of planning skills, has resulted in many countries in a highly centralized, cumbersome, and unresponsive planning machinery. Both of these symptoms have resulted in valid criticisms of central State planning. It is hoped, however, that this book will demonstrate that planning by the State need not be so narrow or restrictive.

ATTITUDES TO HEALTH PLANNING

Given the history of planning as an activity both in our personal lives, and also in pursuit of business and public sector ends as described earlier, one might expect its influence and presence in the health sector to be well established by now. However, the history of planning in the health sector is still relatively short. Furthermore, attitudes to planning differ markedly between health professionals. As has already been noted, even countries such as the UK, with a well-established State-funded and State-provided National Health Service, set up a genuine planning system only comparatively recently. In other industrialized countries with a more fragmented health-care system, health planning may be even less firmly established. In some developing countries — India, for example — there may already be a well-established tradition; others (including some former USSR countries such as the Baltic states, for which planning was carried out in Moscow) may still have only a young planning system.

For some health professionals, planning is often viewed with suspicion, with its practitioners being at best an inconvenience and at worst an unnecessary evil. It is worth reflecting briefly on the source of such attitudes.

Some of these suspicious attitudes can be found in any field dominated by professionals concerned to maintain their controlling position. The medical profession, whose attitudes still form the dominant force within the health sector, is perhaps particularly resistant to the contribution of other non-clinical professional skills such as planning. This arises in part from a strong allegiance to and defence of clinical autonomy — the right of a doctor to make unfettered decisions in the interests of her/ his patient. This perceived right is challenged by some forms of formalized planning.

The concept of clinical autonomy can, however, never be absolute. It can only operate within given bounds. A doctor is only free to make decisions within existing resource and service constraints; for example, s/he cannot take an X-ray if there is no X-ray machine. As such, no decision can ever be totally free. One of the important functions of an allocative planning system is to allocate resources to different health problems according to agreed criteria. In the absence of a formal and open planning system, the ability of individual doctors or specialties to obtain resources is still constrained, but in different ways. Inevitably allocations thus reflect the ability of individual doctors to lobby for funds. By contrast, the role of public sector health planning is to minimize these resource constraints subject to the overriding public interest, rather than solely to the ability of a particular doctor to argue for additional resources. Antagonism to planning that arises from conflict between the priorities of individual specialists and the health sector as a whole is, perhaps, understandable or even inevitable.

Other negative attitudes arise, however, from the lamentable record of health planning in many countries, both developing and industrialized. Planning, as an activity, has failed in a number of ways as we now examine briefly.

The record of health planning

Unfortunately, the record of planning is often not good. Plans often fail to be implemented and remain grand designs on paper. Elsewhere plans may be implemented but fail to respond adequately to the real needs of the population. We argued earlier that the dilemma that gives rise to the need for planning is the gap between available resources and health needs, leading to the requirement to make choices as to how to use these resources. All readers will be able to identify for themselves examples of poor choices made in the past that have resulted in current use of resources which is inefficient or inappropriate. Common examples are the imbalance of resources between hospitals and primary care, between preventive/promotive care and curative care, between different social groups, between different regions or geographical areas, between staff salaries and medical supplies, or between different types of staff such as auxiliaries and specialists. The occurrence of any of these misallocations of resources suggests that previous decisions have been inappropriate — a planning failure. It is important to understand the possible reasons for this, if planning is to be strengthened in the future.

In some countries, emphasis on the formal process of planning has led to its being overzealously viewed as a bureaucratic function. At its worst, planning becomes an end in itself, with its real objective — the achievement of health improvements through strategic changes in the health sector — submerged under the planning process. The (false) identification of planning solely with the production of plan and project documents is a symptom of this. Its real aim, that of effecting change, is often smothered in the reams of planning documents which reside forlornly on the shelves of senior administrators. Such an approach has little observable impact on the health-care or health status of the country. This could be classed as a failure of implementation.

In other countries it has failed not so much through a lack of activities as through a more technical failure to analyse needs appropriately or to estimate resources accurately. It may also fail through attempts to impose plans from the centre in a top-down fashion, without the involvement of both the health-care providers and the communities in the decision. Elsewhere the planning process has been isolated from other decision-making processes (such as budgeting or human resource planning) with resultant inconsistencies. Planning has frequently been ineffective because of a failure to consider the inherently political nature of the process, discussed further below.

The result has been a variety of planning disasters, both small and large. Most people with experience of the health sector can give their own examples of such disasters — ranging from mislocation of facilities in inaccessible sites, through the construction of inappropriate and expensive hospitals, to the failure to open facilities or services because of a lack of trained staff or funds. This should not, however, be interpreted as an inevitable failure of planning, but rather a recognition of the need to develop systems appropriate to the particular health-care needs and resources of a country. However, these understandable criticisms of planning have often led to a rejection of the process without any clear idea of how it will be replaced.

The result of such failures has led to cynicism about and rejection of planning on the part of some health professionals. However, they are not all suspicious of planning; many are more tolerant, and recognize that, considered as an art (or science), in comparison with medicine it is still in its infancy, and can be expected to make such mistakes. Such supporters believe that, on balance, the situation without planning is likely to be worse than that with it.

A significant number of professional health planners are drawn from the ranks of the health professions (medicine, nursing, and public health being common first disciplines), and bring their professional skills to bear on planning problems. Others, though not full-time planners, readily accept the need for planning, and provide important inputs into the process while remaining within their own chosen profession. Indeed, one of the challenges that faces planning today is not so much a matter of trying to develop specialist planners, but rather one of exposing a broad range of health professionals to the importance and concepts of planning in order that they can participate in the process.

Communities who have been ignored by a top-down planning process may also feel understandable alienation from the process, and a second major challenge facing professional planners is to ensure that health planning systems are designed and operated so as to provide real (rather than token) input into the planning process.

It is clear that all is not well with the state of planning in many countries. However, this book is based on the firm belief that the appropriate response is to improve planning processes, rather than discarding them. Decisions about the future cannot be avoided, and a planning process is therefore inevitable unless a totally market-driven approach is to be adopted. Furthermore, planning, as an activity, however viewed, is currently widely practised in both developing and developed countries, and the issue ultimately reduces not to one over whether decisions about the future should be made, but rather by whom and how they should be made. We now turn briefly to these last and crucial questions.

PLANNING AS AN OPEN TRANSPARENT PROCESS

Decisions as to how future resources will be used are made in all organizations, although not necessarily in an open and explicit manner.

- They may, for example, be made by a small elite group within the organization with little reference to the views of users, or other members of the organization. Such decision-making may be carried out in ways that are covert or closed, thereby not only failing to gain useful input from other interested parties but potentially alienating them from the decisions made. Within the health sector, individual specialist doctors have often had a particular influence on decisions about resources, though again often not in a manner that allows open discussion of the merits of particular proposals in relation to alternative uses of the resources.

- Organizations may also shy away from making decisions about the future. In such situations, the status quo will prevail and effectively an *implicit* decision has been made not to change the current situation.

- Lastly, the failure of an organization such as a health ministry to make clear and open decisions about the future allocation of resources may be seen by external donor agencies as an indicator of a situation in which policy is not being formulated and in which they may feel tempted to fill the planning gap with proposals of their own.

All these situations reflect a failure to make clear and open decisions in a manner that allows inputs from all those with an interest (or as they are now commonly termed, 'stakeholders'). This failure can be alienating and is frequently a cause of planning failure. Successful planning, it is suggested, requires the development of an open and transparent process, with widely understood workings, to which interested parties can contribute.

PLANNING AS A TECHNOCRATIC OR AS A POLITICAL ACTIVITY

How planning is carried out within any organization reflects a variety of factors. These include the organizational structure, the stated or constituted aims of the organization, the relative power of different groups within the organization and their own aims, the political or ideological climate of the country, and the relationship between the organization and its users or consumers.

Many examples of planning failure can be traced to a very narrow notion of planning as the application of apparently rational planning procedures, by a small group of technocrats, seemingly oblivious to these broader political factors. Planning involves change; and each change has its opponents as well as its proponents. Which changes occur (if any) will depend to a large extent on the power of those with different values and attitudes, relative to those endorsing the proposed change. The art of successful planning must therefore involve analysis of power structures, alongside its more apparently objective technical aspects.

An example may clarify this. A health service may have as its stated aim the improvement of the health status of the country. A technocratic planner may examine this aim, look at the limited resources available, recognize that the greatest improvements to health status would be made by preventive and primary care services, and suggest a plan to close a number of hospital beds, diverting the resources thereby released to health centres, dispensaries, and preventive services. Such an approach may be apparently rational to the planner, but is unlikely to be achievable. Resistance to such closures is bound to be met from hospital workers, from doctors to auxiliaries. In such a situation, the objectives of such groups clash with that of the overall organization either in terms of their interpretation of health status or their own objectives of career advancement and professional protection and employment. Resistance may also be met from community members who perceive the hospital as the main form of health-care. Whether the apparently 'rational' plan is actually so rational, and indeed whether it is implementable, hinges on whose values or objectives one is concerned with, and where the power lies, both within and outside an organization.

The last point then to be made in this introductory chapter is that planning is very much concerned with the analysis of power structures and values, alongside its use of certain more apparently objective techniques. This point will be emphasized throughout the book.

SUMMARY

This first chapter has introduced the concept of planning as a means of responding to the dilemma of a scarcity of resources in comparison with the demands placed upon an organization. There are many examples of poor planning, but nevertheless some form of explicit decision-making about the future is needed within organizations in order to deal with this dilemma. To be effective, such decision-making needs to combine elements of technique and broader analysis of power relations within the organization and the wider community. It also needs to obtain a balance between the views of central decision-makers and those at the periphery, and between the views of health-care providers and communities. The role of the State within the health sector is likely to vary between countries, depending on a variety of factors, including historical and ideological factors and how health is viewed by different groups, and may include policy-making, regulation, financing, and service provision. Although the record of health planning has not always been good, it is argued that a State role in health planning is essential.

INTRODUCTORY READING

The following are both general introductory readings to the topics covered in this book and to the more specific areas introduced in the first two chapters.

For a good introduction to many of the issues surrounding the dilemma of scarcity and choice and planning see Abel-Smith (1994). A number of different aspects of planning are explored in Akhtar (1991).

The books by Conyers (1982) and Conyers and Hills (1984), though not specific to the health sector, provide a good and practical background to development and social sector planning. Reinke's book on planning (Reinke 1988) is a general health planning text, with particular emphasis on techniques. Collins (1994) provides a good introduction to health management and organizational issues, whereas Amonoo-Lartson *et al.* (1996) focuses on practical issues at the district level. Walt (1994) analyses policy formation processes and illustrates very clearly the political nature of planning. Lee and Mills (1983) is one of the first books on economics related to the health sector in developing countries, and provides a good overview of the subject. Other health economics texts are also suggested, and others are included in Chapter 14. In addition to the above books, a number of journals frequently carry articles in the areas covered by the book. These are listed below.

Increasingly the World Wide Web provides a mechanism for information, and some selected sites are given below.

EXERCISE 1

1. Consider the examples of choices facing the health sector given in Figure 1.1. Are there other key ones that face the health sector in your country? How are these choices currently made?
2. Complete the matrix in Fig. 1.2 for a country well known to yourself, such as your own. Plot on the matrix the positions of the different components of its health system with respect to its financing and provision roles.
3. How might these roles be altered? What would be the effect?

REFERENCES AND FURTHER READING

Abel-Smith, B. (1994). *Introduction to health: policy, planning and financing.* Longman, Harlow.
Akhtar, R. (ed.) (1991). *Health Care Patterns and planning in developing countries.* Greenwood Press, Connecticut.
Amonoo-Lartson, R. *et al.* (1996). *District health care: challenges for planning, organisation and evaluation in developing countries,* 2nd edn. Macmillan, London.

Chowdhury, Z. (1995). *The politics of essential drugs: the makings of a successful health strategy: lessons from Bangladesh.* Zed Press, London.
Collins, C. (1994). *Management and organization in developing health systems.* Oxford University Press, Oxford.
Conyers, D. (1982). *An introduction to social planning in the third world.* Wiley, Chichester.
Conyers, D. and Hills, P. (1984). *An introduction to development planning in the third world.* Wiley, Chichester.
Corrigan, P. (1979). *The World Health Organisation,* p. 7. Wayland Press, Hove.
Gish, O. (1977). *Guidelines for health planning.* Tri-Med, London.
Hogwood, B. and Gunn, L. (1984). *Policy analysis for the real world.* Oxford University Press, Oxford.
Lee, K. and Mills, A. (1983). *The economics of health in developing countries.* Oxford University Press, Oxford.
Mills, A. and Lee, K. (1993). *Health economics research in developing countries.* Oxford University Press, Oxford.
Mooney, G. (1992). *Economics, medicine and health care,* 2nd edn. Harvest Wheatsheaf, Hemel Hempstead.
Reinke, W. (ed.) (1988). *Health planning for effective management.* Oxford University Press, New York.
Walt, G. (1994). *Health policy: an introduction to process and power.* Zed Books, London:
Witter, S. and Ensor, T. (1997). *An introduction to health economics for Eastern Europe and the former Soviet Union.* Wiley, Chichester.

Journals

Bulletin of WHO (World Health Organization)
Health Policy and Planning (Oxford University Press)
Health Policy (Elsevier)
International Journal of Health Planning and Management (Wiley)
International Journal of Health Services (Baywood Publishing)
Public Administration and Development (Wiley)
Social Science and Medicine (Pergamon)
World Health Forum (World Health Organization)

Annual publications and sources of data

Demographic yearbook (UN annual publication)
The state of the world's children (UNICEF/OUP annual publication)
Human development report (UNDP/OUP annual publication)
United Nations year book (UN annual publication)
World development report (World Bank/OUP annual publication)
World health statistics annual (WHO annual publication)

Web sites

There is now a wide variety of websites providing information of interest to planners though these are of varying quality. The following gives some examples of websites of organizations of possible interest to readers. It is intended to provide an introduction to the range available and is not intended to be comprehensive. Readers should note that website addresses are liable to change without notice.

Type and organization	Description	Web address
Multilateral agencies		
UN	United Nations Homepage	http://www.un.org/
Womenwatch	UN Internet gateway on the advancement and empowerment of women	http://www.un.org/womenwatch/un/
World Bank	World Bank homepage	http://www.worldbank.org/
WHO	World Health Organization home page	http://www.who.int/
National government departments and agencies		
UK Department of Health	Homepage of UK health ministry	http://www.open.gov.uk/doh/dhhome.htm
USAID	Homepage of US government aid department	http://www.info.usaid.gov/
IDRC	Homepage of Canadian International Development Research Centre	http://www.idrc.ca/
British Council	Homepage of UK funded British Council	http://www.britcoun.org/index.htm
Non-governmental organizations		
Directory of NGOs in official relations with WHO	List of web links to all NGOs which collaborate formally with WHO	http://www.who.int/ina-ngo/
One World Directory	Internet community of 260 organizations	http://www.oneworld.org/partners/partners_list
Journals		
Health Policy and Planning	Contents and abstracts of articles	http://www.oup.co.uk/heapol/contents/
BMJ	British Medical Journal	http://www.bmj.com/
UK universities		
UK university gateway	Map with links to British universities	http://www.scit.wlv.ac.uk/ukinfo/uk.map.html
Gateways and general resources		
International Development Network	Designed to allow development professionals to link to one site. Contains general planning and management tools and range of relevant links and resources	http://www.idn.org

Type and organization	Description	Web address
ELDIS	Gateway to information sources on development and the environment	http: //www.ids.ac.uk/eldis/eldis.html
SOSIG	Social Science Information Gateway, an online catalogue of thousands of high quality Internet resources relevant to social science education and research	http://www.sosig.ac.uk/
OMNI	Organizing Medical Networked Information: gateway to Internet resources in medicine, biomedicine, allied health, health management and related topics	http://www.omni.ac.uk
Health Link database	The Healthlink Worldwide database is available on subscription and can be searched from this site. Free subscription available for those working in developing countries	http://www.healthlink.org.uk/database.html
Manager's Electronic Resource Centre	Various resources provided by Management Sciences for Health	http://erc.msh.org/index.htm
ID21	Development Research reporting service, a selection of the latest and best UK-based development research	http://www.id21.org/

Discussion lists

Afro-Nets	Provides useful links to organizations both within Africa and outside the region involved in research and various discussion forums	http://www.healthnet.org/afronets/
MSH decentralization forum	Electronic discussion forum on decentralization run by Management Sciences for Health	http://erc.msh.org/forums/decentr.htm
Mailbase	Provides electronic discussion lists for the UK higher education community	http://www.mailbase.ac.uk/

2

Approaches to planning

The last chapter introduced planning. For any organization providing health-care, two types of planning were distinguished — *allocative planning* (the making of decisions relating to how resources will be used and which activities will be undertaken) and *activity planning* (the setting of monitorable implementation schedules). Both of these types of planning are as relevant for a private health-care provider as for a public one, although different priorities are likely to be set by each, resulting in different allocative plans. Chapter 1 also explored a number of scenarios for the State relating to functions as a policy-setter, financer, provider, and regulator of health-care. Different ideologies and historical circumstances will result in different roles and levels of health-care provision by the State, although few if any governments provide no direct health-care or no central funding for health-care. The State, however, has two roles which are quite distinct from those of other health-care providers. These are the policy-setting and regulatory functions, with overall responsibility for health of the nation. How these are interpreted will vary according to the differing views of the nature of health.

We now turn our attention to different approaches to planning. This chapter begins by examining three models of planning. Although none of these is likely to be desirable (or indeed feasible) in its pure form, each throws light on different ways of approaching planning. In practice these models are inevitably combined.

The chapter then outlines one such combination, and introduces the various stages in the planning process, which are further explored in later chapters. The chapter finishes by looking at some of the differences between planning for a single organization and the broader role of planning in the public sector.

PLANNING MODELS

A number of writers have distinguished between three different models of planning: *comprehensive rationalism*, *mixed scanning*, and *incrementalism*. In practice, it is difficult to put any one particular planning process into such neat pigeon-holes; indeed it is rare to find practising planners who are familiar with the terms, let alone making a conscious decision to operate within any one of these models. They are, however, useful as conceptual tools to highlight different aspects of planning. It is with this in mind that the following brief introduction to them is given. Readers wishing to explore them in more depth are referred to readings at the end of the chapter.

Comprehensive rationalism

The definition given in the last chapter referred to planning as an explicit activity that attempts to determine how resources are used to further the specific goals of an organization. Common sense might suggest that any such decisions about the future require a sequence of broad logical steps such as those set out in Fig. 2.1. Such a series of steps is often depicted as a continuous cycle. The first stage analyses the current position or problem to be solved. Next the aims (where we want to be) are decided. All the possible alternative courses of action are listed, and assessed as to their feasibility and capability to achieving the aims. Lastly, having decided on the most appropriate alternative, action is taken to implement it. The cycle then starts again with a reassessment or evaluation of the situation.

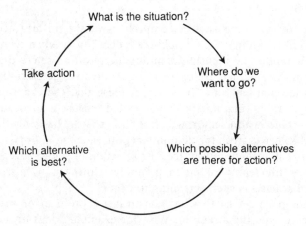

Fig. 2.1   Steps in 'rational' planning

It is difficult to fault such a logical series of steps; and indeed few planners would wish to dispute that in an ideal world such a process (typical of what is known as the comprehensive rational approach) is desirable. In practice, however, a number of difficulties arise with the application of such an approach.

- The approach suggests a chronologically ordered cycle of events, each leading inexorably on from the previous one. In practice a number of sub-cycles are likely to be set up, and indeed various activities may occur in parallel. For example, the targets set may well be altered in the light of the discussion of the resource implications of different options with the realization that the targets were too ambitious or overcautious. Similarly, evaluative activities may occur at any point in the planning process. Such modifications to the simple model do not change the basic assumptions and logic underpinning the model. Rather, they modify the process of the application of the model. The stages remain, albeit in a different and more complex ordering.

- There are more serious difficulties, which question the very feasibility of such an approach. These concerns relate to the impossibility of carrying out, in real life, such a comprehensive and exhaustive list of operations. For example, the full process described above requires all alternative options to be assessed. However, the number of options potentially available in developing, for example, a national health plan is very large (even, it could be argued, infinite). The information requirements of examining the detailed implications of each option are vast, and they are in practice unassessable. A good example of the practical difficulties of such an approach is given by the experience of planners in Latin America who in the 1960s developed an extremely comprehensive system of planning known as the PAHO-CENDES method (see Hilleboe *et al.* 1972). The approach was eventually abandoned as unworkable in its original form, largely as a result of the tremendous requirements of the process itself in terms of information and human resources.

Mixed scanning

The difficulties of operating such a comprehensive system are recognized by proponents of mixed scanning. Here a deliberate decision is taken to narrow down the area of manoeuvrability by focusing planning attention on selected areas of interest. An early stage in the modified cycle (see Fig. 2.2) involves determining the priority or problem areas for planning, and it is within these that the examination of options occurs. Mixed scanning (Etzioni 1967) is so called because it advocates a broad sweep or scan of the whole health sector, which then forms the basis for the more detailed examination of selected areas for planning action. Such an approach is less costly in terms of time and information resources. Its selection of priority areas for alternatives certainly reflects the reality of much planning. However, it raises a fundamental question: on what basis is such screening to occur?

Criteria need to be set as to what constitutes a problem or priority and what, therefore, deserves specific attention. Why, for example, focus on mother and child health, the hospital sector, or the organizational structure of the health system? By

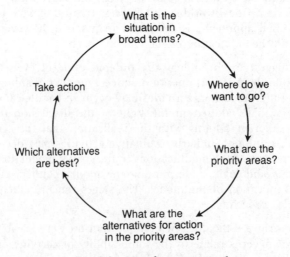

Fig. 2.2   Mixed scanning cycle

their very nature such decisions — made at the stage in the planning process at which detailed examination has not occurred — will involve a large degree of instinct, hunch, or experience. As we shall see in the next chapter, an example of how the selection of priority areas for attention has been contentious can be found in the debate between advocates of a comprehensive and a selective approach to primary health-care. Such decisions ultimately involve subjective judgements as to the priority areas. Consequently, they are no longer the apparently objective rational process suggested by the parent of the process (comprehensive rationalism).

This raises one of the major issues concerning these planning models: the degree to which the assumptions or value systems that underpin planning decisions are made explicit and recognized within the planning process.

Allocative planning is concerned with the possibility of change. If planning was solely concerned with the maintenance of existing situations, then it would be reduced to simple activity planning. Change (and the possibility of change) in most situations will result in both gainers and losers, and so in proponents and opponents of the plan. For allocative planning to succeed, an analysis of the effects on different groups of different proposals, and of the likely consequent degree of support or opposition, is required. Techniques such as stakeholder analysis and political mapping have been developed to assist in this (see, for example, Reich 1994).

Chapter 8 examines the whole process of setting priorities and the values inherent in this in more detail. It argues that planning can never be a purely objective, technical activity but requires basic value judgements on which to rest the techniques. Although this perhaps is more obvious in the mixed scanning approach, through the selection process, it is equally true for the comprehensive rational approach, despite its apparent veneer of objectivity (illustrated by the word 'rationality', which suggests the lack of any value-judgement factor).

Incrementalism

The third approach to planning, incrementalism, recognizes the political nature of planning in a far more overt manner than either of the previous approaches. The term 'political' is used here in a wide sense, and, though inclusive of ideology and party politics, is by no means confined to these. It is used to cover analysis and action that recognizes the nature and effect of different interest groups in society, whether based on class, employment or business, area of residence, professional or trade union association, religion, ethnicity, gender, or any of the other variables which determine an individual's values, loyalties, and actions. Figure 2.3 provides a diagrammatic representation of some of the major groups and sub-groups who are likely to have an interest in planning decisions.

Planning, as it is seen in this third approach, has been described as a process of 'muddling through' (Lindblom 1959) or as a series of 'disjointed steps' moving in an incremental manner towards the set goal, the degree of movement at any time being determined by the political context as defined above.

Incrementalism is, at first sight, more a description of the reality of much planning than a normative prescription of how to plan. It recognizes that in planning which

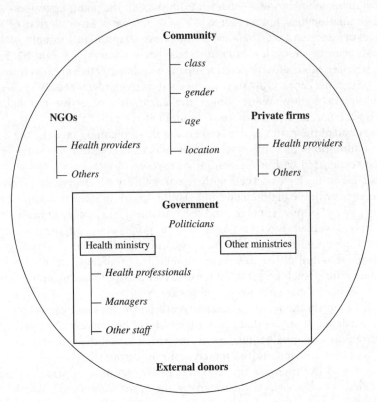

Fig. 2.3   Some groups with an interest in the health planning process

deals with social issues affecting groups of people, there can be no such thing as objectivity, or shared assumptions. Members of different groups (however defined) will have differing views as to the desirability of planned actions. A plan which appears to the decision-maker entirely rational and sensible may be viewed with suspicion, if not opposition, by some groups, who may resist it. Consequently, plans can rarely proceed in a straight line towards a set goal. A current example within the UK, outside the health-care sector, is the clear difference of view between groups who advocate the expansion of the road network in response to traffic congestion and those who see it as destructive to the environment. The conflicting 'rationality' of each group rests on and stems from their different values.

This description of the reality of planning is likely to be familiar to practising planners. However, incrementalism is also viewed more prescriptively by some writers, who suggest that planners should take account of such political forces and adapt their plans accordingly. This can perhaps be compared to wind-powered sailing. The sailor who takes no account of prevailing winds and attempts to steer a straight-line course will soon capsize! The successful sailor is rarely sailing directly towards the desired destination, but rather recognizes the direction of the wind and 'tacks' in a series of steps towards the desired destination, as illustrated in Fig. 2.4. In such a situation it is perfectly feasible to be adopting a plan proposal that appears to be inconsistent with the final goal sought, if such a move is seen as a necessary inter-mediate step to take account of the political context and reality. The degree to which a plan can proceed smoothly in a straight line towards the desired objective without deviation depends in large part on the degree to which the plan has sufficient direct political support to overcome countervailing forces.

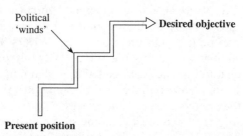

Fig. 2.4   Diagrammatic representation of incrementalism

An example may help to clarify this. Imagine a plan which had analysed that a new cadre of medical assistants was required, because of the cost, inefficiency, and in-appropriateness of using doctors in primary care situations. There may be strong opposition from the medical professionals to such a cadre being formed, on the basis that it is seen to be a competitive threat. In such a situation it may be necessary to sweeten the apparently bitter pill by introducing, at the same time as the new cadre, various inducements to the medical staff (perhaps supervisory allowances, in recogni-tion of their new role of supervising medical assistants). Although such inducements may seem to be inconsistent with the basic aim of improving efficiency, they may be a short-term price to pay for the attainment of a long-term goal — a strong and effective medical assistant cadre. Exercise 2 at the end of this chapter provides an example for group work which may help to demonstrate this point further.

Such an approach can be seen to be at odds with that of pure rationalism, which sees planning as an ordered march towards the set goal, using the shortest distance between the point of origin and the ultimate destination, and which would not recognize the need for short-term diversions from this path.

The incrementalist view of planning may then be a fair description of the reality of much planning activity. Its emphasis on political aspects is a useful reminder of the inherently political nature of planning. However, too much attention to such political analysis may stifle the possibility of the sort of radical change necessary in many countries experiencing very low levels of health status and resources, and saddled with an inappropriate health-care structure. Instead of radical action, it may reinforce the notion of planning as a 'dripping tap' phenomenon. It may be that in such a situation it is all too easy continually to take the line of least resistance, and to lose sight of the long-term objectives of the health sector. In such a situation, plans may simply become a reflection of the relative strength of particular groups, and as such may ensure the maintenance of the status quo, or the enhancement of the position of the powerful.

This contrasts with the PHC philosophy (discussed in Chapter 3), which is predicated upon promoting equity and empowering the weak or dispossessed.

Having reviewed the different models, let us now return to the question of the relationship between these theoretical analyses of different approaches to planning and the reality of planning as practised within the health sector of many countries.

No planning system, in practice, conforms to any one of the above models in its pure form. However, it is possible to analyse planning systems and to recognize within them leanings in one direction or another. PAHO-CENDES, which has already been mentioned, was a highly 'rational' and technocratic approach, and foundered in part because of the demands it made on information and its emphasis on techniques as opposed to process and politics. On the other hand, WHO's Managerial Process for National Health Development (see Fig 2.5; WHO 1981), although proposing a clear sequence of steps which follow the basic skeleton of planning outlined earlier in the chapter, recognizes the inherently political nature of planning through its emphasis on political support at the various stages of the process.

A successful planning approach must combine strong technical skills with a recognition of the political process. A clear understanding of the desired ends of planning is needed, together with a systematic approach to the planning process. At all stages in the process, one eye needs to be kept out for the feasibility of any actions in terms not only of traditional variables (resources and technical factors) but also of the broader

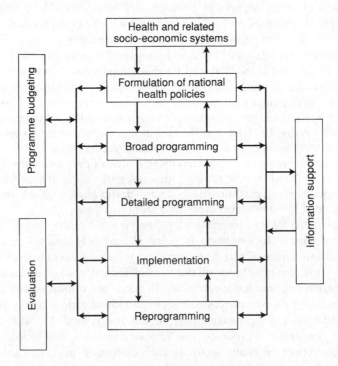

Fig. 2.5   Managerial process for national health development. Reproduced, by permission, World Health Organization

political process. Let us now bring these elements together into a realistic but rational approach to planning.

REALISTIC RATIONAL PLANNING

Figure 2.6 sets out the main stages such a rational process might be expected to follow. The diagrammatic representation of planning as a cyclical set of activities is frequently found. In fact it is perhaps more accurate to describe it as a planning spiral, with the end-point of each cycle forming the start of the next cycle, but at a higher plane. Each of the stages of this spiral is now described briefly.

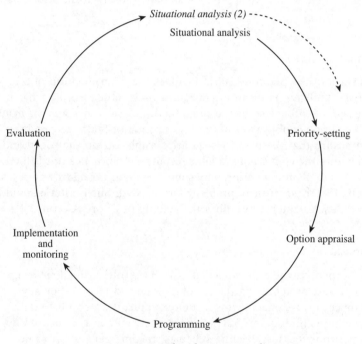

Fig. 2.6   The planning spiral

Situational analysis

The first step in such a process involves an assessment of the present situation. This is often referred to as a situational analysis. This analyses the present situation from various perspectives:

- It examines the current and projected characteristics of the population including its *demography*.

- It looks at the *physical and socio-economic* characteristics of the area and its *infrastructure*.

- It analyses the *policy and political environment* including existing *health policies.*

- An essential part is the analysis of the health needs of the population.

- It would also look at the *services* provided both by the *non-health sector* and by the *health sector* itself. The latter would focus on facilities provided, their utilization and service gaps, together with organizational arrangements.

- The situational analysis would also examine the *resources* used in the provision of services and their current *efficiency, effectiveness, equity, and quality* of services.

It should be stressed that a situational analysis conducted by a public sector plan needs to cover the whole of the health sector, and not just those services provided directly by the public sector. Chapter 7 looks more closely at the situational analysis stage.

Priority-setting

The second stage of the planning spiral involves the determination of a hierarchy of *goals, objectives,* and *targets* of an organization — in other words, what it wants to achieve. This will be influenced by the situational analysis, especially the health needs, and by the broad policy objectives of the organization or State. Any realistic planning system must ensure that the priorities set are feasible within the social and political climate, and within the context of available resources. In practice this is likely to mean that within any one planning period only some problems are addressed. Clear criteria for the selection of these priority problems are needed. Such criteria should include political feasibility. Chapter 8 examines the activity of priority-setting.

Option appraisal

The third stage involves the *generation* and *assessment* (often called *option appraisal*) of the various options for achieving the set objectives and targets. For any target there may be a number of ways of achieving it. For example, if a target is to reduce levels of malnutrition within children by 25% in 5 years, there will be a variety of ways of doing so — such as supplementary feeding schemes, income-generation projects, demonstration gardens, and nutritional surveillance programmes. Although it is often worthwhile and productive at this stage to allow a wide variety of creative ideas to emerge, it is important that this set of options is quickly reduced, without too sophisticated an analysis, to a reasonable shortlist. Such preliminary criteria are in practice often applied subconsciously; for example, options may be discarded at this stage by recognition of their high resource implications, their political or social unacceptability, or their technical non-feasibility.

Each of the remaining options on the shortlist is looked at in turn, and is assessed in three ways:

- The impact of each is examined to see its effect on the health target set. Each alternative approach is likely to have a different impact on the health problem (in terms of both when and how much) — in this example, the levels of malnutrition.

- The resource implications will be examined, both to look at the efficiency with which each alternative could meet the targets (known as its cost-effectiveness) and to determine whether overall the option can be afforded, given resource constraints.
- The feasibility of each approach will be examined to see whether there are other barriers to its success (such as technical or political constraints).

This stage is examined further in Chapter 10.

Programming and budgeting

The option appraisal stage will result in preferred options (or a combination of approaches), which will then form part of the plan. This process will be carried out for each priority area and its associated set of targets. The programming stage translates the results of the earlier decision into a series of programmes, each with a budget. The result of this is the plan document, which is a statement of intent concerning the activities over the plan period. Chapter 12 looks at programming. As planning within the public sector becomes more decentralized (see Chapter 3) the focus of planning is on specific geographical areas each developed within the constraints of their resources. Chapter 11 examines issues of resource allocation from central agencies to lower levels.

Implementation and monitoring

The penultimate stage involves the *implementation* of the plan, a neglected yet essential part of planning which is discussed in Chapter 12. This involves transforming the broad programmes into more specific timed and budgeted sets of tasks and activities, and involves the drawing up of a more operational plan or a work plan. This is the type of planning that we have described earlier as activity planning. An essential part of this process is the *monitoring* of the implementation of these activities.

Evaluation

Lastly, a process of *evaluation* of the plan provides the basis for the next situational analysis, and hence a fresh lead in to the planning spiral just described. Evaluation shares many of the characteristics of appraisal, and is discussed in Chapter 10.

PLANNING AS A POLITICAL PROCESS

The above has suggested a series of tasks which a planner needs to accomplish to develop and implement a plan. The remainder of this book will focus on these stages and the detail of them. However, it is important always to bear in mind that planning is a political process, and is not solely the production of a plan. As Walt (1994) clearly analyses, the process of developing policies is highly influenced by the context in which this occurs and the key actors with a stake in the policy outcome. Planning is concerned with change, and the prospect of change inevitably brings opponents and supporters of the proposal. The means of producing the plan is thus often as important as any final documentation. Many planning systems have suffered (and indeed in some cases still do suffer) from overattention to the bureaucratic formalities of planning and a failure to take account of the political processes. The relationship between planners, policy-makers, service-managers, communities, and other stakeholders in the planning process is critical to the success of planning, and will be discussed further in Chapter 14. One particular group of actors with a high potential ability to influence plans are donors. The development of a robust strategic planning capacity is likely to increase the ability of the State to set its own agenda and resist unwelcome intrusion into the policy-setting processes of a country by external agencies.

The implications of this for planning are, it is suggested, threefold.

- First, it is important that there is open consultation at the time of plan development in order both to ensure relevance of plans and, as far as possible, to develop identification with the plans by different groups.

- Second, planners need to recognize the need to put effort into developing cohesive support for proposals. The support of groups who may have shown little interest in proposals needs, where possible, to be harnessed.

- Lastly, it has to be recognized that there will, inevitably, always be opponents of plans or aspects of plans. Planners need to analyse whether such opposition is strong enough potentially to damage the chances of implementation of proposals. In such situations, planners may need to be pragmatic and look for compromise proposals that will be implementable.

PRIVATE AND PUBLIC SECTOR PLANNING

The preceding sections described general approaches to allocative planning. The general principles and stages of planning outlined above are as valid for a private health-care provider as for a public sector provider. Planning for institutions within the private sector requires a similar combination of technical skills and political analysis. The parameters and value judgements which form the planning framework are, however, bound to be different. The different aims of the private and public sectors will lead to very different contents for their plans.

Comparison of the planning approaches used in the private sector reveals strong similarities, though the terminology employed may differ. These differences reflect the different organizational cultures of the two types of provider. Table 2.1 sets out a typical business planning approach, setting alongside this the comparable public sector approach as laid out in Fig. 2.6. Public sector institutions have, as their primary aim, the improvement of the health of a community by meeting its health needs. Private sector health-care providers, by contrast, have as their objective the making of profits by responding to individuals' health demands.

Table 2.1   Comparison between the business and public sector planning approach

Business planning	Public sector planning
Determination of mission statement	Setting of goals
Analysis of strengths, weaknesses, opportunities, and threats (SWOT analysis) (including marketing)	Situational analysis (including needs assessment)
Determination of strategy	Option appraisal and monitoring
Operational plans	Operational plans
Implementation	Implementation
Feedback	Evaluation and monitoring

In addition to the above, there are two other major differences between private and public sector planning. The first relates to the different aims of the two sectors outlined above. Chapter 1 argued that promotion of health is often affected more by activities outside the health sector than by direct health service provision. This is discussed in more detail in the next chapter. This point has important implications for the planning role of the health ministry, with its overall responsibility for health promotion. Health ministry plans must take account of the role of other sectors in the promotion of health, even though these are not its direct responsibility. Public sector plans provide the opportunity to provide a more holistic and balanced view of health and its promotion. Private firms, by contrast, are concerned only with their own activities.

The second difference stems from the fact that the private firm operates within a context and environment which is controlled by the regulatory function of the State. The State in its planning activity has the dual role of planning its own direct service provision activities together with its regulatory functions towards other health service providers. The planning process provides an important opportunity for the health ministry to influence the type of health-care provided by other agencies. This may include the setting of standards, fee levels, and location of services.

In many health ministry plans, the major emphasis is still placed on the ministry's own direct service provision role. Unfortunately little attention is given to either the activities of other health-related sectors or the regulatory functions of the State, and thus important opportunities are missed. One of the main thrusts of the recent drive to Health Sector Reform (HSR) policies has been to recognize these aspects. This is discussed further in Chapter 3.

The above has focused on differences between the private-for-profit and public sectors. There is of course, a third sector, the voluntary or non-governmental organization (NGO) sector, which sits somewhere between these two. In many ways it shares the objectives of the public sector, though it does not have the wider sectoral policy and regulatory responsibilities, but it has the organizational freedom often associated with the private sector. Its planning processes are likely to be slightly different from both the private-for-profit and the public sector, though again sharing the common underpinning rationale and approach.

Within the planning approach outlined above, there are two particular points at which this wider function can, and should, be deliberately incorporated.

- The situational analysis needs to be far broader than that of a pure service provider, such as the private sector organization. It needs to look at the sector as a whole, rather than just at the ministry's own activities and resources. It also needs to assess the broad causes of ill health, so as to allow the possibility for wider intersectoral strategies to be developed.

- The option appraisal must include the potential contribution that other sectors can be encouraged or required to make to the state's overall health goals. Thus options for health promotion must not be restricted to health service activities, but can include regulatory activity, legislation, and collaboration with other non-health agencies.

LEVELS OF PLANNING

Within the three groups of organizations described above — public, private-for-profit, and NGO — there are likely also to be different levels of planning within the organizations. Figure 2.7 shows diagrammatically the various levels within the health sector at which planning may occur and the different types of plans at each of these levels. Although the principles and broad processes will be similar at each level, as one moves down to the lower levels plans will be more specific with the central plans providing the broad strategic envelope into which they are placed. Each level therefore

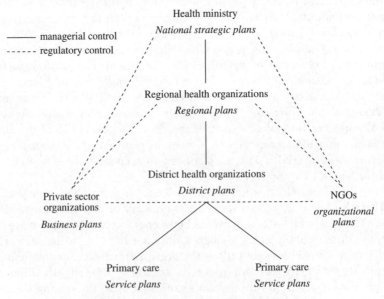

Fig. 2.7 Organizational levels of planning

needs to take account of plans being developed both in other organizations working at the same *horizontal* level and also plans of both higher and lower levels in the system, the *vertical* dimension.

PLANNING, MANAGEMENT, AND POLICY

The terms planning, management, and policy-setting are often closely linked and used interchangeably. This can cause confusion and although there are no 'correct' definitions it is useful to clarify how the terms will be used in this book.

The term *policy* will be used to denote statements of broad intent by an organization. As such it can be used at various levels within an organization. For example, a health ministry may have a policy to encourage the private sector, and a district health management team may have a policy to give greater emphasis to primary and preventive care. At the technical level there may be more precise policies, concerning immunization schedules for example. The realization of such policies will occur through the production of plans which put flesh on the bones of a broad policy and signal the particular intentions for action by an organization. Clearly, however, policy does not arise from a vacuum, but as the result of analysis coupled with value judgements. The planning process, and particularly the situational analysis, thus has a critical role to play in formulating policy.

At each level within an organization plans will be made which are constrained by higher level policies, among other things. For example, there may be a national policy to promote links with traditional practice, and this would have to be taken into account by districts setting their own specific policies and plans.

There is often similar understandable overlap between planning and management. The term *management* has been increasingly used to replace 'administration' in recent years. Management is generally seen as involving greater delegated powers, whereas administration refers to the application of rules and regulations determined at a higher level. Management is the overall decision-making process within an organization. One aspect of this concerns decisions that are taken concerning the future — planning. Management as a whole will also include decisions about present activities. As we shall see, however, planning is only useful if it leads to successful implementation, the latter being an aspect of management! They are therefore overlapping and inextricably linked activities, with the main difference being related to the future nature of planning decisions.

PLANNING ACTIVITIES AND TERMS

This chapter has concentrated on the different broad approaches to planning. The rest of the book deals with the practicalities of combining the technical and political aspects, at the various stages of planning, that have been highlighted into feasible plans. Before proceeding to look in more detail at these planning techniques, we need to introduce a number of planning terms, of which there are many. This chapter ends with a brief review of a number of these alternative planning activities and terms which are employed, in order to make clear their relationship to the broader planning approaches outlined earlier. A summary of these terms is given in Table 2.2.

• The term *development planning* has already been introduced in the last chapter, and is used generally to refer to planning carried out at the national level and concerned with the national context. In the 1960s and early 1970s this was largely synonymous with *economic planning* relating to the control of the economy. The shift in development thinking that occurred in the 1970s in many countries and agencies led to a broadening of the concept of development planning to incorporate the social sector.

• In some organizations *strategic planning* is seen as a separate activity which attempts to provide a broad directional framework for the more detailed plans. Often this strategic view is incorporated in comprehensive health plans.

Table 2.2   Planning activities and terms

Terms	Activity
Economic/development planning	National-level activity aimed at steering the economic or development policies, primarily through public expenditure or fiscal policies
Strategic plan	Document outlining the direction an organization is intending to follow, with broad guidance as to the implications for services or action
Business plans	Strategic plans prepared by business organizations setting out their direction, and usually providing income and expenditure projections
Corporate planning	Term, now not often used, to describe an integrated approach to planning for an organization. Analogous to business plan
Regulatory planning	Activities of State planning bodies that set planning guidelines for private sector activities
Service/programme planning	Planning focusing on the services to be provided. Used to contrast with capital planning (see below)
Capital planning	Plans focusing on the capital developments of an organization such as its building programme
Project planning	Planning focusing on discrete time-limited activities
Human resource/ manpower planning	Plans focusing on the human resource requirements of an organization or country
Physical plans	Plans relating to construction elements
Operational plans	Activity plans detailing precise timing and mode of implementation
Work-plans	Operational plans referring to the activities of a small unit or of an individual

- The term *perspective planning* may be used to refer to long-term strategies over perhaps a 10 year period. Increasingly such a long-term view is used in combination with shorter-term *rolling plans* which have at any one time a shorter (e.g. 3 year) cycle. Such a combination is seen as a flexible response to the need for short-term detailed plans within the context of a longer-term view. This contrasts with, and often replaces, the more traditional sequential 5 *year* plans that have been widely used in many public sectors.

- Although the term *business planning* originated in the private commercial sector and is often used as the basis for obtaining loan funds from outside investors, it is occasionally used in the public sector to describe costed medium-term plans.

- The term *corporate plan* is now less used but was used in the 1970s to describe strategic planning activities relating to an organization.

- *Regulatory planning* may often be a formalized activity carried out by a separate agent of the State to ensure that standards are met by the private sector, and to provide a framework for competition. It often has authority over issues such as the size and location of medical facilities.

- *Service* or *programme planning* is a term used to contrast with *capital* or *project planning*, and focuses change on plans for particular services or programmes.

- By contrast, *capital plans* deal exclusively with changes arising out of capital or development expenditure, typically on buildings or equipment. Chapter 12 deals in more detail with this point; however, it is worth noting at this stage that many planning departments were originally seen as dealing primarily with capital projects and budgets, which were perceived as the major agent for change. Increasingly it is recognized that change can occur through alterations in service patterns not necessarily involving major capital expenditure; and hence the rise of the term service planning.

- *Project planning* is a variant on capital planning, in which change is seen to occur largely through projects, and in particular projects funded and often heavily influenced by outside donors. Again, the dangers of overemphasis on project planning are discussed in Chapter 12.

- *Human resource planning* is a well-established sub-discipline of planning dealing with personnel — a major resource in the health sector. It is still often known as manpower planning, a term which is avoided in this book because of its gender bias. Chapter 13 focuses on this area of planning.

- *Physical planning* is a very separate discipline, and not to be confused with more generic health planning. It is concerned with the overall physical relationships of facilities, and is often the responsibility of local government departments. Although there are relationships between it and more general health planning this book will not deal with physical planning, other than in a very general sense in Chapter 12, where aspects of capital planning are covered.

• *Operational plans* and *work plans* refer to what we have classified earlier as *activity planning*. They are terms used to describe the detailed formulation of specific activities, usually with a monitorable timetable.

SUMMARY

This chapter has introduced the reader to two essential but contrasting aspects of planning. The first is the need for planning to be systematic and to follow a clear sequence of logically ordered activities. This rational component of planning is important to provide a framework for clear decision-making. The second is the recognition that planning deals with issues of power, so that analysis of power-relations is a necessary component of any planner's toolkit. Different approaches to planning that lay different emphases on these various aspects have been discussed. Finally, the approach that this book follows, one which attempts to combine these various aspects of planning, has been outlined.

INTRODUCTORY READING

In addition to the readings of Chapter 1, the following are more specific to the areas discussed in this chapter.

Gilbert and Specht (1977), Cole and Lucas (1979), and Faludi (1973a,b) all provide insights into the different approaches to planning, including the debates between rationalism and incrementalist modes. Different models of planning can be seen in Hilleboe *et al.* (1972), which among other approaches describes in some detail the PAHO-CENDES approach. Further case studies can be found in Jeffery (1986) about India, and Gish (1977) on his work as a health planner in Tanzania. WHO's approach to planning is described in WHO (1981), which is part of a series of publications dealing with different aspects of WHO's Managerial Process for National Health Development. More general discussions of the planning process and its relationship to policy analysis can be found in Hogwood and Gunn (1984).

Chowdhury (1995), Walt (1994), and Reich (1995) provide good insights into the nature of the policy and planing processes. Koivusalo and Ollila (1997) provide a useful overview of international agencies involved in the health sector.

At the more decentralized level of health-care delivery, Amonoo-Lartson *et al.* (1996) and MacMahon *et al.* (1980) both include sections on planning.

EXERCISE 2

Examine the following case study and then consider the questions below. If possible try to do this in groups, and present your results to each other.

In a country heavily dominated by curative hospital-based care, the health plan calls for a switch in resources from such activities to community-based health-promotive activities. In particular the plan calls for:

- a slow-down in the hospital building programme

- the creation of a community health worker cadre, supervised by nurses from nearby clinics

- a training programme for nurses in diagnostic skills

- the development of community health committees

- a variety of health-promoting activities, including a ban on smoking in public places.

Discussion questions

1. Which groups are likely to support the plans, and why?
2. Which groups are likely to oppose the plans, and why?
3. How could analysis of this help in ensuring the implementation of the plans?

Notice how:

- the same group (such as village leaders) may support one element of a plan and not another

- within a group there may be variations of view (for example doctors may be split according to specialty)

- individuals may belong to different groups and thus have divided views (for example a smoking public-health doctor may have mixed views about the ban on smoking)

- groups may not be homogeneous — the 'community' will comprise a variety of views

- identification of this type of information early on in a plan may help to overcome resistance to it through the formation of alliances and the recognition of support for and opposition to particular proposals.

REFERENCES AND FURTHER READING

Amonoo-Lartson, R. *et al.* (1996). *District health care: challenges for planning, organization and evaluation in developing countries*, 2nd edn. Macmillan, London.
Blum, H. (1981). *Planning for health: generics for the eighties*, 2nd edn. Human Sciences Review, New York.
Chowdhury, Z. (1995). *The Politics of essential drugs: the makings of a successful health strategy: lessons from Bangladesh*. Zed Press, London
Cole, S. and Lucas, H. (eds) (1979). *Models, planning and basic needs*. Pergamon, Oxford.

Conyers, D. (1982). *An introduction to social planning in the third world.* Wiley, Chichester.

Conyers, D. and Hills, P. (1984). *An introduction to development planning in the Third World.* Wiley, Chichester.

Etzioni, A. (1967). Mixed scanning: a third approach to decision-making. *Public Administration Review.* Reprinted in Faludi (1973a).

Faludi, A. (1973a) *A reader in planning theory.* Pergamon, Oxford.

Faludi, A. (1973b) *Planning theory.* pergamon, Oxford.

Gilbert, N. and Specht, H. (1977). *Planning for social welfare: issues, models, and tasks.* Prentice-Hall, Englewood Cliffs, NJ.

Gish, O. (1977). *Guidelines for health planners.* Tri-Med, London.

Hilleboe, H. E, Barkhuus, A., and Thomas, W. C. (1972). *Approaches to national health planning.* Public health paper No, 46. WHO, Geneva.

Hogwood, B. and Gunn, L. (1984). *Policy analysis for the real world.* Oxford University Press, Oxford.

Jeffery, R. (1986). Health planning in India 1951–84: The role of the planning commission. *Health Policy and Planning,* 1, 127–37.

Koivusalo, M. and Ollila, E. (1997). *Making a healthy world: agencies, actors and policies in international health.* Zed Press, London.

Lindblom, C. E. (1959). The science of muddling through. *Public Administration Review,* 19, 79–88. Reprinted in Faludi (1973a).

McMahon, R. *et al.* (1980). *On being in charge: a guide for middle-level management in primary health care.* World Health Organization, Geneva.

Reich, M. R. (1994). Political mapping of health policy: a guide for managing the political dimensions of health policy. Data for Decision Making Project, Harvard School of Public Health, Boston.

Reich, M. (1995). The politics of health sector reform in developing countries: three cases of pharmaceutical policy. *Health Policy,* 32, 47–77.

Reinke, W. (ed.) (1988). *Health planning for effective management.* Oxford University Press, New York.

Walt, G. (1994). *Health Policy: An introduction to process and power.* Zed Books, London.

WHO (1981). Managerial process for national health development: guiding principles. World Health Organization, Geneva.

3

The policy context: Primary Health Care and Health Sector Reform

In the last chapter the close interrelationship between planning and policy was touched upon. This chapter traces some of the key policy themes that have been central to the health sector over the last 20 years in particular.

We start by examining the policy of Primary Health Care (PHC) which for many countries was, on paper at least, the foundation of health policies in the 1980s. In the last 5–10 years the emphasis has shifted away from PHC towards issues related to the structure of the health sector. Health Sector Reform (HSR) policies have become a major concern of many donors and health ministries. The key components of such policies are outlined.

The chapter ends by suggesting that despite recent shifts away from PHC, the principles are still valid and indeed that there are strong potential connections between PHC and appropriate HSR policies. It concludes by looking at the implications of these policies for effective health planning.

ORIGINS OF PRIMARY HEALTH CARE

At a joint WHO–UNICEF conference in Alma-Ata, Kazakhstan, in 1978, health ministers from throughout the world agreed a major statement regarding the health policies deemed necessary to achieve the WHO goal of Health for All. The Alma-Ata Declaration, as the statement is widely known, resulted from trends in thinking in relation to health, health-care, and development which had been converging over the previous decade and earlier. The declaration was, however, important in propounding a broad and consistent philosophy and strategy which became known as the PHC approach.

The Alma-Ata Declaration has had a major effect on the thinking of health ministries throughout the developing world (and to a lesser extent on health services in the developed world). Inasmuch as it is, with justification, still the declared basis for the policy of most governments, this book is set firmly within its philosophy. The PHC approach calls for a major change in attitude both towards the concept of health and in our understanding of appropriate actions to improve the unacceptably low health status of many groups in society. It also recognizes the need for a new relationship between health service professionals and members of the community. These fundamental shifts require a concomitant shift both in the broad process of planning for health and more specifically in the way health services are planned.

It is important to recognize that the development of the PHC approach was an evolutionary one. The two decades before 1978 had seen a number of shifts in thinking in the area both of health and of more general development policy that influenced the Alma-Ata Declaration, and these will now be outlined.

Understanding of the concept of health

Chapter 1 has already introduced a number of issues and trends related to the under-standing of the concept of health. These trends included a movement away from 'health' as narrowly defined towards a more positive and holistic concept. Traditional definitions of health were narrow, and concerned with an individual body's mechanical ability and the operation of its constituent parts and organs. An early dictionary definition, for example, defines health as 'soundness of body'.[1] The pattern of health-care (more accurately described as medical care) in many newly independent countries in the 1950s and 1960s followed what is commonly known as the medical model of health. Such an approach sees illness as the result of physiological difficulties and organic deficiencies. Resultant strategies are predominantly interventions at the individual clinical level. These interventions are typically the development of curative services centred round hospitals (which came to be known disparagingly as 'disease palaces', with the health ministry nicknamed the 'ministry of sickness'). The natural extension of 'organic deficiencies' was to see the role of the body in terms of its functional ability. An example of a functionally based definition is:

a person is well if he is able of carry on his usual daily activities. To the extent that he cannot, he is in a state of dysfunction, or deviation from well-being (Fanshell 1972, p. 319).

Various attempts to categorize different states of ill health have been made. For example, Fanshell (1972, p. 319) provides a listing of functionally derived states of health.

Gradually a shift in the perceptions of health occurred which is reflected in the WHO's even broader definition of health. This widens the view by seeing health as:

a state of complete physical, mental and social well-being and not merely the absence of disease or infirmity (WHO constitution, quoted in Corrigan (1979), p. 7).

To the medical notion of health as relating to the physical and mental conditions of an individual were now added two other factors: a recognition of the place of that individual within society, and of the degree of control and choice that individuals should have over their bodies and matters affecting them. This recognition that people are not only individuals, but also members of a family, community, and society, has important implications for the way we view and plan interventions to promote health. One individual's lifestyle and health has repercussions on the rest of the community. Furthermore, the actions of society or a community have repercussions on the health of its individual members. Poverty, unemployment, racism, and gender discrimination, all products of society, reduce the quality of life and hence (in this broader definition) the health of an individual.

---

[1] Pocket Oxford Dictionary, 1942 edn.

The early public health movement in the UK was based on recognition of the effects of wider causes of ill health, and in particular poverty, inadequate sanitation, and poor housing. Thus, though the concept of social health was not new, its genesis, in the public health movement of the nineteenth century, was eclipsed by the rapid growth in high-technology clinical medicine aimed at an individual's physical ill health.

In many colonized countries there was also early recognition of the importance of public health (within the East African context, for example, see Turshen 1984), but its purpose was usually quite clear, and was limited to the protection of the colonizers through a 'cordon sanitaire'. The development of health services in these countries in the post-war period up to and after independence largely followed the pattern of health-care development in the industrialized countries, where the majority of doctors and policy-makers were trained. This emphasized the role of curative services, and in particular of hospitals.

In the industrialized countries there was renewed recognition in the 1960s that many of the advances in health status over the preceding century had occurred as a result of changes in living standards rather than as a consequence of medical advances (documented in McKeown 1976). Furthermore, for many developing countries the pattern of ill health experienced is analogous in terms of its causes to that of Europe in the nineteenth century; high infant, child, and maternal mortality and morbidity resulting from communicable diseases, including malaria and respiratory infections, water-borne diseases, including cholera and gastro-enteritis, malnutrition, measles and pregnancy-related conditions. Table 3.1 shows such a pattern for illustration. This makes the work of epidemiologists such as McKeown particularly salutary. They demonstrated that many of the health advances experienced by the industrialized countries occurred prior to the major medical advances associated with this century, and resulted instead from changes in living conditions and improvement in standards of living. This does not imply that medical interventions are of no importance, but it does suggest that interventions to improve health must identify the underlying real causes of ill health and be prepared to act on them.

Such a pattern implies a major health-promoting role for public health initiatives within the health sector, through immunization programmes for example. It also demonstrates the importance of sectors other than the traditional health service sector. The success of the WHO smallpox campaign in the 1970s provided an impetus for more emphasis on preventive programmes aimed at individuals through immuniza-tions. Beyond that, however, lie the wider causes of ill health, including poor water and sanitation, malnutrition, inadequate housing, and, ultimately, poverty. In develop-ing countries, actions by the agriculture ministry, for example, may well have a greater impact on health status than action by the health-care sector. This is even more true when the broad notion of health is taken to include concepts such as poverty and social justice.

This recognition of the true causes of ill health, and hence of the need for multiple interventions, reinforces the need, already discussed in Chapter 1, to distinguish carefully between health (or medical) care and health itself. No longer can the term 'health' be loosely interchanged with the term 'health-care'.

Table 3.1 Causes of discharge from all general in-patient facilities in Swaziland in 1979 ranked by ease and method of prevention. Figures in brackets are percentages

Normal		Numbers by age (years)				
		0–1	1–14	15–45	45+	Total
	Total	4299	5726	18 516	3903	32 444
Easily preventable technically, of which		2553	2018	4014	696	9281
Communicable, of which		2306	1645	1600	469	6020
Preventable by immunization:		273	704	639	285	1901
Measles		151	361	3	–	515
TB		54	226	581	273	1134
Whooping cough		40	59	5	–	104
Typhoid		3	39	45	10	97
Tetanus		22	3	2	–	27
Diphtheria		1	1	–	1	3
Polio		2	9	–	–	11
Cholera		–	6	3	1	10
Preventable by environmental sanitation		2014	870	752	141	3777
Dysentery, enteritis (food-borne)		1997	723	533	110	3365
Helminthic		3	27	3	2	35
Other parasitic diseases		1	22	31	1	55
Malaria		11	32	98	18	159
Anthrax, brucellosis (pest-borne)		–	–	1	1	2
Bilharzia (water-borne)		2	6	86	9	163
Sexually transmitted and related diseases		12	8 (2)	73	6	99
Others		7	63	136	37	243
	Total	4299	5726	18 516	3903	32 444
Non-communicable, of which		247	373	2414	227	3261
Nutritional diseases		229	322	111	64	726
Complications of pregnancy		18	51	2303	163	2535
Non-easily preventable, of which		1327	3063	6717	1542	12 649
Communicable, of which		978	1293	1246	336	3853
Respiratory diseases (other than TB)		783	819	693	202	2497
Skin diseases		122	316	379	103	920
Others		73	158	174	31	436
Non-communicable, of which		349	1770	5471	1206	8796
Digestive system		45	149	475	151	820
Injuries and poison		140	1014	2941	396	4491
Cardiovascular		13	24	243	202	482
Neoplasms		1	15	217	101	334
Mental disorders, including senility		3	10	75	11	99
Muscular and skeletal		13	93	134	41	281
Other genito-urinary		65	203	1146	225	1639
Others		69	262	240	79	650
		419	645	7785	1665	10 514
Others						
Normal deliveries		–	59	6271	1157	7487
Symptoms and other ill-defined conditions		419	586	1514	508	3027

Source: Green, A. (1980) Table 1.

Closely related to the holistic notion of health is the idea of individuals having a more proactive role in their own health and health-care. In the industrialized world, the 1960s and 1970s witnessed a rise in consumerism, with calls by consumer groups for greater attention to their perceived needs. The role of the professional as not only the provider of services, but also the determiner of needs, was challenged. In some market systems this resulted in more concern for individual attention (often manifested in the 'hotel' aspects of health services). However, there were also calls for the demystification of medicine, and for a greater involvement of service consumers in decisions both about their own treatment and, more broadly, about the general style of health-care provision. In the UK, for example, the 1974 re-organization of the National Health Service included provision for Community Health Councils, composed of community members with rights (albeit fairly limited) to involvement in health-care decision-making. In parallel to this was a growing recognition in developing countries of the importance of involvement in decision-making by communities over matters affecting them. This was manifested particularly through the community development movement discussed in more detail below. However, it had important effects on the philosophy of PHC, with its emphasis on community participation as an important component of the wider definition of health.

Shifts in development policy

Shifts in development thinking were also occurring in the decade leading up to Alma-Ata; for an account of different development theories see Hunt (1989). Development policies in the 1950s and 1960s had been dominated by the thinking of economists for whom development was seen as a process through which all countries would pass provided conditions were right. Thus less developed countries would, by imitation, follow in the footsteps of the developed industrial economies.

The barriers to such modernization were seen as a lack of capital, foreign exchange, trained personnel, and what might now be termed an 'enterprise culture'. The intention of development strategies (such as import substitution industrialization, and development of local industries to conserve scarce foreign exchange) was to close these gaps. The indicator of success was seen as growth of the gross national product (GNP); and ministries of economic development and planning produced development plans that largely reflected this approach.

It would be simplistic to suggest that promotion of GNP was the only goal of the development planners of that period. It was seen rather as the necessary precursor to social development — the generator of resources to allow the social sectors including health and education to grow. However, by the early 1970s there was increasing recognition that any growth in GNP which had occurred was not having concomitant effects on social indicators (such as infant mortality, literacy rates, and income distribution). Furthermore, health and other social sector ministries in some countries had instituted strengthened planning units. These were increasingly vocal in arguing the case for additional development funding. In some cases such arguments were formed in the language of the growth theorists, suggesting that the poor health status of the workforce was a barrier to growth. Health-care, it was argued, could itself be seen as a means to promote economic production. It could be viewed as an investment good.

Elsewhere, health planners argued for increased spending on health-care as a development end in itself. By 1978, the strategies had shifted in many countries to focus greater attention on the social ends of development. Allied to this was increasing concern about the distribution of wealth in developing countries. This concentration of wealth in the hands of a few was compounded by a lack of access to services for the many, both in the rural areas and in the rapidly growing peri-urban areas. Commitment to basic rights, including health-care, as propounded by the International Labour Organization (ILO), became a feature of the preamble to many development policy statements.

The opposing school of development theory to that of the modernists argued that the situation in which developing countries found themselves was the direct result of the earlier and ongoing 'development' of the industrial powers. This occurred originally through their position as colonial exploiters, and continued subsequently through their role as controllers of the world's economic (and military) centres, and through their dominant position as trading partners. For the dependency school, under-development of former colonies is the direct result of the development of other countries. The spectacular gains of the North, achieved over the last century, were only possible at the expense of the continued underdevelopment of former colonies. As such they are unrepeatable, under the present economic structure, for the under-developed countries. Development will not occur without a shift in the economic power balance.

Dependency theory has also been applied specifically to the health-care field. In particular Navarro (1974) has argued that the underdevelopment of many Latin American health-care systems is the direct result of dependency on the industrialized countries.

Alongside these broad changes in development thinking were attempts to promote development at the village level through community development initiatives, often with wide-ranging objectives. Some of these were little more than attempts to impose centralist strategies under a new guise. Others saw community development as a means to raise additional resources, through self-help schemes. However, there were instances of genuine attempts to facilitate the empowerment of communities, and to provide the means for their active participation in the development process.

In the health-care field, the slogan 'Health by the People' was coined (Newell 1975), reflecting the idea that improvements in health required the involvement of communities as active partners rather than as passive recipients. Such an approach could be seen in developments in a number of countries. China, for example, with initiatives such as the barefoot doctor scheme, was often quoted as an example of how communities can contribute on their own terms to their own health development. The use of community (health) workers (see Walt *et al.* 1990 for an account of the development of community health worker programmes) began to be seen not only as an important way of involving the community in health-care decision-making, but also as a relatively cheap way of providing basic services, in situations where the State had very limited budgets. A related approach to resource shortages, both financial and professional, was the use of paramedicals, such as medical assistants in Tanzania, to perform many of the tasks traditionally carried out by doctors.

Such community health workers and paramedicals were, with the exception of the feldshers (school leavers trained to provide care to rural populations) in the USSR, largely unknown in industrialized countries. They were seen, however, both as a realistic response to the extreme resource limitations of the health sector and as a more appropriate and acceptable way to deal with many of the major endemic health problems, such as malaria and gastroenteritis. The inappropriateness of much of the medical model was increasingly being challenged. Seminal books, such as *Medical care in developing countries* (King 1966) and *Paediatric priorities for developing countries* (Morley 1973) argued for a major shift in emphasis from expensive high-technology medicine to more cost-effective interventions.

The development of health centres and under-fives clinics was seen as a more appropriate and relevant response to the health needs of the vast majority. Concern about the appropriateness of a number of medical interventions were echoed in the North, for example by Cochrane (1972). He argued that the efficacy or effectiveness of many medical interventions had never been scientifically tested. Other writers, notably Illich (1977), went much further, arguing that current medical care was often dangerous for people's health.

THE ALMA-ATA DECLARATION

The preceding outlined a number of themes: the broadening of the concept of health, an understanding of the wider causes of ill health, a desire to incorporate a greater involvement of communities in decision-making, a shift in development thinking towards social ends, and a recognition of the inappropriateness of many of the health-care structures inherited by developing countries to tackling their predominant health problems. These themes formed the backdrop to the 1978 Alma-Ata Conference. (The Alma-Ata Declaration itself can be found in WHO (1978). For an analysis of it see Walt and Vaughan (1981).) The resultant declaration endorsed PHC as the means of attaining the WHO goal of Health For All.

The Declaration is important on at least two levels. Firstly, it expresses a philosophy of thinking about health and health-care. Thus, running through it are five themes. These are:

- the importance of equity as a component of health

- the need for community participation in decision-making

- the need for a multisectoral approach to health problems

- the need to ensure the adoption and use of appropriate technology

- an emphasis on health-promotional activities.

In addition, since Alma-Ata, two further themes have has emerged, which were implicit within the declaration. They are decentralization and the involvement of a variety of health sector agencies (as distinct from other sectors such as education) The principles of PHC are universal, in that they are considered relevant for any country at any point in time. They are discussed below, as they have important implications for the planning approach adopted.

However, at a second level the declaration listed particular essential service interventions. These are:

- education concerning prevailing health problems and the methods of prevention and control
- promotion of food supply and proper nutrition
- adequate supply of safe water and basic sanitation
- maternal and child health-care, including family planning
- immunization against the major infectious diseases
- prevention and control of locally endemic diseases
- appropriate treatment of common diseases and injuries
- provision of essential drugs.

All of these elements are again universal basic requirements, although many higher-income countries have already attained basic levels. As a result the Alma-Ata Declaration was for a long time, unfortunately, associated primarily with the needs of developing countries.

The declaration was perhaps also unfortunate in its choice of the term 'Primary Health Care'. This term already had connotations. It had been used in many countries such as the UK to refer to the first level of care. As a result, the spirit of the declaration regarding the principles referred to above has been applied in some instances to primary care *services* alone. Both the principles of appropriateness of technology and equity imply the need for the development of such an infrastructure of basic services. However, this is a limited interpretation of PHC without reference to the whole of the health system, other sectors, or the need to involve communities in decision-making. Within this book a broader view of PHC, as relating to the application of the five principles to the whole of the health and related sectors, is taken. Each of these will now be briefly discussed, before examining their relevance for planning approaches.

EQUITY

Equity is a term frequently used, though usually extremely loosely. It is often confused with equality. Equity, however though related, is different, in particular through its incorporation of the idea of social justice. A variety of possible definitions of equity exist, including the following:

- equal health
- equal access to health-care

- equal utilization of health-care

- equal access to health-care according to need

- equal utilization of health-care according to need.

The first of these at first sight accords most closely with the WHO goal; however, it has to be recognized that it is unattainable. Although possibly a desideratum, it is of little practical use to the planner seeking criteria against which to develop plans. The second and third definitions are also unworkable, and possibly undesirable. One would not, for example, regard a situation as equitable where everyone used health-care the same number of times (equal utilization), irrespective of their degree of ill health. Similarly, equal access to health-care, in a world of limited resources, may imply unequal access relative to need. Given the importance of social justice in the concept of equity, it is fair to suggest that the last two definitions come closest to the philosophy of PHC.

Which is closer depends in part on how broadly 'access' is defined. If it is defined narrowly to imply physical access alone (although it is impossible to envisage a health system where everyone with equal needs lives at exactly the same distance from health facilities!), then the presence of any other factor inhibiting the take-up of health-care is likely to make 'access' alone an unacceptable definition. If the health system charges a fee, for example, then utilizable access is dependent on ability to pay as well as on proximity to the service.

The alternative definition to that concerned with access concerns utilization. Utilization of services is recognized to be related to a variety of factors, including distance from the service. These are outlined in Box 3.1. Analysis of such factors suggests that three overall underlying factors incorporating various of these more specific factors are the class, ethnicity, and gender of an individual. Social epidemiological studies have been conducted to examine the importance of these factors. In the UK, for example, one study (Townsend *et al.* 1982) demonstrated marked difference in

---

Box 3.1 Some factors affecting utilization of health-care

Physical distance from the health facility
Cost involved in using the health facility:

- fees charged
- travel to and from facility
- drug costs

Lost income during time spent in attending
Attitudes of employers to absence from work
Perceptions of need and of the utility of health-care
Cultural constraints on the use of medical care
Attitudes of health professionals

Table 3.2   Use of heath services by children under 7 by occupational class of father (Great Britain, 1965). All figures are percentages

Class	I	II	IIIN	IIIM	IV	V
Had never visited a dentist	16	20	19	24	27	31
Not immunized against:						
smallpox	6	14	16	25	29	33
polio	1	3	3	4	6	10
diphtheria	1	3	3	6	8	11

Reproduced from Townsend *et al.* (1982), Table 17, with the permission of the Controller of Her Majestys Stationery Office.

the utilization of health services between different classes. Table 3.2 shows one example of this.

Studies in Zimbabwe (Segall 1983; more recent work in Zimbabwe related to equity can be found in Loewenson *et al.* 1991) and South Africa also showed differences in both health status and utilization according to race, as exemplified in Tables 3.3 and 3.4.

Table 3.3   Ratios of some indices of inequality

Population sub-group	Infant mortality rate	Mean family income per head	Mean cost of health-care received
White	1.0	39	36
Urban black	3.5	5	8
Rural black	10.0	1	1

Reproduced from Segall (1983) with permission.

Table 3.4   Indicators of health and income in South Africa by racial group during apartheid

	Indians	Whites	Coloureds	Africans
Maternal mortality per 100 000 in 1989	5	8	22	58
Percentage of population below minimum living level in 1989	10.7	1.6	28.1	52.7
Infant mortality per 1000 births 1980–85	18.9	13	56	82

Source: Rensburg *et al.* (1992); ANC (1994).

If access is more broadly defined to incorporate such factors, then both definitions of equity, whether couched in terms of utilization or of access, are likely to have similar implications. The difference between them is reduced to individual decisions to utilize health-care. The importance of this depends on the degree to which one believes such decisions are affected by one's environment.

A useful distinction has been made between vertical and horizontal equity (West 1981).

- *Horizontal equity* implies equal treatment for equal need. For example, all pregnant women without complications would receive similar care.

- *Vertical equity* implies the unequal treatment of unequal need. It suggests that differing levels of health provision be made available for pregnant women expecting no complications from those with likely complications. It also suggests different levels of care for pregnancy as compared to other health needs, such as coronary patients.

In planning services it is relatively easy to understand the concept of horizontal equity, although it may be difficult to achieve. However, the concept of vertical equity is far harder to apply, requiring a working definition of need, and value judgements about how to react and how to prioritize services for relative needs. To continue the example above, similar provision of services for all pregnant women with no complications is easy to understand and to monitor. However, decisions as to the relative emphasis (and hence resources) to be placed on services for pregnant women compared with coronary care require a judgement as to the relative needs of and priority to be given to each group of patients. This is discussed further in Chapter 8.

In planning for PHC, the first key essential must be a clear, well defined, and workable understanding of equity, and resultant criteria for monitoring movement towards it. If, for example, the utilization-based definition is employed, horizontal equity would suggest that utilization rates by different groups (by class, location, occupation, gender, or race) should be similar for similar health needs.

Planning for equity requires the identification of those groups currently disadvantaged in terms of health status, or access to or utilization of services. This may, for example, be in terms of location. Emphasis in many health plans in the 1970s lay on services for rural populations, which were seen as the most disadvantaged. There is now increasing recognition that such a broad categorization was perhaps simplistic. There are increasingly large numbers of urban dwellers (in particular in the peri-urban areas), whose health status and health service access is as least as bad as that of those in the rural areas, if not worse. This is often compounded by the lack of an established and supportive social structure. Within the rural areas, blanket assumptions of need are also not helpful. Rural populations often include significant differences in income levels and health status.

Another of the major groups consistently disadvantaged in many countries is women. Where health plans have taken specific interest in the health of women, it has been largely through their reproductive role, with emphasis on 'maternal' services. Far more attention needs to be given to issues of gender more widely within the context of planning. (For a discussion of gender and planning see Moser (1993), and Leslie (1989). Other references related to gender and health are given in the bibliography.) Even within the area of reproduction, however, a gender-sensitive analysis might lead to far greater emphasis on the roles and responsibility of men within the area of family planning. At the level of planning structures it is also essential that the

Table 3.5 Selected key indicators for regions and development groupings

	Under 5 mortality 1996 (No. of deaths under 5 years per 1000 live births)	Infant mortality 1996 (No. of deaths under 1 year per 1000 live births)	GNP per capita 1995 (US $)	Life expectancy at birth 1996 (years)	Maternal mortality rate 1990 (No. of deaths of women from pregnancy-related causes per 100 000 live births)
Sub-Saharan Africa	170	105	501	51	980
Middle East and North Africa	65	50	1 701	65	320
South Asia	119	80	345	61	610
East Asia and Pacific	54	41	1 043	68	210
Latin America and Caribbean	43	35	3 271	69	190
CEE/CIS and Baltic states	36	29	2 086	68	85
Industrialized countries	7	6	25 926	77	13
Developing countries	97	66	1 101	62	470
Least developed countries	171	109	220	51	1100
World	88	60	4 812	63	430

Source: UNICEF (1998).

process ensures the full participation of women both through community processes and professionally. Planning units, for example, have a responsibility to ensure full and real representation of both sexes within them.

Lastly, it is important to recognize the major inequities that exist between countries and regions of the world. Table 3.5 sets out some key health indicators which illustrate the significant differences that still exist, and which development policies should be focused on.

A planner therefore needs to identify the disadvantaged groups and regions, and ensure that any plans developed take specific account of their needs. One role of the planner is as an advocate for these groups, ensuring that their voice is heard.

COMMUNITY PARTICIPATION

The second principle underlying PHC is that of community participation. (See Rifkin (1985) and Zachus and Lysack (1998) for discussion of the whole relationship between community participation and health planning.) A variety of different inter-pretations as to what is meant by the term have emerged since Alma-Ata. These include:

- the individual's responsibility for her/his own health

- individual or community involvement in decisions about health-care

- the individual's contribution to resources or community 'self-help' schemes.

All the above can be detected in the Alma-Ata Declaration, although varying emphases have been placed on them since. For example, the last one has been used by propo-nents of community financing of health-care as a justification for such initiatives as the World Bank's policies in health-care financing and UNICEF's Bamako Initiative. The interpretations of the term 'community participation' are in fact quite different, each with differing implications for the type of planning system adopted.

The individual's responsibility for health

The Alma-Ata Declaration recognized the need to empower individuals in their relations with the health professions. The consumer movement of the 1960s had highlighted the passive relationship that often exists between the doctor and her/his patient. Furthermore, there was increasing recognition of the importance of non-medical factors such as lifestyle in the promotion of health. These were seen as the responsibility of individuals rather than of health professionals.

Strategies that recognize the responsibility of the individual may emphasize areas such as health education in transmitting information about factors that affect health. They also recognize the need to change attitudes and develop skills in the health professions towards 'their' patients. Some analysts suggest that the market (or, as in some State health-care systems, a surrogate market) is an appropriate way to ensure greater accountability of the medical profession to the individual, on the basis that a patient will go elsewhere unless satisfied with her/his doctor's attitude. This of course assumes the existence of alternative choices, but for many this is unrealistic.

In some countries the failure of existing institutional health-care has led to the development of community-based groups providing alternative forms of health-care. These may remain as such, or may develop into pressure groups for changes in the State health sector in service provision. In many countries this has been closely related to the development of the women's movement, representing more fully the broader interests of women and their empowerment in society.

Individual or community involvement in decisions about health-care

A second interpretation of the concept of community participation concerns involvement in decisions about the general type and pattern of health-care (as opposed to the application of this in individual cases). This approach is promoted for at least two reasons. Firstly, the concept of the accountability of public services suggests that the funders of public health-care should be entitled to some say in how these are provided. Secondly, at a more pragmatic level, it is recognized that involvement of potential users of the services is likely to increase the possibility of the services being acceptable to (owned by), and so used by, them.

Each of these two rationales for community participation in decision-making has implications for the type of participation it will encourage.

- The first requires the need to demonstrate that broad-based accountability occurs. This may lead to the setting up of new structures such as health committees, or to the modification of existing decision-making processes. Whichever it is, it requires a recognition by planners of the need to gain genuine acceptance of plans. Consultation processes become an important part of the planning timetable.

- The second requires the early involvement of those affected by any potential development, and continued interaction with them through the various planning stages. Formal accountability is less important here than ensuring that the community views expressed are representative of the wider community.

It is important to distinguish between participation by users and by communities. These two groups are, of course, different, the first being a subset of the second. Consultation processes that focus on users (for example by clinic-based surveys) may fail to reflect the attitudes of the wider population towards services and in particular those who do not use it because of dissatisfaction with it.

Individual or community involvement in self-help and financing schemes

The third interpretation of community participation concerns the mobilization of additional resources, either financial or in kind. The latter may include the involvement of community members in the construction of buildings or maintenance activities, the donation of materials or labour, or the 'paying' of a community member to be trained and to work as a community health worker. The former involves a variety of community financing schemes, ranging from revolving drug funds to village insurance schemes. These are discussed further in Chapter 5; but it is important to note that most community members already contribute in one form or another to the financing of State health services. In addition, neither of the above approaches necessarily implies that the community or individual will have a voice in decision-making. Consequently they offer a very different model of community participation from that of the first two approaches. Although such involvement is not to be decried, its implications for planning are not the same as those described earlier, and indeed are less in the spirit of PHC.

An appropriate planning structure compatible with PHC requires an understanding of which type of participation is aimed at. The first two definitions are closest to the concept of PHC, and have implications for decentralized forms of decision-making, involving a variety of community groups at an early stage of the planning process.

The whole area of community participation in planning is complex; it would be naive to suggest that it is an easy process to develop. The concept of 'community' implies a group of people sharing something in common. However, communities are rarely easy to define. Geographical communities inevitably comprise a population with varying class, gender, and age composition, and are unlikely to be homogeneous in their views about health-care needs. Seeking views or decisions from communities carries implications in terms of the weight given to one group compared to another. It is all too easy in developing community participative structures to reinforce existing power structures that may be exploitative of, or ignore, various groups, such as women or the landless. Community participation can be subverted into an extremely manipulative process.

Furthermore, the notion that all individuals are necessarily either interested in decisions about health-care or have the free time, energy, or resources to attend meetings or donate labour is again naive.

The challenge for a planner, then, is to develop a structure that is neither exploitative nor ignorant of the needs of sections of the community. Where there are strong democratic structures, these may provide the appropriate mechanism at different levels. However, where such structures are weak, alternative mechanisms may be necessary, which may, of course, be seen as threatening to established power bases and consequently difficult to establish. There are no universal solutions to these dilemmas, and each health system needs to develop, within its own context, its own response to the general principle of community participation.

A MULTISECTORAL APPROACH TO HEALTH*

The third theme in PHC recognizes the multifaceted nature of the causes of ill health. It has already been pointed out that many health problems endemic in developing countries are the product of factors related to poverty or the environment. The solutions to these problems also lie in that direction. Planners need to recognize

---

* Some writers define multisectoralism to include the involvement of multiple agencies within the health sector. This, a separate issue, is discussed later in the chapter.

the limitations of health services, and the potential for other sectors in the area of health promotion. Three examples may clarify this.

- Promotion of good feeding practice may be an important element of a nutrition policy. However, a more fundamental cause of malnutrition may be a lack of food itself, resulting from poverty, or inadequate farming conditions or practice. These are unlikely to be alleviated through the activities of the health sector.

- The use of oral rehydration solutions may be an important means to rehydrate children suffering from gastroenteritis. However, a more long-lasting solution is likely to involve improvement in sanitation and water supplies, and control of the promotion of commercial feeding milks.

- Health education activities aimed at parents/carers in clinics may be a useful way of transmitting messages. However, involvement of the education sector in conveying information to children (using for example the Child to Child teaching approach; Child to Child Trust 1991) may result in wider changes in habits.

And so the list can continue. Traffic accidents, violence against women, asthma, heart disease all have causes that lie outside the domain of the health sector. The message of PHC is that the health (care) ministry may not be the most important provider of the inputs needed for sustained improvements in health. The role of the health ministry, rather, is one of a catalyst, or of a co-ordinator of health-related activities. The health planner needs to take account of this in the development of strategies, by involving representatives of other sectors in the planning process. At what level and how this is best achieved depends largely on the health-care structure. However, one of the arguments for greater decentralization stems from the need to bring agencies together — which is further discussed below.

APPROPRIATE TECHNOLOGY AND SERVICE MIX

The fourth principle of PHC concerns the need to employ appropriate technologies. The term 'technology' here refers to the combination of skilled personnel and other resources, including equipment and can be widened to suggest the need for an appropriate service mix (for example the balance between different hospitals and first-level care) and method of service provision (for example integrated versus vertical services). An appropriate technology therefore is such a combination that takes account of both the health-care needs and the context of a country including its socio-economy. This would include consideration of:

- cost

- efficacy and effectiveness in dealing with the health problem

- acceptability of the approach to both the target community and health service providers

- broader social and economic effects

- the sustainability (including the capacity to maintain equipment) of the approach.

High-technology solutions to health-care problems may require very skilled personnel and/or sophisticated equipment. *Appropriate technology* has often been seen as the opposite, and hence interpreted to mean 'low' or basic technologies. However, this is a misinterpretation. The appropriateness of a technology cannot be determined universally. In some situations and contexts, high-technology solutions may be the most appropriate. However, often the adoption of particular technologies has not been carefully scrutinized. Indeed the choice of particular technologies is often the result of practices adopted in training courses designed for different health and health-care contexts, rather than a conscious planned decision. Yet the technologies adopted can have major implications for the ability of a health service to sustain them. It is essential therefore that assessment of the technology is incorporated into planning decisions. This has important implications in particular for the way in which appraisals of options are made during the planning process. These are further discussed in Chapter 10.

A HEALTH-PROMOTIVE AND PREVENTIVE APPROACH

The final principle of PHC relates to the importance of adopting, where possible, a promotive approach to health problems. Such an approach sees health as a positive attribute (and not merely the 'absence of disease'). Given the nature of health pro-blems in developing countries, to a large degree this stems from the principle of appropriate technology: prevention and promotion are the appropriate approaches to many of the health problems, and particularly through the involvement of other sectors. This can be seen in Table 3.1 (p. 46) in which in-patient morbidity is analysed by means of prevention. The incorporation of the principle in PHC reflects the need to shift thinking in the traditionally curative-oriented health sector so that promotive approaches are at least always considered.

   This emphasis on promotion has been viewed in some quarters as an attack on curative services. However, it does not minimize the role of curative health-care. For many health problems there are no feasible preventive approaches; and even where there are, they cannot be expected to prevent all cases of particular diseases. It recognizes rather that for many countries there is at present a major skew towards curative care. One of the important and politically difficult tasks for a planner, there-fore, is to redress this imbalance, enhancing the role of and resources available to prevention and promotion.

DECENTRALIZATION

Many health-care structures, in particular in developing countries, are of a highly centralized nature (often as a result of the structures set up by former colonial powers) with decisions, both those of a broad policy nature and more detailed operational decisions relating to service delivery, being made nationally. Since Alma-Ata, decentralization has come to be closely associated with the principles of PHC.

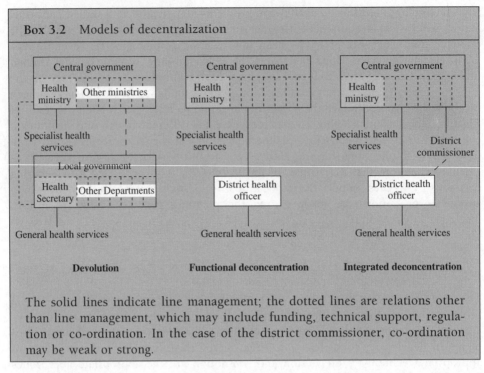

Box 3.2　Models of decentralization

The solid lines indicate line management; the dotted lines are relations other than line management, which may include funding, technical support, regulation or co-ordination. In the case of the district commissioner, co-ordination may be weak or strong.

Decentralization as a term is used very loosely to cover a number of different forms of decision-making structures, including delegation of powers and devolution. There are various different models of decentralization (see Collins 1994). These are summarized in Box 3.2.[2]

There are various arguments for the adoption of decentralized forms of structure and decision-making.

- Firstly, it is argued that decentralization away from the central or national level brings decision-making closer to the communities served. As such it accords with the principle of community participation.

- Secondly, it brings decision-making closer to the field-level providers of services, and hence may make it more appropriate.

- Thirdly, it is argued that there is greater potential for multisectoral and multiagency collaboration at the lower service delivery levels than through centrally controlled structures.

- Fourthly, it has been suggested that decentralization may enhance the ability to tap into new forms of finance-generation.

- Lastly, it is suggested that by breaking down the large monolithic decision-making

---

[2]　Assistance from Charles Collins in developing Box 3.2 is acknowledged.

structures typical of many national service ministries, decentralization may lead to greater efficiency in service provision.

Against these positive potential attributes of decentralization are various negative ones; see Collins and Green (1994) for a discussion of some of the pitfalls surrounding decentralization. The most serious, perhaps, is that decentralization can lead to inequity between different areas — particularly when it is linked to a local resource-generating mechanism. There is also concern that decentralization can lead to different levels of technical standards between different areas.

Other concerns relate to the speed and process by which decentralization can occur. A lack of sufficient skilled staff, for example in areas such as financial management, has often been used as an argument against the decentralization of financial management powers.

If handled inappropriately, decentralization can also result in a shift away from the principles of PHC. Some of these approaches may, ironically, lead to less community involvement in decision-making, or to the enhancement of the power of certain elites.

Decentralization should not therefore be seen as an objective in itself. Handled appropriately, it is likely to be a necessary, though not a sufficient, criterion for the achievement of the other principles of PHC. For a planner, one of the available options which needs consideration during the development of a plan is whether the current decision-making and administrative structures are likely to enhance or hinder the achievement of PHC. Modification of such structures can be an important component of any health plan as will be argued later.

MULTIAGENCY COLLABORATION

The final theme associated with PHC is that of collaboration between different agencies involved in the health sector (as distinct from collaboration between different health-related sectors). At the time of the Alma Ata Declaration, the main (perceived if not actual) actor in the health sector was the State. Since then there has been increasing recognition of the role of other agencies, including NGOs, private-for-profit organizations, industrial health services, and traditional practitioners. The role of other providers is discussed further in Chapter 4. The PHC approach suggests the need for collaboration between these organizations in view of the overall limited resources available to the health sector, in order to maximize their impact. Decentralization may provide one of the mechanisms for achieving this.

For some analysts from the New Right, however, competition between providers is seen as a healthy relationship leading to higher standards and greater efficiency; the evidence for this is minimal. This approach is discussed later in the chapter as it constitutes one of the elements of HSR policies.

OBSTACLES TO THE IMPLEMENTATION OF A PHC APPROACH

The preceding paragraphs outlined the major principles of PHC. Before summarizing the implications of these for the planning process, we should look at some of the obstacles associated with the adoption of PHC strategies. 20 years after the adoption of the Alma-Ata Declaration, many countries still have not fully internalized the philosophy in such a way that it is reflected in their planning systems and strategies. Various different reasons can be put forward to explain why the early optimism following Alma-Ata has not always been justified.

Misinterpretation of the PHC concept

It has already been suggested that the philosophy of PHC has been misunderstood by some. This has led to emphasis on the primary level of care, or to particular components of the strategy, such as community health workers, frequently called PHC workers, to the exclusion and neglect of other parts of the health system. Other misinterpretations centre around the principles of community participation, with undue emphasis being given to resourcing and community financing rather than empowerment.

Selective PHC strategies

A second reason for the failure to adopt the PHC philosophy fully can be traced to suggestions that it was not feasible in the short term with the resources available. An alternative to what became known as *comprehensive PHC* was promoted, and became known as *selective PHC*.[3] The strategy of selective PHC suggests that priority diseases be chosen for intervention, based on centrally predetermined criteria. This has resulted in some countries in vertical disease-led approaches which run counter to the idea (central to PHC) of integrating services. The use of centrally determined criteria for the selection of these health problems also reduces the possibility of community involvement in setting priorities. It also implies a return to a medical model of health, and ignores the importance of development in its widest sense. Lastly, at a practical level, it fails to recognize the importance of building up an adequate infrastructure from which particular programmes can be built.

A more recent version of selective strategies has arisen with the advocacy by agencies such as the World Bank of basic packages of care as part of HSR policies (World Bank 1993). This is discussed later in the chapter.

Resistance to change

The third and most significant factor which has constrained the development of PHC is the resistance encountered from a variety of groups. Various groups have felt (rightly in some cases) threatened by the philosophy of PHC. Some health professionals have been concerned at the erosion of their power. Commercial interests, such as the drug industry, have been concerned at a potential loss of markets.

---

[3] Initially proposed by Walsh and Warren (1979), but later taken up by agencies such as UNICEF with its GOBIFF programme. See Rifkin and Walt (1988) and Unger and Killingsworth (1986) for an introduction to the debate.

More fundamental, however, is political resistance. Some politicians have seen the emphasis on social justice, equity, participation, and empowerment as challenging existing political structures and their own position within them. PHC has been described as a revolutionary philosophy; and indeed, if taken to its logical conclusion, it would require a complete change in the political structure and situation of a number of countries. The principles of PHC have far greater significance than to the delivery of health services alone. The broader concept of health that we have outlined, and which includes social justice, is immensely challenging to the political structures of many countries.

In each of these groups, professional, commercial, and political, there are examples of resistance to the philosophy of PHC and the changes it could bring. The last chapter emphasized the need for planning systems to recognize the reality of such resistance.

Centralized management and planning infrastructure

Lastly, the failure of some countries to implement PHC policies can be attributed in part to the failure of the planning and management infrastructure. Attention in a number of countries in recent years has focused on policies to decentralize health management decision-making structures. Such policies, as we have seen, may stem from the principles of community participation and multisectoralism. In recent years increasing attention has been paid to decentralization as part of wider interest in the health system structures, and we turn now to looking at HSR policies.

HEALTH SECTOR REFORM

By the early 1990s, a new policy theme of similar global significance to PHC was emerging. This arose as a response to concerns over the failure of health sectors in many countries to respond adequately to the health challenges they faced. The health sector was seen as typically centralized, inert, inefficient, and ineffective. Furthermore the public sector, which had been seen in many countries as the main provider of health-care, was facing increasing pressure to contain public expenditure as a result of recessionary pressures and in some countries as part of Structural Adjustment Programmes.

Just as with PHC policies, the widely accepted elements of a HSR package were the product of policy themes developed over a number of years. Many would see the publication of the 1993 World Development Report (World Bank 1993) as the first major statement of HSR policies, although it echoes many themes that had been developed in the 1980s and before. In the early days of interest in HSR there appeared to be a universal model to which many donor agencies subscribed; see Collins *et al.* (1994) for a discussion of the dangers of such universalism. However, the experience of implementation of HSR has led to a greater understanding that there can be no single 'right' model of how the health sector should be structured. Universal solutions are unlikely either to work or to be appropriate for different health-care contexts. Various readings which examine the experiences of HSR in different countries and ideologies are suggested at the close of the chapter. For reform to lead to an improvement in the operation of the health sector, the structures need to be appropriate to the country context. This is further discussed below. Despite this rejection of universalism, there are, however, a number of elements common to most HSR programmes. Though they are interlinked, for the sake of analysis they are outlined separately below.

Separation of functions of the health sector

Underpinning many of the specific components of HSR is a recognition of the functions that need to occur for the health sector to operate effectively. Chapter 1 described these functions as policy-setting, health-care provision, financing and regulation. There are two important implications of this.

- Firstly, some of these functions have been undeveloped in some countries — in particular regulation.

- Secondly, some governments have also failed to recognize that these functions do not need to be carried out by a single agency and indeed may be best performed by different organizations.

Historically many countries have viewed the public sector as the main actor in the health sector and have not adequately recognized the actual or potential role of other organizations, such as NGOs.

One of the results of this has been the development in some countries of what has become known as the *purchaser–provider split*. For example, the UK NHS reforms led to the development of health authorities (purchasers) responsible for setting up contracts for the provision of secondary services by different hospital trusts (providers). This is seen both to enhance competition between the trust hospitals and to allow the health authorities to focus on strategic planning rather than the management of health-care provision.

Enhanced role for non-State organizations

Arising from the above, HSR initiatives often promote an enhanced role for organizations outside the public sector. The rationale for this may differ between countries and indeed may be mixed. Other organizations may be perceived as having a comparative advantage over the public sector in carrying out one or more of the key health sector functions. Most commonly, private-for-profit and non-profit organizations have been perceived as more efficient health-care providers than the public sector, though there is little evidence to prove this. The use of the private sector is also seen to be a way of allowing a reduction in the role and size of the public sector, part of the broader agenda of many Structural Adjustment policies.

Strengthening of market approaches to management and organizational relationships

The third element arises from a belief that the existence of competition enhances efficiency. The rise of the New Right in the 1980s led to the development in a number of industrialized countries of market approaches to health-care. This may occur in a variety of ways. The most obvious are the opening up of the possibility of private organizations competing directly with public organizations for contracts to provide care (for example hospital care for a defined catchment area) and the development of *internal* or *quasi markets* within the public sector, in which different public sector organizations compete for work. Less obvious ways include the introduction of mechanisms previously associated with the private sector, such as performance-related pay, into public sector personnel management.

The evidence that competition enhances long-term efficiency is disputable, however, and concerns have been raised as to the unfeasibility or negative effects of such approaches. Competition requires at least the possible existence of other organizations against which to compete (*contestability*) which frequently is not the case. The negative effects include the potentially high costs associated with competition (known as *transactions costs*) which arise, for example, through the development of bids, and the legal arrangements for contracts. There is also concern that the information systems in many countries may require massive investment solely to feed the competitive process. Too great an emphasis on competition may lead to a shift within organizations away from long-term health objectives to shorter-term income generation objectives.

Decentralization

The next approach often associated with HSR is decentralization. As pointed out earlier in the chapter, the move to decentralize has a long history in many countries. Within HSR initiatives, this is seen as a critical element in reducing what is seen as cumbersome centralized bureaucracy and to allow greater local control and flexibility. The various decentralization models were outlined in Box 3.2 and the arguments for and against decentralization are highlighted on p. 60–61.

Clinical packages, evidence-based medicine, and explicit prioritization

The resource constraints facing the health sector has led to a greater recognition of the need to set clear priorities. The World Development Report (World Bank 1993) proposed a means of priority-setting which brought together information about the impact of interventions (the Disability Adjusted Life Year — DALY, further discussed in Chapters 8 and 10) in reducing the Burden of Disease with their cost and which then ranked them to provide a minimum set of clinical services to be provided. Priority-setting is at the heart of planning, and this recognition of the resource constraints is critical to any planning process. However, the criticisms that have been raised against DALYs as a priority-setting mechanism (Anand and Hanson 1997, Barker and Green 1996) echo many of those brought against the selective PHC approach discussed earlier.

The broader message of HSR has been the need to measure both the effectiveness of particular interventions together with their cost. The growth in interest in both *evidence-based medicine* and *economic appraisal techniques* reflects these.

Integration of vertical programmes

The health sector in many countries contains various parallel vertical programmes, dealing either with specific diseases or groups of diseases. Common ones include TB control, an expanded program of immunization (EPI), communicable diseases, and AIDS programmes. Although the vertical nature of these programmes has some advantages (including clear programme focus, staff specialization and expertise, and ability to attract specific funding) there are also various potential disadvantages. These include inconvenience to users, inefficiency arising from duplications, competition for funding, and lack of local control. The heightened interest in decentralization has been one of the factors behind attempts to integrate these separately managed programmes into the general service.

Orientation to users

Some HSR packages include attempts to make the health sector more user-oriented. The health sector can often be criticized as being oriented to the needs of its staff rather than its users and mechanisms have been sought to redress this. User charges (see below) are seen by some as a means of enhancing consumerism within the health service; decentralization (with, for example, representation by patients on hospital boards) is also seen as bringing services closer to users, whereas specific devices such as marketing and user charters are perceived as means of finding out users' wants and setting out minimum service standards. The important distinction between users and communities made on p. 56 needs to be borne in mind.

Shifts in funding approach

Lastly, HSR initiatives have often included new funding mechanisms. In resource-poor countries the severe constraints on the public sectors ability to fund health-care adequately led to increased interest in new approaches in the 1980s. In particular there were advocates of the (increased) use of user charges (World Bank 1987), community financing (UNICEF 1995), and social insurance systems (Abel-Smith 1992). User charges in particular were viewed by some as fitting the market model well. These approaches are discussed further in Chapter 5.

HSR, PHC, AND PLANNING

The preceding sections have outlined the key issues arising from the two broad sets of policy that have been of global importance over the last two decades. There have obviously been policy initiatives in specific health areas, such as TB or AIDS, but we are concerned here with broader system issues. In many countries, HSR has taken over from PHC as the key policy issue. Indeed, in some donor agencies it even appears to be slightly embarrassing to talk about PHC, which is regarded as somewhat old-fashioned and out of date. However, there has been little open debate about the relationship between HSR and PHC. This book, though not concerned about the semantics of which term is used, considers that the objectives of PHC policy remain as important today as 20 years ago. This is based partly on a value judgement about, for example, the importance of equity over other more market-oriented principles such as choice.

There is undoubtedly a need for reform of the health sector in many countries. However, reform can take many shapes and the choice of which approach to take needs to be set against clear sectoral objectives. Box 3.3 sets out a set of such criteria against which a health sector might be judged.

Box 3.3 Possible criteria for assessing the appropriateness of the health sector

---

Health enhancement
Equity and lack of discrimination
Cost-effectiveness of resource usage
Participation of communities in decision-making
Transparency and accountability of decision-making
Localized decision-making
Choice of service provision
Equality of opportunity for health service staff

Though we may understand the gut sense of these criteria, they are not easy to define nor to put into operation. They may even pull against each other, requiring trade-offs to be made. Thus, for example, the introduction of blanket user charges may produce additional funding which might lead to health enhancement but would have negative equity implications. Each society is likely to make different decisions about how they make such value judgements. Indeed, as societies change, so are the judgements they are likely to make. This dynamic nature of societies is, of course, one of the strong arguments against universalist solutions to health sector structural deficiencies. The choice of these criteria has implications for both the structure of the health sector which is chosen and the planning system.

Firstly, they should form ongoing criteria against which the content of plans are developed and assessed. As we have argued, all plans are the product of technical analysis and value judgements. A clear understanding throughout the planning process and actors of these values is essential. Secondly, the planning process itself needs to be sensitive to the chosen criteria. For example, if transparency of decision-making is seen to be of great value, then the planning process needs itself to be open and clear.

In many countries, planning was seen as the vehicle for delivering PHC policies, and the 1980s saw the development of planning systems. However, the record of such policies has not been resounding. Although some of this failure can be attributed to contextual constraints such as recession, planning has also often not lived up to its expectations. In some countries this has led to what amounts to almost a rejection of planning processes, which have been identified closely with the centralized bureau-cratic decision process, and a desire to set up structures that provide other means of setting priorities and making decisions about the future. It is argued here that this would be short-sighted: the planning process needs to be improved rather than rejected. It needs to respond to the objectives of the health sector and use these criteria as parameters to frame the planning process. For example, decentralization implies the need to rethink central and peripheral planning roles. The centre needs to move away from the imposition of top-down detailed plans, to a role of setting broad policies and strategies and leaving the detailed implementation to lower levels of the service and to other non-Sate agencies. As part of this changing role, it therefore also needs to develop its regulatory and quality assurance role. This is further discussed in Chapter 14.

SUMMARY

This chapter has set the scene for the rest of the book by looking at key issues in the policy context — the PHC approach and HSR — both of which have implications for the appropriate approach to planning. It has argued that clear sectoral objectives are needed against which HSR occurs, and which build on the important foundations set by the PHC approach. Planning systems need to respond to these objectives and to reform their own processes appropriately.

INTRODUCTORY READING

For a general introductory reading on the concepts of PHC, see Walt and Vaughan (1981). The debate on selective PHC is not only important in itself but is illuminating in terms of wider issues of policy formation. See Unger and Killingsworth (1986) for a critique of selectivism; and the issue of *Social Science and Medicine* of 1988 edited by Rifkin and Walt (1988) contains a number of articles discussing selectivism. Werner *et al.* (1997) provide a very readable account of policy shifts including a strong critique of the World Bank policies. MacPherson and Midgley (1987) provide a more general introduction to social policy, and Doyal (1979) provides a very readable introduction to political analysis of issues in health, though not specifically within the context of developing countries. For a similar approach written from the Zimbabwean context see Sanders (1985). Readers wanting an introduction to economic theories of development should refer to Hunt (1989).

Zwi and Mills (1995) provides, in a special edition of *Journal of International Development*, a review of health policy trends and Barker (1996) outlines key specific issues in policy. There is a significant body of literature now written about different aspects of HSR including Cassells (1994) and Creese (1994) and Frenk (1994) on the broad principles of HSR, Bennett *et al.* (1977) on the private sector, Green and Matthias (1997) and Hulme and Edwards (1997) on NGOs, Broomberg (1994) on the health-care managed market, McPake (1996) on semi-autonomy for hospitals, Mills (1998) on contracting, Smith (1997) on decentralization. Sen and Koivusalo (1998) provide a useful critique of HSR against the PHC policy objectives. Various case-studies of aspects of reform in specific countries are also provided. In addition to the key 1993 World Development Report on the health sector, a more recent one (World Bank 1997) looks at the role of the State.

EXERCISE 3

1. Assess for a country well known to you:

   - the major health problems of the country

   - how these could be best tackled

   - the role of sectors other than health in overcoming these problems.

2. Consider a health project or programme which has recently started.

   - Were communities involved in the decision?

   - If so how? Was it genuine or token involvement?

   - If not, how could they have been?

   - Which social group in the country experiences the worst health?

   - Why?

   - What particular steps should the health service take to improve this?

REFERENCES AND FURTHER READING

Aas, I. H. M. (1997). Organisational change: decentralisation in hospitals. *International Journal of Health Planning and Management,* 12(2), 103–14.

Abel-Smith, B. (1992). Health insurance in developing countries: lessons from experience *Health Policy and Planning,* 7(3) 215–26.

Adeyi, O. *et al.* (1997). Health status during the transition in Central and Eastern Europe: development in reverse? *Health Policy and Planning,* 12(2), 132–45.

African National Congress (1994). *A National Health Plan for South Africa.* African National Congress. Johannesburg

Alberts, J. F. (1997). Socio-economic inequity in health care: a study of services utilization in Curacao. *Social Science And Medicine,* 45(2), 213–20.

Anand, S. and Hanson, K. (1997). Disability-Adjusted Life Years: a critical review. *Journal of Health Economics,* 16, 685–702.

Barker, C. (1996). *The health care policy process.* Sage, London.

Barker, C. and Green, A. (1996). Opening the debate on DALYs. *Health Policy and Planning,* 11(2), 179–83.

Bennett, S, McPake, B. and Mills, A. (eds) (1997). *Private health providers in developing countries.* Zed Books, London.

Bloom, F. and Xingyuan, G. (1997). Health Sector Reform: lessons from China. *Social Science and Medicine* 45(3), 351–60.

Bloom, G. (1997). *Primary care meets the market: lessons from China and Vietnam.* IDS Working Paper 53, Institute of Development Studies, Brighton.

Bobadilla, J-L. *et al.* (1994). Design, content and financing of an essential national package of health services. *Bulletin Of The World Health Organization,* 72(4), 653–62.

Broomberg, J. (1994). Managing the health care market in developing countries: prospects and problems. *Health Policy and Planning* 9(3), 237–51.

Bryant, J.H. *et al.* (1997). Ethics, equity and renewal of WHO's health-for-all strategy. *World Health Forum* 18(2), 107–15.

Cassells, A. (1994). Health sector reform: key issues in less developed countries. *Journal of International Development* 7(3), 329–47.

Cheema, G. S. and Rondinelli, D. A., (eds) (1983). *Decentralisation and development.* Sage, Beverly Hills, CA.

Child to Child Trust (1991). *Doing it better: a simple guide to evaluating Child to Child approaches.* London University Institute of Child Health and Institute of Education.

Cochrane, A. (1972). *Effectiveness and efficiency: random reflections on health services.* Nuffield Provincial Hospitals Trust, London.

Cohen, J. M. and Hook, R. M. (1987). Decentralised planning in Kenya. *Public Administration and Development*, 7, 77–93.

Collins, C. D and Green, A. T (1994). Decentralisation and Primary Health Care: some negative implications in developing countries. *International Journal of Health Services*, 24(3), 459–76.

Collins, C. (1994). *Management and organisation in developing countries.* Oxford University Press, Oxford.

Collins, C. *et al.* (1994). International transfers of National Health Service reforms: problems and issues. *Lancet*, 344, 244–50.

Conyers, D. (1983). Decentralisation: the latest fashion in development administration? *Public Administration and Development*, 3, 97–109.

Corrêa, S. (1994) *Population and reproductive rights: feminist perspectives from the South.* Zed Press, London.

Corrigan, P. (1979). *The World Health Organisation.* Wayland, Hove.

Cosio, P. (1996). An era of change and reform in health and social security in Mexico. *World Hospitals and Health Services*, 32(3), 10–14.

Craft, N. (1997). Women's health is a global issue. *British Medical Journal*, 315, 7116, 1154–7.

Creese, A. (1994). Global trends in health care reform. *World Health Forum* 15(4), 317–22.

Curtis, S. *et al.* (1997). Caught in the traps of managed competition? Examples of Russian health care reforms from St. Petersburg and the Leningrad region. *International Journal of Health Services*, 27(4), 661–86.

Dejong, J. (1990). Ten best readings in structural adjustment and health. *Health Policy and Planning* 5(3), 280–2.

Donaldson, C. (1995). Economics, public health and health care purchasing: reinventing the wheel. *Health Policy,* 33(2), 79–90.

Doyal, L. (1996). The politics of women's health: setting a global agenda. *International Journal of Health Services*, 26(1), 47–65.

Doyal, L. (1995). *What makes women sick: gender and the political economy of health.* Macmillan, Basingstoke.

Doyal, L. (1979). *The political economy of health.* Pluto Press, London.

Ensor, T. (1993). Health Sector Reform in former socialist countries of Europe. *International Journal of Health Planning and Management,* 8, 169–87.

Ensor, T. (1997). Reforming health care in the Republic of Kazakhstan. *International Journal of Health Planning and Management,* 12(3), 219–34.

Evans, R.G (1997). Health care reform: who's selling the market. *Journal of Public Health Medicine,* 19(1), 45–9.

Fanshell, S. (1972). A meaningful measure of health for epidemiology. *International Journal of Epidemiology,* 1, 319–37.

Fiedler, J. L (1996). The privatization of health care in three Latin American social security systems. *Health Policy and Planning,* 11(4), 406–17.

Freire, P. (1972). *Pedagogy of the oppressed*. Penguin, Harmondsworth.

Frenk, J. (1994). Dimensions of health system reform. *Health Policy,* 22, 19–34.

Gilson, L. (1995). Management and health care reform in sub-Saharan Africa. *Social Science and Medicine* 40(5), 695–710.

Gilson, L. and Mills, A. (1995). Health sector reforms in sub-Saharan Africa: lessons of the last 10 years. *Health Policy,* 32, 215–43.

Giusti, D. *et al.* (1997). Viewpoint: public versus private health care delivery: beyond the slogans. *Health Policy and Planning,* 12(3), 193–8.

Gonzalez-Block, M. A. (1997) Comparative research and analysis methods for shared learning from health systems reforms. *Health Policy,* 42, 187–209.

Green, A. (1980). Health, population and development, *Report of National Symposium on Population and Development,* pp. 104–124, Ministry of Agriculture and Co-operatives, Government of Swaziland.

Green, A. and Matthias, A. (1997). *Non-governmental organizations and health in developing countries.* Macmillan, Basingstoke.

Grogan, C. M (1995). Urban economic reform and access to health care coverage in the Peoples Republic of China. *Social Science and Medicine,* 41(8), 1073–84.

Gu, X. Y, Tang, S. L and Cao, S. H (1995). The financing and organization of health services in poor rural China: a case study in Donglan county. *International Journal Of Health Planning and Management,* 10(4), 265–82.

Hardiman, M. and Midgley, J. (1982). *The social dimensions of development — social policy and planning in the Third World.* Wiley, Chichester.

Hesketh, T. and Zhu, W. X. (1997). Health in China: the healthcare market. *British Medical Journal* 314, 7094, 1616–18.

Horn, J. (1969). *Away with all pests.* Monthly Review Press, New York.

Hulme, D. and Edwards, M. (1997). *NGOs, states and donors: too close for comfort.* SCF, London.

Hunt, D. (1989). *Economic theories of development: an analysis of competing paradigms.* Harvester-Wheatsheaf, Hemel Hempstead.

Illich, I. (1977). *Limits to medicine.* Penguin, Harmondsworth.

Jeffery, R. (1988). *The politics of health in India.* University of California Press, Berkeley.

Kanji, N. *et al.* (1995). Quality of primary outpatient services in Dar-es-Salaam: a comparison of government and voluntary providers. *Health Policy and Planning,* 10(2), 186–90.

King, M. (ed.) (1966). *Medical care in developing countries.* Oxford University Press, Nairobi.

Koivusalo, M. and Ollila, E. (1997). *Making a healthy world: agencies, actors and policies in international health.* Zed Press, London.

Leslie, J. (1989). Women's time: a factor in the use of child survival technologies? *Health Policy and Planning,* 6, 1–19.

Lindbladh, E. *et al.* (1998). Equity is out of fashion? an essay on autonomy and health policy in the individualized society. *Social Science and Medicine,* 46(8), 1017–25.

Loewenson, R., Sanders, D., and Davies, R. (1991). Challenges to equity in health and health care: a Zimbabwean case study. *Social Science and Medicine,* 32(10), 1079–88.

MacPherson, S. (1982). *Social policy in the Third World.* Wheatsheaf, Brighton.

MacPherson, S. and Midgley, J. (1987). *Comparative social policy and the Third World.* Wheatsheaf, Brighton.

Mckee, M., Figueras, J., and Chenet, L. (1998). Health Sector Reform In The Former Soviet Republics Of Central Asia. *International Journal of Health Planning and Management* 13(2), 131–47.

McKeown, T. (1976). *The role of medicine: dream, mirage or nemesis.* Nuffield Provincial Hospitals Trust, London.

McPake, B. (1996). Public autonomous hospitals in sub-Saharan Africa: trends and issues. *Health Policy,* 35, 155–77.

McPake, B. and Ngalande Banda, E. (1994). Contracting out of health services in developing countries. *Health Policy and Planning,* 9(1), 25–30.

Midgley, J., Hall, A., Hardiman, H., and Narine, D. (1986).*Community participation, social deprivation and the State.* Methuen, London.

Mills, A. (1998). To contract or not to contract?: issues for low and middle income countries. *Health Policy and Planning,* 13(1), 32–40.

Mills, A. *et al.* (1997). Improving the efficiency of district hospitals: is contracting an option? *Tropical Medicine and International Health,* 2(2), 116–26.

Montoya-Aguilar, C. and Marchant-Cavieres, L. (1994). The effect of economic changes on health care and health In Chile. *International Journal Of Health Planning and Management,* 9(4), 279–94.

Morley, D. (1973). *Paediatric priorities in the developing world.* Butterworth, London.

Moser, C. O. N. (1993). *Gender planning and development: theory practice and training* Routledge, London.

Navarro, V. (1974). The underdevelopment of health or the health of underdevelopment: an analysis of the distribution of human health resources in Latin America. *International Journal of Health Services,* 4, 5–27.

Newell, K. (ed.) (1975). *Health by the people.* WHO, Geneva.

Nittayaramphong, S. and Tangcharoensathien, V. (1994). Thailand: private health care out of control? *Health Policy and Planning,* 9(1), 31–40.

Oakley, P. and Marsden, D. (1984). *Approaches to participation in rural development.* International Labor Organization, Geneva.

Okojie, C. E. E. (1994). Gender inequalities of health in the Third World. *Social Science and Medicine* 39(9), 1237–47.

Rensburg, H. C. J. *et al.* (1992). *Health care in South Africa: structure and dynamics.* Academica, Pretoria.

Rifkin, S. (1985). *Health planning and community participation: case studies in South East Asia* Croom-Helm, London.

Rifkin, S. and Walt, G. (eds) (1988). Selective or comprehensive primary health care? *Social Science and Medicine,* 26 (special issue).

Rosenthal, G. and Newbrander, W. (1995). Public policy and private sector provision of health services. *International Journal of Health Planning and Management,* 11(3), 203–16.

Sanders, D. (1985). *The struggle for health: medicine and the politics of underdevelopment.* Macmillan, Basingstoke.

Sauerborn, R. (1997). Health Sector Reform: can research make, a. difference? *Research Into Action,* 10, 2–3.

Schmidt, D. H and Rifkin, S. F. (1996). measuring participation: its use as a managerial tool for district health planners based on a case study in Tanzania. *International Journal Of Health Planning and Management,* 11(4), 345–58.

Segall, M. (1983). Planning and politics of resource allocation for primary health care: promotion of a meaningful national health policy. *Social Science and Medicine,* 17, 1947–60.

Sen, K. and Koivusalo, M. (1998). Health care reforms and developing countries: a critical overview. *International Journal of Health Planning and Management,* 13, 199–215.

Smith, B. C. (1997). The decentralisation of health care in developing countries: organisational options. *Public Administration and Development,* 17(4).

Smyke, P. (1991). *Women and health.* ed Press, London.

Standing, H. (1997). Gender and equity in Health Sector Reform Programmes: a review. *Health Policy and Planning,* 2(2), 1–18.

Stock, R. (1986). Disease and development or the underdevelopment of health: a critical review of geographical perspectives on African health problems. *Social Science and Medicine,* 23, 689–700.

Tatar, M. and Tatar, F. (1997). Primary health care in Turkey: a passing fashion? *Health Policy and Planning,* **12**(3), 224–33.

Thomason, J. (1994). A cautious approach to privatization in Papua New Guinea. *Health Policy and Planning,* **9**(1), 41–9.

Townsend, P., Davidson, N., Black, Sir D., and Smith, C. (1982). *Inequalities in health — the Black Report.* Penguin, Harondsworth.

Turshen, M. (1984). *The political ecology of disease in Tanzania.* Rutgers University Press, New Brunswick.

Unger, J.-P. and Killingsworth, J. (1986). Selective Primary Health Care: a critical review of methods and results. *Social Science and Medicine,* **22**, 1001–13.

UNICEF (1995). *The Bamako Initiative: rebuilding health systems.* UNICEF, New York.

UNICEF (1998). *The state of the world's children.*UNICEF/OUP, New York.

Walsh, J. A. and Warren, K. S. (1979). Selective primary health care: an interim strategy for disease control in developing countries. *New England Journal of Medicine,* **301**, 967–94.

Walt, G. ed. (1990). *Community Health Workers in National Programmes: Just another pair of hands?* Open University Press, Buckingham.

Walt, G. (1994). *Health policy: an introduction to process and power.* Zed Books, London.

Walt, G. and Gilson, L. (1994). Reforming the health sector in developing countries: the central role of policy analysis. *Health Policy and Planning,* **9**(4), 353–70.

Walt, G. and Vaughan, J. P. (1981). *An introduction to the primary health care approach in developing countries: a review with selected annotated references.* Ross Institute of Tropical Hygiene Publication No 13. London School of Hygiene and Tropical Medicine, London.

Watkins, K. (1995). *The Oxfam poverty report.* Oxfam Publishing, Oxford.

Werner, D., Sanders, D. and Weston, J. (1997). *Questioning the solution: the politics of Primary Health Care and child survival.* Health Wrights, Palo Alto.

West, P. (1981). Theoretical and practical equity in the National Health Service in England. *Social Science and Medicine,* 15c, 115–22.

Whitehead, M. (1987). *The health divide: inequalities in health in the 1980s.* Health Education Council, London.

WHO (1978). *Primary Health Care Alma-Ata 1978: Report of the International Conference on Primary Health Care, Alma-Ata, USSR.* Health for All Series No 1. WHO, Geneva.

WHO (1981). *Managerial process for national health development: guiding principles.* WHO, Geneva.

WHO (1997). *The contractual approach: new partnerships for health in developing countries.* Technical Document, WHO Geneva.

WHO (1998). *Gender and health.* Technical Paper, WHO Geneva.

Williams, S. *et al.* (1994). *The Oxfam gender training manual.* Oxfam, Oxford.

Witter, S. (1996). 'Doi Moi' and health: the effect of economic reforms on the health system in Vietnam. *International Journal of Health Planning and Management,* **11**, 159–72.

World Bank (1987). *Financing health services in developing countries: an agenda for reform.* World Bank, New York.

World Bank (1993). *World Development Report 1993: investing in health.* Oxford University Press, New York.

World Bank (1997). *World Development Report: the state in a changing world.* Oxford Universiy Press, New York.

Zachus, J. D. and Lysack, C. L. (1998). Revisiting community participation. *Health Policy and Planning,* **13**(1), 1–12.

Zwi, A. and Mills, A. (1995). Health policy in less developed countries: past trends and future directions. *Journal of International Development,* 7(3), 299-328.

4

Planning for health

Chapter 3 emphasized two areas critical for the promotion of health, but frequently neglected by public sector health planners. The first is concerned with health-care providers, outside the direct control of the public sector. The second relates to the wider set of forces which may affect health, and hence the potential role of agencies other than direct health-care providers. A planning process truly concerned with *health*, and not just either *health-care* or even more narrowly, *public sector health-care*, needs to deliberately broaden its focus to incorporate these two areas.

Figure 4.1 illustrates these two elements. The horizontal axis of the matrix represents the spectrum of organizational type, ranging from State organizations through NGOs to private-for-profit companies. On the vertical axis is represented the type of activity in which they are engaged. At the bottom lie those activities that may affect health (positively or negatively), but are not directly health-care provision. At the top are those activities related to direct health service provision. From the perspective of the health ministry, other organizations have characteristics which will affect its relationship with them. Other State organizations, such as the agriculture ministry, will share similar methods of working — a common civil service culture. Indeed, their broad welfare-promoting objectives are likely to be similar, although their areas of activity are very different. On the other hand, although other health-care organizations have the common factor of being health service providers, they may have very

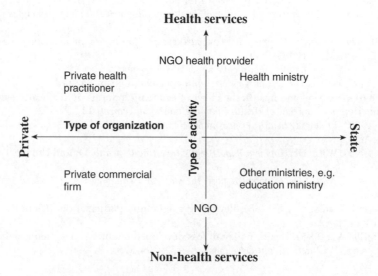

Fig. 4.1   Matrix of different agencies with an impact on health

different aims. Thus, while private practitioners may superficially seem to share characteristics with government health services, their profit motives may cause them, in reality, to operate very differently. Both of these types of difference are compounded in private commercial firms, which share neither 'State objectives' nor the common bond of being health-care providers.

For many countries, the principal roles of the public sector have been in the areas of financing and direct service provision. Planning activity has reflected this; and, in many health plans, the emphasis still lies on the direct planning of health-care services provided by the public sector. In recent years, however, there has been increasing recognition of the *de facto* scale of the role of health-care providers outside the immediate public sector. and of the need to look at wider health promotion strategies. This chapter looks in turn at each of these different components. It starts by examining the implications of taking a sectoral perspective on health-care — the horizontal axis of Fig. 4.1

PLANNING FOR THE HEALTH-CARE SECTOR

The organizations involved with health-care can be classified into five groups. These are:

- *The State*, including both government ministries and quasi-governmental organizations such as State-run social security institutions. Government ministries which may directly provide health-care include the health ministry, the prison service, and the army. In many respects this last in effect acts as an independent occupationally-based health system.

- *Non-governmental organizations (NGOs)*. This term is usually reserved for particular non-profit organizations outside government, although their definition, as we shall see, is rarely precise. Their best-known roles in the health sector are as health-care providers or as policy advocates.

- *The private-for-profit allopathic sector.* This group typically comprises private urban-based medical practitioners providing clinic-based services, although in some countries it may also function on a larger scale, and include secondary hospital-based care.

- *Occupational health-care providers.* This includes health-care provided by firms for their employees, and in some cases for their employees' dependants.

- *Traditional practitioners.* The last group is that of traditional practitioners practicing a wide variety of skills, including, for example, traditional birth attendants and bone-setters.

For many countries, the bulk of health-care is provided by the non-State sector, although there are also likely to be significant differences in the particular population groups served by the different providers. It remains also likely, however, that the State is still the largest single provider of health-care, thus giving an impression of dominating health-care provision.

The detailed characteristics of these providers differ from country to country. Furthermore, in many countries the boundaries between the groups may be hard to define. For example some countries (such as Tanzania) have for some time had a policy of 'designating' certain mission hospitals as district (quasi-governmental) hospitals, and providing them with financial subsidies for the performance of this function — a form of purchaser–provider split. The distinction between these hospitals and government-owned hospitals is thus blurred.

However, despite this, there are several common characteristics of each of these groups which it is important to note. Examples of these are given in Table 4.1. An outline of the characteristics of each group outside the public sector, the prime focus of this book, is set out below.

Non-governmental organizations

There is no clear definition as to what precisely constitutes an NGO, and considerable differences exist from country to country; see Green and Matthias (1997) for a more detailed discussion of the NGO sector. In some countries the term used is itself different, other terms in use including 'private voluntary organizations' (PVOs), 'voluntary organizations', and 'charitable organizations'. Although such inter-country differences are not important for the purpose of setting internal government policy, it is important that at least within a country a workable definition is adopted and adhered to.

For the purposes of this chapter NGOs are defined as organizations having three major distinguishing characteristics:

- their motives are welfare-promoting rather than profit-making

- they are largely autonomous from government in their decision-making

- they are formally constituted organizations.

None of these criteria is, of course, absolute, or indeed easy to operationalize. For example, no organization can ever be completely autonomous from government as the supreme legislative body. Nor is it easy to operationalize the concept of profit in some situations. However, while perhaps leaving some organizations not clearly defined as falling into or out of the NGO grouping, these criteria will allow a distinction to be made among the majority of the non-State-sector health-care providers. Such a definition essentially allows the inclusion in the category 'non-governmental organizations' of all organizations, other than government, the private sector, informal organizations, and company services.

NGOs have been a significant part of the health sector for many years. Indeed, in a number of countries the development of allopathic health services can be traced back to early missionary-provided health-care, which often had the dual motives of providing care for missionaries and their employees (and later their congregations), and of serving as a vehicle for evangelism.

In many countries, church-related health-care still forms a significant part of the

Table 4.1 Some characteristics of major health-care providers

Characteristics		State	Non-State			
		Health ministry	NGOs	Occupational health-care providers	Private-for-profit	Traditional practitioners
Motivation		Welfare of citizen	Welfare promotion Evangelism Promotion of members' interest (e.g. trade unions)	Contributions to profits through health of workers	Profit maximization	Profit Welfare of community
Types of activity	Policy formation	✓				
	Public health services	✓	✓			
	Personal preventive services	✓	✓	✓		
	Curative services	✓	✓	✓	✓	✓
	Advocacy		✓			
Location of services		Throughout	Throughout	Urban, mines, estates	Urban	Rural

overall sector, although the evangelical motive has often been played down or replaced by wider concerns such as providing health-care to disadvantaged groups. A more recent addition has been the growth of secular NGOs. Initially these were pre-dominantly international organizations, such as the Red Cross and Red Crescent societies, Oxfam, Save the Children Fund, and CARE. Increasingly, indigenous country-based organizations (albeit often with strong international links) have become significant. Such organizations are often less involved in the broad main-stream delivery of health-care through hospitals, health centres, and clinics, in the way that church-related organizations had often been. Instead, they may target specific functions, roles, and groups which have been seen to be otherwise neglected.

In practice, in many developing countries there is a wide spectrum of activities in which NGOs are engaged. Table 4.2 gives examples of the type of activities that NGOs may be involved in within the health sector.

Table 4.2   Activities of non-governmental organizations

Activities	
Service provision, including:	The provision of health-care services either to the population at large or to particular groups of the population. Examples include
General health-care	• Hospital, health centre, and clinic-based delivery of health-care to the population of an area
Specialist care	• Health-care to target groups, such as mental health-care or care of AIDS patients
Pilot, innovative	• Small-scale projects designed to test new forms of health-care delivery
Politically sensitive	• Provision of services that may or may not be acceptable to the government, but which are considered to be politically sensitive and impossible for the government to be directly associated with, e.g. refugee health-care, or family planning within certain cultures
Public educational	• Health education programmes to the public
Research	Research-based activities which may be linked to pilot programmes or to advocacy work as described above
Advocacy to government	Provision of advice to the government on particular areas of policy. Such organizations may act as pressure groups on behalf of certain causes
Fund-raising	Raising of funds from the public, either for the organization itself or to provide grants for other organizations (e.g. service club organizations such as the Rotary Club)
Co-ordination of other NGOs	A variety of different co-ordinating bodies exist, providing a range of functions, from policy co-ordination to training, provision of support services, joint purchasing, and advocacy to government on NGO matters

Private allopathic practitioners

The other element of the non-State sector considered here comprises those organiza-tions (often described as the private sector) whose primary motivation is the genera-tion of profits for their owners. Such organizations may vary from large-scale hospitals through to small back-street private clinics. In some countries health professionals may be allowed to practice privately alongside their public sector responsibilities. Depending on the regulatory powers (both actual and applied) there may be a range of health professionals practicing independently including medical doctors, nurses, clinical officers, medical assistants, and untrained 'quacks'. Although the bulk of such practice is to be found in the urban areas, reflecting the greater concentration of higher incomes necessary to purchase private health-care, rural-based private practice is not uncommon.

Although private practice may not be a major part of the health sector in many countries, its impact is often disproportionately significant. Its ability to offer higher salaries enables it to attract staff from the public sector, discussed in Chapter 13; its quest for profits may lead to cost-cutting or overprovision of low priority or unnecessary services and questionable quality. Furthermore the combination of neo-liberal economic policies which encourage the growth of the private sector generally together with the low pay of public sector health professionals is leading to uncontrolled growth of this sector in some countries (see, for example, Bennett and Tangcharoensathien 1994).

Occupational providers

Medium to large employers may take on the responsibility for the health-care of their employees. Where this is voluntary, the motive for it is predominantly commercial, being based on a recognition that the productivity of the workforce is likely to be affected by its state of health. Time may also be lost from work owing to ill health in members of the employee's immediate family, and health cover may be extended to such dependants. Health cover may also be viewed as a fringe benefit as part of the overall remuneration of the workforce. A distinction needs to be made between occupational health-care which deals with occupationally-related health-care, and schemes of health-care provision which apply to all forms of ill health of employees and their dependants, whatever the cause. In some countries legislation exists to ensure that firms above a certain size are required to provide, at a minimum, cover for occupationally-related health problems.

Health cover provided by employers may be in the form of directly provided services (for example clinics and even hospitals) or in the form of reimbursement of fees for health-care provided at other institutions. In the case of the former, where the employer is not only the financer of the health-care, but also the provider, there are a number of planning issues (in addition to regulatory inspection roles). In particular, fragmentation of the health sector can cause such services to be inefficient, and the government may wish to encourage or even require collaboration. Where firms provide health-care facilities in areas not covered by public facilities, the health ministry may also wish to develop arrangements for such facilities to be made available to the wider public — perhaps financed by government. This is again an example of split function between purchaser and provider.

One of the major planning issues relating to this sector which faces a government is the impact on equity that the development of such a sector can have. There is a danger of a stratified health sector arising from employment-related health-care, and the health ministry will need to consider this in developing its policies and plans.

Traditional practitioners

The last group are traditional practitioners, who in many countries may often be the first point of health-care contact. For a planner, many of the difficulties about fragmentation and an incomplete information base that were discussed above apply to this sub-sector as well. However, one significant difference from the planner's perspective is that there are three major policy differences between the private and traditional sectors.

- Firstly, the philosophy of Primary Health Care (PHC), and in particular its emphasis on appropriate forms of health-care, suggests the need to respect, if not incorporate, traditional health-care within wider State health policies.

- Secondly, the traditional sector, because of its different professional base, does not have the same syphoning effect on State-sector personnel as the private sector.

- Lastly, the distribution of, and access to, traditional practitioners in many countries, although by no means restricted to the rural areas, is more even than that of the predominantly urban-based and expensive private sector.

Given both the potential size of the non-State sector (often over 50% of the whole health sector), and the differences in characteristics between the various elements of it, there are two main responsibilities of the State towards that sector.

- Firstly, the State has a duty, as the custodian of the health of the population, to ensure that the quality of any health-care provided meets minimal standards. This regulatory role is not usually viewed as a planning function, but rather as one of an inspectorate. Its strength will depend on the socio-political and legal context, the ruling ideology, and the levels of resources available to be allocated to the task.

- Secondly, depending on the ideological stance of the ruling group, and in particular where there is a concern for equity, there may also be a desire for a more interventionist policy which aims to ensure not only a basic level of quality, but also that resources are as efficiently and equitably allocated as is possible in line with government policies. This book is set within the context of the PHC principles to underpin such a policy framework. The present chapter will therefore assume the more interventionist view of planning this sector which has just been outlined.

DEVELOPMENT OF GOVERNMENT POLICIES AND PLANS
TOWARDS NON-STATE ORGANIZATIONS

The process of development of policy towards any of the elements of the non-State sector can most easily be conceptualized as a series of steps or questions to be answered for each subsector of the non-State sector. These are outlined in Figure 4.2.

The answers to these questions will, naturally, differ between countries and within any country at different times. They need to be set against the broad policy objectives of the State. Thus, for example, a country that sees equity as a paramount policy parameter will assess the private sector differently from a country which assigns great importance to the development of a market economy.

This book is not primarily about policy alternatives as such, but rather about the planning process, and how this goes about setting and implementing policy. As an example of this process, the rest of this chapter focuses first on how this policy flowchart can be applied to the non-State sector focusing on the NGO and private-for-private organizations, as an example of its wider application.

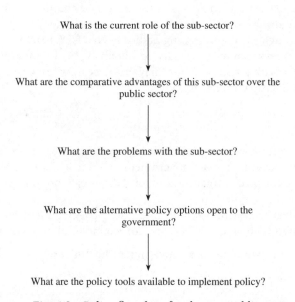

What is the current role of the sub-sector?

What are the comparative advantages of this sub-sector over the public sector?

What are the problems with the sub-sector?

What are the alternative policy options open to the government?

What are the policy tools available to implement policy?

Fig. 4.2   Policy flowchart for the non-public sector

Current role and state of sub-sector

The first task of a health planner developing government policies towards the non-State sector is to draw up a broad inventory of organizations within the sector. Such an inventory should include information on:

- the policies and type of activities carried out by such organizations

- the location of these activities

- whether there were any specific target groups for these activities

- what were the levels and sources of funding available to the organizations

- their organizational characteristics.

For the purpose of developing a national policy a broad picture of the sector is necessary. At the decentralized level, a more precise set of information is necessary to develop district-specific policies towards the non-State organizations operating within the area.

In many countries this information is not readily available. One of the frequent difficulties for the health planner arises from an inability to obtain detailed information about the activities of the private-for-profit sector, and about the plans both of its practitioners and of future entrants into the sector. To ensure the flow of accurate and comprehensive information, legislation about reporting requirements may be necessary. This in itself reflects a previous neglect of the development of policy in this area. In some countries information is available within ministries other than the health ministry that have specific responsibility towards the non-governmental sector, although it may not always be fully documented. Elsewhere some of the information may be available through the co-ordinating bodies of NGOs. Where information is not readily available, surveys may be necessary to obtain it. In the long term, however, legislation about reporting requirements may be necessary to ensure the flow of accurate and comprehensive information.

Comparative advantages of non-State organizations

The second step involves assessing whether, and in what areas, such organizations have a comparative advantage over government. In particular, are there inherent reasons why private-for-profit organizations or NGOs can provide either a better-quality or more efficient service?

The last decade has seen a burgeoning interest in NGOs. Much of this has been uncritical praise-singing of NGOs. NGOs are, for example, often cited as:

- being more efficient than equivalent government health services

- having a more committed workforce

- being more flexible than government

- being able to work more closely with communities

- having, through shared international experience, specific expertise

- able to generate or to gain access to resources that government cannot

- prepared to work in unpopular fields or locations, or with unpopular target groups.

Similar assertions have been made about the private-for-profit sector, with particular emphasis on its supposed efficiency and consumer responsiveness.

There have, however, been few country studies to test these broad assertions. Moreover, there is no evidence to suggest that *all* NGOs or private organizations possess some of these characteristics, even if some do. The second stage of the development of policy therefore requires an assessment of the actual and potential comparative advantages of the sector. For policy-making purposes, assessment of the reasons for any such comparative advantage is also necessary. Is any comparative advantage the direct result of the inherent nature of the sector, or is it purely a reflection of the current position? For example, it is possible that a church hospital currently provides services more efficiently than an equivalent government one. However, this in itself does not prove that this situation is either inevitable or sustainable. It may, for example, be the result of particular characteristics of the NGO (such as motivation). Alternatively, it may reflect current weaknesses in the operation of the government hospital, through mismanagement for example, which could be rectified. The following treatment sets out some of the areas in which the private sector and NGOs are often claimed to have a comparative advantage.

Efficiency

Organizations within the non-State sector are often paraded as paragons of efficiency; and indeed in many instances this may be so. However, it is important to remember that efficiency is a measure of the relationship between input and output. Some NGOs may have access to resources (often hidden, in the form of subsidies, donations, or 'free' personnel from abroad) which, if costed into the input–output equation, would reduce their perceived efficiency.

However, even discounting such factors, the non-State sector may still claim to be more efficient than the apparently cumbersome bureaucracies of some governments. It has been suggested that there are several reasons for this, including the following.

- Firstly, the *motivation and quality* of staff is often regarded as being higher than that of equivalent staff within the government sector, leading to willingness to work longer hours, and to higher productivity. Some NGO staff may be motivated by the objectives of their organization. However, not all NGO staff identify with the aims of the organization. Like staff in the private sector, they may simply see their organization as an alternative, and possibly a more remunerative, employer. Similarly, staff working within NGOs and the private sector are not necessarily better trained than their equivalents in government. Indeed, the latter may have better access to training programmes.

- Secondly, it is suggested that the *nature of NGO and private organizational and management structures* allows fast and flexible responses to specific situations, and that their *smaller size* also allows greater flexibility of response. It should be noted, however, that some NGOs (and in particular some of the international ones) are large organizations, with bureaucratic procedures almost as cumbersome as those of the government sector.

Careful consideration suggests that the above positive features are not necessarily characteristics of all non-State organizations, nor do they indeed necessarily lead to more efficient organizations than those of government bodies. For example, it is possible, with the right incentive structures and selection processes, to recruit highly motivated staff to the government service. Furthermore, the small size of some non-State organizations may lead to reduced rather than improved efficiency, owing to their inability to reap the rewards of economies of scale in areas such as procurement, training, and support services in general.

Lastly, a distinction needs to be made between the internal efficiency of a single institution (such as a hospital) and that of the sector as a whole. Although the market theory discussed in Chapter 3 suggests that competition may enhance efficiency, there are arguments within the health sector that overall sectoral efficiency may be better served by collaboration. Individual institutions may, within the constraints under which they are operating, be working as efficiently as possible. However, where the health sector is fragmented into unco-ordinated isolated institutions overall efficiency may be reduced. For example, supervision of (or referrals from) primary care facilities may be made by (or to) hospitals run by the same organization rather than by or to the nearest technically competent unit. Also purchasing may not be co-ordinated, and thus may not achieve economies of scale from bulk-purchase discounts.

Indeed, it is conceivable that, with suitably developed policies of decentralization, the public sector may be able to combine the benefits of size with those of the flexibility of small operations.

Resource generation
The private-for-profit sector has traditionally relied on user charges as its main source of income. Although until recently many governments have been understandably reluctant to use this funding mechanism, due both to the equity implications and to its unpopularity, the situation is changing, partly due to external pressures. This apparent comparative advantage of the private sector is thus disappearing.

NGOs may be in a position to generate resources (either financial or in kind) denied to government. These might accrue through public fund-raising, or, in the case of NGOs with international links, through assistance from sources abroad which would not have been available to governments. In addition they may be less constrained by central policies in areas such as cost-recovery.

Use of volunteers
Related to the above is the use by some NGOs of volunteers, either at the policy-making level (for example, as members of the board or management committee) or at the direct or support service provision level. Volunteers are, in fact, a particular example of resource-generation to which NGOs may have access, but which government or other sectors may find less easy to recruit.

Politically sensitive service provision
Some governments prefer other organizations to offer certain services which they may want to see provided, but which for political reasons they are not prepared to provide

themselves. Examples of such facilities include the provision of services to political refugees, or the provision of family planning services within certain cultures. In some cases government may even 'contract out' these activities to NGOs by providing them with grants to carry out the work on their behalf.

Specialist fields of work

It is possible that some NGOs may gain experience through their international operations which can then be applied elsewhere. Some NGOs (for example the Red Cross and Médecins sans Frontières) have gained a reputation for working in the field of emergency relief. In countries which are not exposed regularly to disasters there may be little in-house experience of such work within the government, and international specialist NGOs may, therefore, have a clear comparative advantage in this field.

Willingness to work in unpopular fields

NGOs are often cited as being prepared (and indeed in some instances mandated by their constitutions) to work in unpopular areas or fields. Thus certain organizations may work with particular target groups otherwise neglected (for example, the mentally handicapped or AIDS patients), or in remote, underserved areas. This is less likely to be the case with profit-seeking private organizations.

Multisectoral approach

Non-State organizations may be less constrained by the sectoral boundaries placed around government ministries, which may limit their ability to develop multisectoral strategies for health promotion. A number of NGOs which have a broad objective of community development, for example, may include within this a mix of activities ranging from income generation, through education and housing, to health-care. It is however, less likely that the private-for-profit sector would take this broader holistic view of health, given its objectives.

Grass-roots organizations

NGOs have a reputation for being able to get closer to communities, and hence for being more effective both in broad health-promotional activities and in achieving genuine community participation. Furthermore, a number of NGOs are explicitly committed to working with, and to empowering, disadvantaged members of communities. However, although this is clearly true of a number of organizations, there are others which are very centralist. It is again impossible to make general statements of this kind about all NGOs.

Private sector organizations are often viewed as being more responsive to their users' demands as an essential component of attracting custom. The distinction between users and the wider community which has already been made, needs reiterating.

Problems of non-State sector organizations

To set against the above potential comparative advantages, there are also a number of potential problems. These include the following.

Motives
Perhaps the most fundamental difficulty with the private-for-profit sector stems from their profit-seeking motives, which may clash with broader community health objectives. Some NGOs may also have motives which lead to activities or services inconsistent with government policies — for example, church health services primarily motivated by evangelical rather than health aims may clash with overall government policies. An example of such differences may be an unwillingness on the part of certain churches to work with traditional practitioners, or in the field of family planning.

Fragmentation within the sector
We have already discussed whether competition between providers leads on balance to greater sectoral efficiency or inefficiency. Whilst the profit motive of private organizations is likely to lead to such competition, this may also be true for NGOs whose motives are different. One potentially negative spin-off from the individualistic nature of many NGOs is the possibility of competition rather than collaboration between them. In some countries in the past this has been particularly true of evangelical church facilities, each vying for converts. In a situation of acutely scarce resources, such competition is likely to be counterproductive rather than inducing efficiency, as economies of scale and the benefits of planned distribution of facilities are missed.

Managerial and organizational inefficiency
Some of the apparent efficiency of non-State organizations may be the result of their small size and their consequent ability to operate informal management structures. Such structures are likely to be ill-suited to larger organizations, however, and as the small successful organizations grow they may face difficulties in making the necessary transition to the managerial and organizational requirements of larger-scale operation.

Personnel syphoning
The ability of some non-State organizations to offer more attractive salaries or fringe benefits has led in some countries to serious outflows of staff from the public sector. These will be discussed in Chapter 13.

Diversity of experience

The above lists of comparative advantages and problems are not exhaustive, but are intended to be illustrative. More importantly, each of the examples should be seen as only a potential advantage or disadvantage. Each country, and indeed region and district within a country, is likely to have different experiences of the private sector and NGOs. Indeed, it is this diversity of experience which makes it both difficult to generalize about policy and essential that each public sector health planner examines the specific characteristics of the sector, both as a whole, and for each of its constituent members, prior to developing policy and plans.

Policy alternatives for health ministries

Once a planner has carried out the above assessment, at either the national or local level, the next step is the development of policy alternatives.

There are essentially five broad policy options open to health ministries regarding their relationship with the non-State sector. With the exception of the first they are not mutually exclusive options. Each of these is briefly outlined.

Laissez-faire

This option involves leaving the sector completely alone. Although this may be the policy currently followed in some countries, it is often more by default than by design. Such a policy would rationally follow from an analysis which suggested a natural complementarity between public and non-State services, and that there was no need to interfere in this 'natural' arrangement. There appears, however, to be no *a priori* reason why such a complementarity should exist.

Regulatory controls

The second option involves tighter control on the sector, through a variety of tools (discussed below). This is a policy option which a government might wish to employ where it was felt that the sector as a whole or individual organizations were providing inappropriate, inefficient, or low-quality services.

Support for the sector

Thirdly, there is the possibility of providing broad-based support, including financial support. Such a policy, again, can either be targeted at specific organizations that are considered to be providing appropriate services consistent with or necessary to government policies and plans, or at the sector as a whole.

Devolution of government services

A further policy option involves the transfer of existing government services to non-State organizations. This would be appropriate where it was felt that they had a clear and sustainable comparative advantage over government in the provision of particular services. Such a policy may be coupled with the previous one, with government, which would act as the major financer, essentially contracting with organizations to provide services on its behalf.

Transfer of existing services to government

The converse of the previous policy would be the transfer of services currently provided by the non-State sector to the government, where it was felt inappropriate for the sector to provide the services. This might be because of the nature of the services, or because it was felt that the government had a comparative advantage.

It should be stressed again that such policies may be specific to individual organizations, or to the sub-sectors (private-for-profit and NGO), or may be related to the sector as a whole. Policies towards the private sector will depend largely on the government commitment to the principles of PHC, and in particular to that of equity.

The diversion of scarce resources, and particularly human resources, has clear implications for the public sector's access to such resources, and hence to the overall distribution of health-care throughout a country.

It is important, however, that the policy should be based on the analysis described earlier. It, and the detailed policy tools (see below), also need to be tested against the political feasibility of implementation, again in part a product of the context.

Policy tools

Having developed a policy or set of policies towards the non-State sector, the final step is to set up specific policy tools to implement the policy. A health ministry may have a variety of potential policy tools at its disposal to further its policies towards other sectors (Bennett *et al.* 1994). Some of these are more easily targeted at individual organizations than others, and some have different cost implications and effects. These policy tools include:

- provision of supplies
- inspection of facilities
- registration of and requirements for reporting procedures
- mechanisms for the co-ordination of NGOs
- provision of recurrent grants or subventions
- provision of capital grants
- tax concessions
- access to government training
- membership of management boards for government officials
- membership of government policy committees for non-State sector officials
- provision for unified staff between government and non-State sector
- development of contracts between the health ministry and other service providers
- foreign exchange controls
- control of foreign aid brought into the country.

The resource implications, feasibility of implementation, and short- and long-term impact of such policy tools need to be carefully assessed

PLANNING FOR HEALTH PROMOTION

The first part of this chapter concentrated on the relationship between the health ministry and health-care providers who function outside the direct managerial control of the State.

We now turn to those agencies who are not health-care providers, but whose actions have an impact on health (the vertical axis of Fig. 4.1). Chapter 3 stressed the need to take account of the important health effects of factors outside the direct control of the health sector, including the positive and negative effects of other organizations. Health-care provision alone (however defined) would not lead to the major shifts in health status that are required. A genuine health strategy needs to examine and impinge on the underlying causes of ill health — factors ranging from poor nutrition, through tobacco-related cancers to social inequalities, The activities of other organizations may be positive or negative in their impact. For example, in the field of agriculture, they may be positive, through the nutritional impact of an agricultural extension programme, or negative, through the harmful effects of the use of pesticides. This group of agencies is even more heterogeneous than those operating outside the State's ambit but within the health-care field, which were discussed in the earlier part of this chapter. They can, however, be classified into groups in a similar manner according to their 'ownership', and in particular into private-for-profit organizations and not-for-profit. However, there are two major differences from the preceding analysis of health-care providers. Firstly, this second group will include other government (non-health-care) departments, such as agriculture, education, or community development. Secondly, the range of activities which potentially has an impact on health is almost infinite — particularly when a broad definition of health is taken. (See WHO (1986) for an introduction to some of the issues around intersectoralism.)

At a superficial level, the process of planning for health promotion (rather than solely for health-care) in this wider sense involves the processes of identifying priorities and looking for options to meet them. These options, however, include the possibility of action from outside the direct control of the public health sector; it is partly as a result of this that the reality of planning for health from within the health sector is not easy. However, there is a further and possibly more serious reason for the common failure to develop a real multisectoral approach. Indeed, there are many examples of countries that, in genuinely attempting to develop a multisectoral approach to the promotion of health, have been disappointed by the lack of response from other sectors. This second reason underlying the difficulties of uniting sectors in a common health-promotion strategy is, however, not hard to find. Other organizations, including other parts of the government services, have their own objectives, which may not always accord with the demands of a specific health objective. An example from within the UK illustrates this well. An article published in the *British Medical Journal* (Smith 1982) looked at the politics of alcohol from the perspective of the objective of reducing alcoholism as a health problem. The article demonstrated the different interests of government departments, and indeed of the ruling political party, in this area. Some of the key interests are summarized in Table 4.3. These show that not all the organizations involved will necessarily support anti-alcohol policies.

In terms of Fig. 4.1, therefore, the further one moves away from the health ministry's position, the less likely there is to be accord with its objectives. The implication of this is not that health planners should abandon the objective of developing a multisectoral approach. However, the illustration does call into question the naivety of some of the early attempts to promote even limited multisectoralism between government

Table 4.3   Different government-related organizations in the UK with interests in alcohol

Organization	Interest in alcohol
Health ministry	To reduce alcoholism and alcohol-related deaths
Home Office	To reduce offences related to drunkenness
Department of Transport	To reduce drink-related accidents
Treasury	Tax revenue on sales of alcoholic drinks: £3597 million in 1980
	Contribution to GNP: 7.7% of consumer expenditure is on alcohol 3.4% of working population is employed in drinks industry
Department of Trade	International trade in alcoholic drinks: positive balance of trade of £449.3 million in 1980
Conservative Party	Donations from drinks industry in 1979 of £107 000

Source: derived from Smith (1982).

departments through the setting-up of interministerial committees led by the health ministry. Such committees, which sprung up after Alma-Ata in a number of countries, were often doomed to become talking-shops, with little demonstrable action flowing from them. To combat this problem there are, it would appear, various tactics that planners can adopt.

• The first, and most important, relates to the lesson already discussed earlier in the book. Planners need to recognize the political realities of planning, and to analyse the objectives of different interest groups, whether they are professional groups, government departments, or private organizations.

• Secondly, planners must recognize that, unless there is a very strong political force behind the health ministry, at the national level, its power on its own is likely to be fairly weak in influencing other government departments. It therefore needs to find allies around specific health objectives, and, where possible, to interest other senior politicians in health interests. However, planners are increasingly realizing that often multisectoral collaboration is more easily achieved at district rather than national level. Indeed, this fact is itself a powerful argument for decentralization.

• Thirdly, planners need to recognize that the change that plans need to effect can be brought about in many ways. The way on which most health planners concentrate is, understandably, through effecting changes to the health-care services under the direct control of the State. However, planners need to look for other means to bring about change in organizations over which they do not have control. These approaches can be grouped into three broad categories — the regulatory, the suasive, and the incentive.

- The *regulatory* approach means making use of the legislative framework — an often underused policy tool of health ministries.
- *Suasive* action implies trying to persuade organizations to adopt a desired course of action. This is clearly the best approach if possible, in that it results in an organization which is itself committed to the action, and not performing it under duress.
- The last approach involves the use of various *incentives* — including financial.

• Lastly, planners need to ensure that they develop plans in such a way as to provide a broad policy framework that encompasses not only other health providers, but other actors on the health stage as well.

We conclude the chapter by looking at the stages of planning to see how public sector planning can be adapted to encourage both a genuine multisectoral and health sectoral approach.

PLANNING FOR HEALTH

Chapter 2 set out the major stages of planning in the form of a planning spiral. At each of these stages, health planners need to take a broad perspective and consider both the contribution that can be made to the achievement of the plan's objectives, and the constraints that may be imposed upon that achievement, by these elements outwith the health ministry. We will now look briefly at the way in which the other parts of the health sector are incorporated at each of these stages.

Situational analysis

At the situational analysis stage, it is important that information on all the activities related to health is incorporated. Earlier in this chapter we have saw that there is often a shortage of information about the parts of the health sector not directly controlled by the health ministry, but it is important that this is not used as a reason for ignoring these areas. This is equally true for health-related sectors. Indeed, it is perhaps particularly important in such situations, as the scarcity of information is itself likely to be a symptom of policy neglect in the past.

Setting objectives

Chapter 8 discusses the process of setting priorities, and argues that it is important that, where possible, these are set in broad health terms, rather than solely in terms of narrow service objectives, and with as full an involvement of the community as possible. Given the specialist interests of some NGOs and of traditional practitioners, it is often important to consult them as part of the process of professional consultation. Although consultation with other parts of the health-provision sector, and particularly the private-for-profit organizations, may also be useful, it should be remembered that their objectives are likely to be based on different values from those of the State. For example, they are unlikely to see promotion of equity as an important objective. At the wider level, other organizations may not, at first sight, see health as an objective of theirs at all. Advocacy, in explaining both the broader understanding of health now being employed and the relationship between health and other activities, may become a necessary planning function.

Option appraisal

The option appraisal stage of a planning process is crucial in terms of planning both the non-State health sector and other health-related activities. Option appraisal involves generating and assessing alternative ways of meeting objectives. These alternatives are often viewed within the narrow constraints of direct health service provision by the public sector. However, the most significant long-term effects on health status are likely to come from actions by agencies which are not direct health-care providers. It is important that at the appraisal stage such agencies are involved in developing possible options for action. Furthermore, as we have seen, the non-State sector is already a significant contributor to the health sector, and assessment of any possible changes in its role should form part of the discussion at the option appraisal stage. It is important that the full range of tools available to the health ministry, including legislative regulatory mechanisms, is considered.

Programming

Once the alternative options, including the use of (or restrictions on) the non-State sector, have been assessed, these will be developed at the programming stage. The full use of policy tools, as different options, is likely to lead to a very different set of programmes at this stage than would be the case in a conventional health plan. It may, for example, include provision for new statutory regulations or for financial support to NGOs, to contracting, or for co-ordinated joint programmes with other agencies, such as the agriculture ministry.

Implementation and monitoring

Some of the actions programmed in the previous stage may demand very different roles and skills from health ministry staff from those to which they are accustomed. For example, the inspectorate function that has been discussed requires skills that, although related to the supervisory skills of a senior health manager, are not identical. Similarly, the drafting of any legislation as part of the application of policy tools will require specific skills.

Evaluation

The last conceptual stage of planning involves evaluation. The principles involved here are the same irrespective of the sector. However, the information base of the non-State sector may need strengthening to provide the sort of data required.

SUMMARY

This chapter has argued that in many countries the health services provided by agencies outside the State may be very significant. In addition, the role of agencies which may have an impact on health, though they are not health-care providers, is critical. Any health plan developed by the State, whether at the national or local level, therefore needs to take account of the existing and potential roles of these agencies at all stages of the planning process. The strategic role of the health ministry does not necessarily require it actually to provide for all the health-care needs of the nation, but it does require it to co-ordinate and provide an overall planning framework for those agencies that do, and one which is consistent with the PHC-based aims and objectives of the government.

INTRODUCTORY READING

Despite the recent upsurge in interest in NGOs, there are still few rigorous studies of NGOs in the health field. The book by Green and Matthias (1997) provides an introduction to the key issues. Bennett *et al.* (1997) provide a useful overview of the private sector. The WHO (1986) and De Kadt (1989a,b) and Lambo (1993) texts are useful introductions to issues of multisectoralism and the more recent Carrin and Polit (1997) text explore this further. A number of the general PHC texts referred to in Chapter 3 are also important in terms of the role of other sectors, particularly within a decentralized framework: see for example Cheema and Rondinelli (1983).

EXERCISE 4

Complete the following table by putting a different NGO operating in your country into each of the boxes.

Main functions	International		Indigenous	
	Church-based	Secular	Church-based	Secular
Service provision				
Training				
Advocacy				
Co-ordination of other NGOS				
Fund-raising for other NGOs				

- Which ones have a comparative advantage over government? Why is this?

- What is government's attitude to them?

- Use the policy flowchart in Fig. 4.2 for a sub-sector in your country to assess current government policies towards it.

REFERENCES AND FURTHER READING.

Bennett, S. (1992). Promoting the private sector: a review of developing country trends. *Health Policy and Planning*, 7(2), 97–110.

Bennett, S, Dakpallah, G., Garner, P. *et al.* (1994). Carrot and stick: state mechanisms to influence private provider behaviour. *Health Policy and Planning*, 9(1), 1–13.

Bennett, S. and Tangcharoensathien, V. (1994). A shrinking state? Politics, economics and private health care in Thailand. *Public Administration and Development*, 14, 1–17.

Bennett, S., McPake, B., and Mills, A. (ed.) (1997). *Private health providers in developing countries: serving the public interest?* Zed Books, London.

Bhat, R. (1993). The private/public mix in health care in India. *Health Policy and Planning*, 8(1),43–56.

Bhat, R. (1996). Regulation of the private health sector in. *India International Journal of Health Planning and Management*, 11(3), 253–74.

Brugha, R. and Zwi, A. (1998). Improving the quality of private sector delivery of public health services: challenges and strategies. *Health Policy and Planning*, 13(2), 107–20.

Carrin, G. and Politi, C. (1997). *Poverty and health: an overview of the basic linkages and public policy measures*. Technical Briefing Note, WHO Geneva.

Cheema, G. S. and Rondinelli, D. A. (ed.) (1983). *Decentralisation and development*. Sage, Beverly Hills.

Commonwealth Secretariat (1988). *Strategic issues in development management: learning from successful experiences*. Proceedings of the Roundtable held at Livingstone, Zambia, 9–13 May 1988. Commonwealth Secretariat, London.

Conyers, D. and Kaul, M. (1990). Strategic issues in development management: learning from successful experience, Part II. *Public Administration and Development*, 10, 289–98.

De Kadt, E. (1989a). Making health policy management intersectoral: issues of information analysis and use in less developed countries. *Social Science and Medicine*, 29(4), 503–14.

De Kadt, E. (1989b). Better health than health care: moving up down and out. *Institute of Development Studies Bulletin*, 14(4), 10–16.

Green, A. and Matthias A. (1997). *Non-governmental organizations and health in developing countries*. Macmillan, Basingstoke.

Hulme, D. and Edwards, M. (1997). *NGOs, states and donors: too close for comfort*. SCF, London.

Koivusalo, M. and Ollila, E. (1997). *Making a healthy world: agencies, actors and policies in international health*. Zed Press, London.

Lambo, E. (1993). The economy and health. *Health Policy*, 23, 247–63.

Lerer, L.B. *et al.* (1998). Health for all: analysing health status and determinants. *World Health Statistics Quarterly*, 51(1), 7–20.

Segall, M. (1983). Planning and politics of resource allocation for primary health care: promotion of a meaningful national health policy. *Social Science and Medicine*, 17, 1947–60.

Smith, R. (1982). The politics of alcohol. *British Medical Journal*, 284, 1392–4.

Streefland, P. and Choudhury, M. (1990). The long term role of national non-governmental development organizations in primary health care: lessons from Bangladesh. *Health Policy and Planning*, 5, 261–6.

WHO (1986). *Intersectoral action for health: role of intersectoral co-operation in national strategies for HFA*. World Health Organization, Geneva.

5

Financing health-care

As we have seen, the basis for planning is the dilemma of scarce resources coupled with vast health-care needs. The focus of the rest of this book is on how the best decisions can be made, within a planning process, to meet priority needs. However, the planner also has a responsibility to look for means of increasing the resource base. The present chapter is concerned with this aspect of planning.

In recent years there has been a sharp increase of interest in the issue of how the health sector should be financed. For many countries the financing of health-care is heavily dependent on tax revenues and social insurance. However, a number of factors have led governments and international agencies to consider alternative funding mechanisms. The World Bank in particular has increasingly advocated the introduction of direct user-charge finance mechanisms (World Bank 1987). UNICEF (1988, 1995) has also encouraged the use of community financing mechanisms including Revolving Drug Funds.

The form and level of health-care financing are now major policy issues and it is essential that planners operating within this context have a clear understanding of the implications of alternative courses of action. This chapter firstly outlines the pressures that have led to the current interest, and argues that country-specific analysis of these pressures need to be undertaken by planners as a basis for policy formulation. Criteria for assessing funding mechanisms are then introduced, and the major alternatives for financing health-care are described.

THE CONTEXT

There is increasing interest in how health services are funded, both in industrialized and in developing countries. Countries have very different mixes of health-care financing mechanisms as a result of various factors. These include the following:

- *Historical reasons.* Financing systems are not easily changed and as such history plays an important role in explaining current patterns. In particular, systems set up by colonial powers often remain as dominant feature of the financing pattern. For an account of the historical development of financing systems, see for example Abel-Smith (1976).

- *Economic basis.* Countries which have developed industrially may be more likely to have developed systems such as social insurance, which are difficult to implement in informal economies.

- *Ideology.* Different ideologies may be more attuned to different financing mechanisms. For example, neo-liberal ideologies are likely to favour individual systems such as user charges over more collective systems such as taxation.

- *International pressures.* International agencies may advocate particular financing systems. For example, the World Bank favours user charges, UNICEF community financing, and ILO social insurance.

The unique combination of the above factors in a particular country gives rise to its financing mix. As the context of a health system changes so the financing system may need to adapt to respond to the new environment. The following outlines a range of pressures which may lead to the need for new health financing approaches.

Demographic changes

Demographic changes have three major effects on health-care provision. First, they may lead to variations in the size of the population covered. In some countries the population growth rates are such that sharp increases in population are still occurring — often expressed through indicators such as the population-doubling time, which may be as short as 24 years in countries with a growth rate of 3% per annum. Such growth rates can cause tremendous strains on the provision of social services, including health-care.

The other two factors relate to the composition of the population. High growth rates have another important effect — an age structure with a high percentage of children. By contrast, countries with low growth rates will, over time, develop a high percentage of elderly population. Higher health service unit costs are associated with the young and the old. The antenatal, obstetric, and under-five age groups are all relatively heavy users of health-care, as are the elderly, with their higher incidence rates of chronic (and expensive to treat) illness. Figure 5.1 shows a typical profile of the unit costs associated with different age groups.

The third demographic factor relates to the relationship between economic producers and dependants in a country. If the ratio between dependants and producers rises, an increasing burden is placed on the producers to provide the means for funding health-

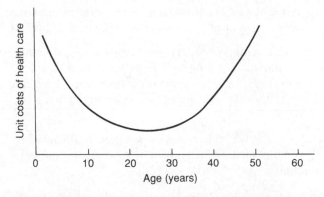

Fig. 5.1   Health-care costs by age (illustrative)

care. High dependant–producer ratios are found in countries with high growth rates, where commonly up to 45% of the population may be less than 15 years old. It should of course be noted that in many societies children and the elderly have an important productive role. The situation is complicated further by the fact that, for many developing countries, there may be extensive unemployment and underemployment, leading to even greater strain on the 'producers'.

Recession

The global recession has been devastating for many developing countries, who have experienced low or even negative growth rates, increasing debt burdens, and high inflation rates. This has severe implications for the ability of governments to maintain, let alone expand, expenditure on health-care. Such effects on the supply of health-care are exacerbated by the increased need for health-care brought about by the recession itself, through the links between poverty and ill health. Indeed it has been argued that the structural adjustment programmes required by the International Monetary Fund (IMF) as a precondition for economic support have themselves increased health-care needs, for example through devaluation and increased import prices.

Rising expectations

A third broad pressure on health-care provision derives from rising expectations about the potential of medical care. In particular, pressure from the middle classes to provide high-technology (and often therefore high-cost) medical care, similar to that available in the industrialized world, is likely to grow as such groups are exposed to the levels of provision in the North. An extreme example of this is Thailand which has 2.0 CT scanners per million population (Bangkok has 10 per million) compared to the UK with 2.3 per million (Bennett and Tangcharoensathien 1994).

Concerns about equity

Significant sections of many countries are currently unserved by any form of organized health-care, and even greater numbers have access to only very basic limited health-care. Governments committed to equity have a major responsibility to improve levels and depths of coverage. This needs viewing alongside the above urban-based pressures for more sophisticated care. To extend and improve basic health-care at a time when there is such strong middle-class pressure may be achievable only by providing substantial additional resources to the health sector.

Disease-pattern changes

As income levels rise, and basic health problems associated with absolute poverty become less significant, they are replaced by different disease patterns. The current major preventable health problems in developing countries are relatively cheap to deal with in comparison, for example, with the chronic health-care problems, such as cancer and age-related conditions, currently faced by the affluent and longer-living countries. Thus, as standards of living rise and morbidity patterns change, these changes are likely to have an effect on health-care costs.

In addition to shifts in disease patterns, the advances of medical technology have led to the possibility of treatment for health problems previously accepted as untreatable. This again places further pressures on health-care providers. Medical advances have also led to the 'discovery' of new diseases such as AIDS, some of which may be genuinely new diseases, although others may have existed previously but have hitherto been inadequately differentially diagnosed.

Cost escalation

Overall health-care expenditure is rising, for two main reasons. Firstly, the pressures described above imply that there is corresponding pressure to increase spending on health-care. Indeed, in some cases this pressure can be linked to the form of the financing mechanism itself, and in particular to some forms of insurance system. In addition, however, health-sector inflation tends to be higher than the rise in the average retail price index, partly reflecting the drug-cost element of health-care. Elsewhere, where health sector pay settlements have been higher than average inflation rates, the labour-intensive nature of the health sector has resulted in severe cost escalation.

Cross-country longitudinal studies show that the higher the gross national product (GNP), the greater is not only the overall expenditure on health-care, but also the percentage of GNP spent on health. In some industrialized countries, cost escalation within the health sector has become a major economic and political issue. In the USA, for example, rising health-care costs have led to attempts to carry out a fundamental overhauling of the health-care system, as the percentage of GNP spent on health continues to rise; the failure of these effots, due to opposing vested interests, provides a salutary lesson in the real politics of planning.

ALTERNATIVE STRATEGIES TO INCREASE EFFECTIVE RESOURCE LEVELS

Individual countries are likely to experience most, if not all, of the above pressures at some point, albeit in differing degrees. The long-term planning process of a country needs to analyse which pressures are likely to be significant for that particular country, in order that appropriate policy responses can be devised. Currently, a frequent response to such pressures is emphasis on how additional resources can be generated. Although such an analysis is important, it is also essential to recognize that some of the above pressures may also be appropriately dealt with in alternative ways. Before considering the option of increasing total resources through the financing mechanisms, three other possible strategies are outlined.

Improving technical efficiency

One means of increasing the effective resources available within existing cash limits is to look for ways of improving the technical efficiency of existing services. *Technical efficiency* refers to the optimal relationship between the inputs and outputs of a particular service (and is different from allocative efficiency which is described below). A variety of techniques and policies have been suggested in various contexts to do this, including the following:

- *Appraisal.* Techniques such as cost-effectiveness analysis may suggest alternative approaches to particular health problems which are more efficient.

- *Contracting out.* Buying-in of services from outside sources (such as catering or cleaning), where these are shown to be more efficient than internal provision.

- *An internal market.* Development of internal budget systems within an organization which is constituted as a quasi-market, with different budget or cost centres selling services (such as radiography) to each other. The assumption behind such a strategy is that such a simulation of the market will improve efficiency.

- *Information dissemination.* Dissemination of comparative information on the performance of different parts of the health service or of an organization, in the expectation that either peer-group pressure or management incentives will lead to changes in practice.

- *Involvement of clinicians in management.* Clinicians are typically the individuals who, through their decisions, have most influence on how resources are spent. Increasing their involvement in budgeting and management may be important as a means of developing greater awareness of cost and greater efficiency.

All of the above should, of course, be routinely examined as part of the ongoing planning and management process. However, although tactics aimed at improving efficiency levels may be, at first sight, the most attractive option, there are limits to the extent to which they can be applied. Indeed, if pursued too far, they can prove to be counterproductive in the short term if a manager's attention is focused too narrowly on efficiency-oriented tactics (which may have diminishing returns), to the exclusion of alternative approaches to the more general problem of underfunding (World Health Forum 1994).

Reallocation of resources within the health sector

A second approach involves trying to improve the *allocative efficiency* of the health sector. Current imbalances between the allocation of resources to different health problems suggest that there is significant scope for improving the allocative efficiency of the sector. Indeed, as we have seen, this is a fundamental activity of planning. Furthermore, such an approach is particularly appropriate where disease patterns are changing and resources can be switched. An example of this is the transfer of resources from smallpox campaigns as the disease was controlled and finally eradicated. In countries where demographic shifts are leading to an increasing proportion of elderly people within the population, resources may be shifted from child services to those for the elderly. A further example, is the decline in the incidence of leprosy globally, which is likely to free up resources for other health problems.

Harder to implement is the transfer of resources from the resource-hungry urban hospital sector to starved primary care services, as a short-term response to inequity. However, as we shall see in Chapter 11, shifts in balance may be possible through differential rates of resource allocation to different services.

Reallocation of resources to the health sector from other sectors

A third alternative open to governments to increase health-sector budgets without new financing mechanisms lies in giving higher priority to the health sector at the expense of another government sector. The amount provided for the health sector is clearly a political decision, to be taken after consideration of the country's overall social and economic needs. Although the health sector is bound to argue its corner for increased funding, it should be remembered that such funds may have an equal (if not greater) impact on health through other ministries (such as agriculture or education — the other major service ministries in developing countries). It is often argued that in many countries the defence sector is one potential source for funds for reallocation, use of which, it has been argued, would not adversely affect the development prospects of the country (see, for example, Dunlop 1983).

CRITERIA FOR CHOOSING A FINANCING SYSTEM

The preceding has outlined the major pressures which countries face to expand health-care financing. These pressures have resulted in interest in alternative forms of health-care finance. The choice of funding systemis not neutral, however, and involves a major policy decision. It is important that in deciding between alternatives, clear criteria for choice are set out. The first three criteria discussed below hold true for any financing system. The last three have particular importance within the context of a PHC approach.

Viability and ease of use of the system

A basic requirement of any financing system is that it can be made to work, and, although this appears a rather obvious prerequisite, it is important that it should be carefully considered. A number of user charge systems have encountered difficulties, for example, over the practical application of exemption procedures. Elsewhere, social insurance systems have encountered difficulties in obtaining information about employees to ensure employer contributions. Careful consideration of technical feasibility is therefore essential. Linked to this is the ease of use of the system. Some systems may be made workable, but only at the expense of complex, often bureaucratic, and costly mechanisms. Lastly, it is essential to consider the social acceptability of a system. Certain financing systems may not be culturally acceptable within a particular society.

Revenue-generating ability

A second criterion relates to the ability of a system actually to generate funds. Furthermore, it needs assessing in terms of its net revenue-earning ability — that is, the difference between the total revenue generated and the cost of operating the system. A good example of this was the licence fee on dogs in the UK, which was abolished on the grounds that it cost more to administer than the revenue it generated. It is easy to point to an apparently successful scheme while ignoring the costs of its administration. The administration of user charges, for example, may include the costs of billing, accounting, and the safe storage and collection of funds. Cashiers, clerks, and accountants may need to be employed, printing costs may be incurred, and vehicles and safes may have to be purchased. Even where additional staff are not employed, and existing staff are used, this implies an opportunity cost to the health service in terms of alternative activities which staff could have been engaged in, had they not been involved in the revenue scheme. This may be particularly relevant where charges are seen as nominal.

Effects on health-care supply

A third criterion relates to the effects of a financing system on the service itself in terms of its effectiveness and efficiency. Financing systems may have (dis)incentive effects on the pattern of service provision which make them, as a service, less cost-effective. For example, systems of financing which involve three parties — the patient, the health service, and an insurance company — may lead to overprovision of certain (well-rewarded) services — which may not be the most appropriate response to particular health-care problems. Financing mechanisms may lead to such *perverse incentives*. One of the criteria therefore relates to the supply-side effects of a financing mechanism.

Demand-side effects including equity

Financing mechanisms are also likely to have effects on the demand for and utilization of health-care. Some systems may be designed to ensure particular patterns of utilization. For example, user charges may be applied heavily at the outpatient department of a hospital where alternative primary care facilities exist (for example in peri-urban clinics), to discourage its use as a primary care centre. Referrals to the hospital outpatient department from clinics in such instances would not incur this heavy charge. Alternatively, systems which differentiate between the cost to users of preventive and curative care may alter the relative pattern of uptake in a way which makes the service more or less cost-effective.

It is essential also that the effects on equity of alternative financing systems should be carefully considered. Two considerations are important here. Chapter 3 looked at alternative definitions of equity, and suggested that a working definition of equity is 'equal access to care for those in equal need'. It is important firstly, therefore, that the effects of systems on access by different groups (interpreted broadly) should be analysed. User charges may, for example, deter lower income groups from service uptake. Social insurance schemes may favour the higher-paid urban worker. A distinction was also made in Chapter 3 between vertical and horizontal equity. It may be possible to reflect this in the financing system, whereby, for example, user charges differentiate between different types of health need.

It is important however, to distinguish between the effects of the system itself on access and utilization, and any possible redistributive policies which may be feasible with the proceeds of any financing system. As the World Bank argues, it may be possible to plough fees generated at urban-based hospitals back into the system, but this is not an effect of the financing mechanism *per se* but of the additional funding generated.

A distinction needs to be made also between *willingness to pay* and *ability to pay* (Russell *et al* 1995). When faced with life-threatening health needs, individuals may, appear willing to pay for health-care; furthermore, they may *appear* to have the cash to pay. However, the long-term effects of raising this cash may be devastating to a family — for example, where assets such as livestock have been sold to generate the cash.

A second consideration relates more deeply to the broader socio-economic consequences of different systems. Economists make a distinction between those methods of raising funds which are *regressive* and those which are *progressive*, depending on the relative income effects on the individual being taxed. A tax is regarded as progressive if it takes a greater proportion of income from a higher-income person; it would be regressive if it took a higher proportion from a lower-income person. Box 5.1 gives an example of this.

Box 5.1   Tax and equity

Three taxes are being considered, to raise a total of £10 000 from a community of 100 people of whom 50 earn £2000 p. a. and 50 earn £500 p. a.

Annual income	50 people @ £2000		50 people @ £500		Total raised (£)
Type of tax	*Amount per person (£)*	*% of income*	*Amount per person (£)*	*% of income*	
Poll tax*	100	5	100	20	10 000
Proportional income tax	160	8	40	8	10 000
Progressive income tax	180	9	20	4	10 000

*By raising the same amount per person the poll tax is *regressive*, as it effectively levies a different percentage for each income group.

Taxes on sales may be regressive or progressive depending on who buys the goods. Where they are essential goods, such a tax is regressive. Where they are luxury goods, they are progressive. Taxes on agricultural goods produced by low-income farmers are similarly regressive. Financing systems within health-care, therefore, have at least two sets of considerations: the differential effects between different income-groups, and between different levels of 'ill health'. This is perhaps best explained by a comparison of two financing systems — a progressive income tax-based system and a user charge system.

Under a tax-based system, collective financing of health-care is carried out in such a way that there is a transfer of resources from the richer elements of society to the poor and sick group. Under user charges, however, the sick are expected to pay for their own ill health, with no cross-subsidy. Thus, even if under the latter the poor and sick did utilize health-care, there are wider implications of social justice in such a system. This is illustrated in Box 5.2.

Participation in decision-making

It has been argued that some financing mechanisms provide greater potential for participation in decision-making than others. In particular, it has been suggested that user charges, through strengthening the direct relationship between the consumer and the provider, provide an opportunity for this. However, this is an individualistic concept of participation, based on market principles of interaction between supplier and demander and ideas of consumer sovereignty. It is a different concept to that which stresses community participation. As we have already seen, there is an important distinction to be made between users and communities (see p. 56).

Multisectoralism

Lastly, the choice of financing systems may make the process of multisectoralism easier or harder. For example, a system based on user charges which develops a very clear relationship between the user of the health service and the provider, based on clinical services, may not encourage the use of funds raised in this manner for alternative health-promoting uses such as water supplies. Alternatively, tax-based systems which have no connection with the health-care system itself allow greater freedom for wider application.

ALTERNATIVE APPROACHES TO FINANCING HEALTH-CARE

Having considered possible criteria for assessing health-care financing, we now turn to an examination of the principal means of raising finance. We consider here the following the major approaches to financing health-care:

- fees for service and private insurance
- tax revenue and social insurance

Box 5.2   Redistributive effects of alternative funding systems

Imagine a community of four people, two with annual incomes of £2000 and two of £1000. In the course of a year one of the richer pair and one of the poorer pair fall sick. Their health-care needs are identical, and cost £150 each. Three means of financing the health-care are considered

- the sick individuals each paying directly for their own health-care
- spreading the costs over the four people equally though use of a poll tax
- spreading the costs on the basis of an income tax.

The effects of these are illustrated in the table below. Each column of the table shows the amount paid by each individual, and the percentage of their income this represents. The different methods have effects of between 0% and 15% on different incomes.

Effect of different payment methods

Individual	Income	Direct payment	Poll tax	Income tax at 5%
A (well)	£2000	0 (0%)	£75 (3.8%)	£100 (5%)
B (ill)	£2000	£150 (7.5%)	£75 (3.8%)	£100 (5%)
C (well)	£1000	0 (0%)	£75 (7.5%)	£50 (5%)
D (ill)	£1000	£150 (15%)	£75 (7.5%)	£50 (5%)
Total	£6000	£300	£300	£300

The matrix below illustrates the different effects of user charges (direct payments) and a collective charge. The axes are wealth (vertical) and health (horizontal). The graphs show the position of the four individuals and the effective direction of transfers.

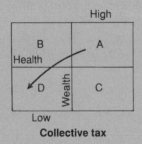

Collective tax

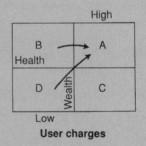

User charges

Note that although funds may not actually be transferred, user charges that take no account of income levels are regressive in impact.

- community financing

- loans and grants.

Each of these need to be assessed separately against the criteria set above and within the specific country context.

Fees for service and private insurance

The most basic form of health-care financing is that of fees for service, where a fee is charged to cover all or part of the cost of the service provided. (The term cost recovery is often used, but is a misleading and unhelpful expression and will be avoided here.) In many developing countries a fixed fee for service, known as a user charge, is used by government health services, both as a means of raising revenue, and as a means of discouraging what may be viewed as 'unnecessary demand'. The World Bank (1987, 1993), among others, suggests that user charges should be applied differentially by type of service; for example, public preventive services being free, and curative primary contact services (but not necessarily referral services) having user charges. Personal preventive services could also be charged, but at a lower rate. Arguments against user charges are discussed below, but focus on the costs of collection, the equity implications, and the dangers of discouraging 'real' need. The degree to which take-up is discouraged is a function of the price and income elasticity of demand for different types of health-care. See Box 5.3 for an explanation of the economic concept of elasticity.

Box 5.3   Economic concept of elasticity

The concept of elasticity as used within economics refers to the effect of one variable on another. In particular the price-elasticity of demand refers to the changes in demand resulting from price-changes. The more elastic a particular service or product is to price-changes, the more its take-up will be affected by price-changes.

Within the health sector, the concept is important in assessing the likely changes in utilization of health-care arising from the imposition of or increases in charges. It is also important in assessing the impact of using sales taxes for public health purposes, such as attempting to reduce consumption of cigarettes.

Fees for service are the normal basis of a private system, including traditional practice. Because of the possibility of very high and unpredictable medical costs, many users of such systems arrange cover through insurance schemes, where the risk of illness is pooled among the insured group. Within insurance schemes, there are a number of alternative combinations, with variations of the type of cover (including in-patient or out-patient cover, with or without obstetric cover, and with possible exclusion of cover for chronic conditions), and the premium payable will depend on various factors.

- Firstly, on the type of cover required — for example, what medical conditions will be provided for, and whether preventive services will be included.

- Secondly, it will also depend on the present health status of the insuree. This will be estimated either on the basis of proxy indicators, such as age, occupation, and lifestyle, or as the result of a medical examination. In order to minimize the amount that they pay out in claims, insurance companies will attempt to identify potential insurees whom they consider to be particularly 'at risk' and, therefore, likely to use and claim for health-care. In such cases they may either refuse to provide cover or set very high premiums. Such at-risk groups may include the elderly, those working in particular industries, or those with a particular lifestyle considered to be unhealthy. For example, individuals considered to be at particular risk of contracting AIDS through their lifestyle may find themselves unable to receive insurance cover.

- Lastly, the premium will depend on agreement to co-payment by the insuree of a proportion of any resultant medical costs. A willingness by the insuree to pay a greater proportion of any medical bill will result in a lower initial premium. The actual payment for the service may be made initially by the individual, who then claims reimbursement, or directly by the insurance fund. The fees charged are usually on a standard agreed rate.

Systems of this kind have a number of disadvantages. The direct payment of fees for service is regressive in that it causes the greatest hardship for the poor, and may cause major difficulties in payment for waged labourers, who are unpaid during sickness. There are also particular difficulties for farmers, for whom income is highly seasonal, with the pre-harvest period being not only the time when cash is shortest, but also when ill health is highest. Exemption schemes have been attempted to overcome some of the most severe equity implications. However, there are difficulties with these which revolve around questions of the following types:

- *Who should be exempted?* Is exemption based on income levels, and if so at what level? Some exemption schemes, set up on the grounds of equity, have been inappropriately used as a vehicle to include other groups, such as government civil servants.

- *What is the process, and who decides the exemption?* This is related to the above, particularly in a situation where individual or family incomes are not known — perhaps because of their semi-subsistence nature. Under such circumstances determination of the status of an individual as exempt or not is more complex, and its results may be very dependent on who is carrying out the assessment. Related to this is whether such decisions should be made prior to initial contact with the health service, or at the point of first contact. In practice it is clearly unacceptable for a health provider to turn someone away for lack of either funds or an exemption certificate; this being so, it is very difficult to isolate the health professional from the process of exemption. Lastly, the means of conducting the exemption process itself can be a major disincentive to utilization of health-care, if it is seen as stigmatizing.

- *What forms of health-care are appropriate for exemption?* Some exemption schemes differentiate between different types of health-care. Exemption may apply, for example, to the use of primary care facilities, but not to primary care at secondary care facilities.

Many schemes have seen the design of the exemption scheme as a matter of detail, yet it often raises fundamental questions of both principle and process and is critical to the success and the overall equity effects of a scheme.

Private insurance schemes which attempt to spread the risk of illness over all insurees also have a number of disadvantages. Firstly, they may result in a stratified health-care system, with different types of cover being held by different groups depending on their ability to pay different levels of premiums. Secondly, they may not spread the risk between individuals who have different likelihoods of illness. Premiums may depend, therefore, on the health risk. Those in greatest potential need have to pay the highest premiums. Thirdly, there are administrative costs in running the scheme (including medical examinations, advertising, and the paperwork involved in claims). This may make them inefficient as resource generators. There may also be a tendency to emphasize curative rather than preventive health services. One of the major concerns about insurance systems, however, is that there are often difficulties in controlling overall medical costs.

- Once individuals are in a scheme, it appears free to them, and they may demand more services than they otherwise would (leading ultimately, of course, to higher premiums). This is known as *moral hazard*.

- Furthermore, there may be no incentive for the doctor who decides on the need for diagnostic tests and treatment to minimize the number or costs of these. Indeed there may be incentives to maximize these, if the income of the doctor is related to the number of medical procedures or tests carried out.

- Lastly, insurance policies within industrialized countries may be tied to employment through block schemes as a fringe benefit, which may have implications for the ease of changing jobs and for the type of policy instituted.

One variant in the general insurance spectrum is that of the Health Maintenance Organization (HMO), in which members pay an annual amount to a medical practice which provides the services required, either directly or through a third party. Within this system the practice acts essentially as the insurance company, and, therefore, has incentives to reduce its own costs by preventive medicine and by minimizing unnecessary medical procedures. Such HMOs have been regarded as a possible solution to the cost escalation in USA, although their actual performance has been questioned on a number of grounds, including the possibility that they may discriminate against members of HMO schemes who, perhaps because of lower educational backgrounds, are less likely to push for their full rights under the scheme.

Tax revenue and social insurance

Social insurance schemes widen the base of private schemes with payments tied to wage-levels, and are often compulsory. In contrast with private insurance, in which individuals pay either a flat rate premium or one related to their health status and risk, payments are fixed as a percentage of income and as such are more equitable. There may be several social insurance schemes in operation, or a single, national one. Health-care is often part of wider social security schemes, which include benefits in time of sickness, retirement, death, maternity, or unemployment. Contributions to the scheme are made by employees, employers, and in some cases the State. Social insurance schemes differ in many respects from private insurance systems. Most importantly, within any scheme cover is identical, and the premiums are based on income rather than health status. However, where there are several social insurance schemes, there may may still be a stratified system depending on coverage. Collection systems for contributions are most easily organized within an industrialized setting. Semi-subsistence agricultural economies are difficult to cover, though there are a number of innovative attempts to develop schemes appropriate for such situations. One of the most famous of these is the card scheme in operation in Thailand, where annual payment allows certain benefits. This is still a flat rate system, but is State rather than privately organized. An example of one in Africa is given in Arhin (1994). The level of actual coverage in such a less industrialized country has implications for the equity of the approach in such situations. The resulting stratified health system may lead to different levels of cover being available for different people. In some situations, the problem of what has become known as 'paper rights' has arisen. This term is used to describe a situation where a person is covered in theory by a social insurance scheme, but in practice no facilities are available.

The social insurance systems in some countries face difficulties arising from the demographic and economic shifts. As life expectancy increases, funds are required to provide cover for people living longer. As the producer–dependant ratio drops (see p. 96–7) the strains on the funds resources may increase. Where this has led to a reduction in quality of care, there may be pressure in compulsory schemes to allow individuals to opt out and seek private insurance, particularly from those with high incomes and good health status. Where this is allowed, this leads to even greater pressure on the remaining funds, as these who are left in are likely to be net contributors.

In some countries social insurance systems have been the forerunners of national systems through either national insurance or tax. Tax-based systems provide a greater opportunity for comprehensive cover through inclusion of those not in formal employment. The degree of comprehensiveness varies; but in the most comprehensive national health systems the services are provided at no — or minimal — direct cost to all citizens.

One advantage social insurance systems have over financing derived from general taxation relates to the ability in the former to earmark funds for health-care in a way that ensures greater consistency of funding from year to year. General tax funds are vulnerable to shifts in political priority from health to other sectors. Hypothecated taxes which are specifically for health (for example a proportion of income tax, or sales on cigarette sales) are one means of overcoming this.

The degree to which a tax-based system is equitable depends on two factors — the means of raising finance, and the means of rationing and distributing the health-care resultant from the 'free' service. Where finance is raised from income tax, this is progressive (individuals receiving higher income pay more tax) as long as all income can be assessed and tax collected. However, where the funding is raised from an indirect tax, this may be regressive, depending on the goods on which such taxes are levied (and, in particular, whether these are essentials or luxury items). Other tax options include payroll taxes, import duties, and export levies. In many developing countries revenue is heavily dependent on trade-based taxes. Secondly, the equity of a tax system will depend on how the (scarce) health-care is rationed. This may be on the basis of queueing, the allocation of resources to different types of service, or accessibility.

Public health and preventive services are usually financed from the public purse in this way, both because of their nature as a public good, and because of a concern that take-up would be low should fees or premiums be attached to them.

Systems financed by tax revenue or national insurance are sometimes criticized as being inefficient. It is argued that the lack of links between the finance mechanism and expenditure leads to a lack of incentives to minimize costs. Furthermore, there are clearly administrative costs involved. Whether these costs are greater or less than the administrative (including billing) costs of a private system will vary from case to case. However, one advantage of a comprehensive system lies in its potential for reducing unit costs through economies of scale and co-ordination of services, though this is most likely to be achieved where the funding and purchasing functions are combined.

Community financing

Alternative methods of raising finance, at the community level, are often suggested, by agencies such as UNICEF under its Bamako Initiative (UNICEF 1988). Some of these are linked to service use (for example, Revolving Drug Funds, which are essentially a form of user charge with the income retained at the level of the facility), whereas others are genuinely community-based such as a community-based levy. Other mechanisms include lotteries and income generation schemes.

Community financing is argued by some to provide a means for participation. However, this can be a very limited view of participation. It is also argued that by linking income and expenditure closely at the point of service delivery, there is greater incentive for efficiency. The degree to which such community-based schemes are equitable will vary. Ultimately the bulk of such schemes can be seen either as being pre-paid community taxes, or as individually-based user charges. As such they are subject to the inherent advantages and disadvantages of these two approaches.

The major equity issue surrounding community financing, however, relates to the proportion of the net resources available to a community that come from the community itself — and hence to the distributive effect of such financing between communities.

Loans and grants

Resources may be provided in the form of loans or grants, either in cash or in kind, through means such as technical assistance or the supply of free drugs. In the case of grants, this has the effect of directly subsidizing the service. In the case of loans, such means of deficit financing in theory imply later repayments. Loans are more usually used for capital financing. The usual source of such loans and grants for the State health sector is through donor funding. Although such aid is often viewed as being a 'gift', it is important to recognize that there are often costs involved, some of which may not be immediately obvious. In the case of loans, these costs may be financial, in terms of repayments. World Bank projects are predominantly funded on the basis of soft loans, for which the repayment terms are easier than those of the commercial banking sector, in terms of both interest charges and repayment period. However, the increasing debt burden that many developing countries face is compounded by such loans. Health ministries must recognize the need to appraise such projects in terms of their effect not only on health-care, but also on the economy as a whole. Some countries are encouraging greater partnership with the private sector through mechanisms such as Private Finance Initiatives. Examples of such arrangements include situations where the private sector provides the capital for new buildings and arranges the construction and even ongoing management of the service in return for payment by the health authority.

Loans and grants may also be 'tied' in different ways. Conditions may be placed on how the money is to be spent, and in particular on where it is to be spent. Thus, for example, donors may require equipment to be purchased from the donor country. This may have hidden costs where there are difficulties with maintenance or spare parts. There may also be costs in terms of particular monitoring and reporting requirements that are separate and different to those already existing. Lastly, Chapter 8 refers to the possible distorting effects of certain types of aid programmes. One development being tried by some donors is the use of 'basket funding' or Sector Wide Approaches (see Cassels 1997) in which donors pool resources in support of a government sectoral strategy. It is too early to see whether the individual priorities, practices and indeed prejudices of different agencies can be overcome in favour of a joint approach, but it offers considerable potential for overcoming some of the deficiencies associated with a series of donors acting independently.

It should also be noted, as we have seen in Chapter 4, that many private and NGO health systems may receive either direct or indirect subsidies from the government and from other organizations.

PLANNING AND FINANCING

The preceding paragraphs have examined alternative forms of raising finance. We conclude now with a brief look at the relationship of finance to the planning function. The reader should recall the distinction made in Chapter 1 between the various roles of the State. As we saw there, it is possible for the State to take on the responsibility for financing health-care without being the actual service provider. The use of other agencies in the provision of health-care is one of the options that may need to be examined.

Within the planning process, the major point at which financing systems need explicit consideration is at the situational analysis stage. At this point it is important to assess the current financial situation and the likely future levels of finance under current arrangements. Often such information may not be readily available (particularly information related to spending in the private sector), and a survey of health financing may be necessary to compile this information. (See Griffiths and Mills 1983 for an example of the methodology of health financing surveys.) It is important also that this analysis applies the criteria introduced earlier to assess the degree to which the current financing system meets set criteria. Table 5.1 summarizes some of these issues in relation to the major forms of finance for recurrent programme expenditure. In any health-care system there is likely to be a mix of financing health-care, and indeed different forms of health-care may be most appropriately funded in different ways. For example, public-health measures are unlikely to be successfully funded through user charges, but require collective financing.

In general, however, it is unlikely that there will be an unambiguous best mechanism for financing. Hence trade-offs between these criteria are necessary. Indeed, the heated debates about financing frequently relate to the different weightings being placed on the various criteria. Some, for example, regard equity as paramount, whereas others see revenue generating capacity as critical. As we have stressed throughout the book, planning involves such value judgements.

SUMMARY

Planning is concerned with developing means of meeting the priority health-care needs with the limited resources available. One option that should be explored is the possibility of increasing these resources. This chapter has looked at the major forms of finance for the health-care system in developing countries, and has suggested criteria for their assessment. However, it should be recognized that there will always be a shortfall between resource availability and needs, and changing financing mechanisms will not therefore obviate the need for prioritization of needs. Financing health-care can be a separate function to the provision of health-care, which may be carried out on behalf of the State by a variety of agencies.

INTRODUCTORY READING

There is a large number of articles and books written about the issue of health financing, reflecting the widespread interest in the topic. Given the importance of the World Bank in terms of influencing policies, its 1987 and 1993 publications are an important starting-point. Leighton (1995) provides an overview of financing in Africa, There are numerous articles concerning aspects of user charges. Much of the debate

Table 5.1 Examples of criteria applied to financing methods

	Fees	Private insurance	Social/national insurance	Tax
Viability and ease of use	Easy if flat rate, costly if not	Easy unless co-payments are part of the system	Difficult unless concentrated waged labour force	Requires adequate tax base
Revenue-generating ability	Depends on elasticity of demand Costs of collection and billing may be substantial		Dependent on size and income growth of labour force	Dependent on size of the tax base; relationship of tax to GNP growth; few marginal costs of collection
Supply side effects	May have perverse incentives for physicians to provide 'unnecessary, tests May lead to emphasis on curative services; difficulties with chronic and 'predictable' care		Dependent on whether services are directly provided or 'bought' and on methods of control More amenable to central needs-based planning	
Demand side effects	Equity effects of transfers from sick to well; and regressive	Regressive; health risks pooled	Inter-fund equity differences; inequity between fund members and others Paper rights problem	Dependent on method of taxation and service provision
Participation effects	Promotes individual involvement		Potential for collective involvement	
Multi-sectoralism	May be a barrier to transfer of 'health funds' to other health-related users		Easier to allow shifts of funds from health services to other services. This can be negative or positive	

has centred round the actual effects of user charges on utilization; a number of articles, such as that of Mbugua (1995) and McPake (1993) examine the evidence. Russell (1996) looks specifically at the issues of willingness and ability to pay. Community financing schemes have also become popular, though these are often no more than disguised user charges. See Stinson (1984) or Abel-Smith and Dua (1988) for examples of these approaches. The Bamako Initiative (UNICEF 1988, Hanson and McPake 1993) has been influential in pushing such initiatives. A different approach is that which follows the social insurance or national insurance path. Ron *et al.* (1990) and articles by Abel-Smith and colleagues (1988, 1992) provide a useful review of such approaches, together with short case studies from a number of countries. Normand and Weber (1994) provide a guide book for social insurance. The connections between different financing and political systems are well illustrated by Viveros-Long (1986) in a case study of Chile. There are a number of articles focusing on changes in the Chinese financing system and its impact on the health system. Articles by Cassels (1997) and Peters and Chao (1998) examine SWAPs.

EXERCISE 5

- What are the major sources of finance for health-care in your country?

- Construct a matrix such as that in Table 5.1 and consider the effects of each of the criteria on each type of financing source in your country.

- Using the user-charges policy flowchart outlined below, consider the effects of the introduction of or increase in user charges.

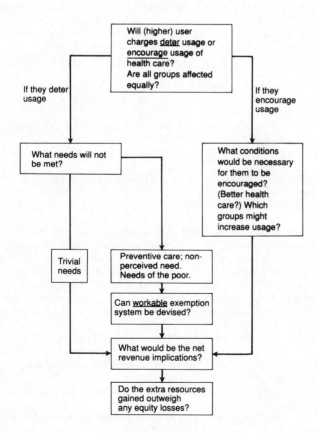

REFERENCES AND FURTHER READING

Abel-Smith, B. (1976). *Value for money in health services*. Heinemann, London.

Abel-Smith, B. (1992). Health insurance in developing countries: lessons from experience. *Health Policy and Planning*, 7(3), 215–26.

Abel-Smith, B. and Dua, A. (1988). Community financing in developing countries: the potential for the health sector. *Health Policy and Planning*, 3, 95–108.

Abel-Smith, B. and Rawal, P. (1992). Can the poor afford 'free' health services? Case study of Tanzania. *Health Policy and Planning*, 7(4), 329–41.

Arhin, D. C. (1994). The health card insurance scheme in Burundi: a social asset or a non-viable venture? *Social Science and Medicine*, 39(6), 861–70.

Asenso-Okyere, W. K. (1995). Financing health care in Ghana. *World Health Forum*, 16, 85–91.

Bennett, S. and Tangcharoensathien V. (1994). A shrinking state? Politics, economics and private health care in Thailand. *Public Administration and Development*, 14, 1–17.

Berman, P. and Dave, P. (1996). Experiences in paying for health care in India's voluntary sector. *International Journal of Health Planning and Management*, 11, 33–51.

Cassels, A. (1997). *A guide to sector-wide approaches for health development: concepts, issues and working arrangements*. WHO, Geneva.

Cassels, A. and Janovsky, K. (1997). Sectoral investment in health: prescription or principles? *Social Science and Medicine*, 44(7),1073–6.

Cham, M.K. *et al.* (1997). The impact of charging for insecticide on the Gambian National Impregnated Bednet Programme. *Health Policy and Planning*, 12(3), 240–7.

De Bethune, X., Alfani, S., and Lahaye, J. P. (1989). The influence of an abrupt price increase on health service utilisation: evidence from Zaire. *Health Policy and Planning*, 4, 76–81.

Dunlop, D. (1983). Health care financing: recent experience in Africa. *Social Science and Medicine*, 17, 2017–25.

Ensor, T. (1995). Introducing health insurance in Vietnam. *Health Policy and Planning*, 10(2), 154–63.

Fiedler, J. L (1996). The privatization of health care in Three Latin American social security systems. *Health Policy and Planning*, 11(4), 406–17.

Gilson, L. (1988). Government health charges: is equity being abandoned? A discussion paper. EPC Paper No 15, London School of Hygiene and Tropical Medicine.

Goodman, H. and Waddington, C. (1993). *Financing health care*. Practical Health Guide No. 8, Oxfam, Oxford.

Griffiths, A, and Mills, M. (1983). Health sector financing and expenditure surveys. In *The economics of health in developing countries* (ed. K. Lee and A. Mills), pp. 43–63. Oxford University Press, Oxford.

Hanson, K. and McPake, B. (1993). The Bamako Initiative: where is it going? *Health Policy and Planning*, 8, 267–74.

Huff-Rouselle, M. and Akuamoah-Boateng, J. (1998). The first private sector health insurance company in Ghana. *International Journal of Health Planning and Management*, 13(2), 165–75.

Huff-Rouselle M., Lalta, S. and Fiedler, J. L. (1998). Health financing policy formulation in the Eastern Caribbean. *International Journal of Health Planning and Management*, 13(2), 149–63.

Korte, R. *et al.* (1992). Paying for health sector. a review and annotated bibliography of the literature on developing countries. EPC Publication No. 12, London School of Hygiene and Tropical Medicine.

Lafond, A. (1995). Improving the quality of investment in health: lessons on sustainability. *Health Policy and Planning*, 10, Suppl. 63–76.

Leighton, C. (1995). Overview: health financing reforms in Africa. *Health Policy and Planning*, 10(3), 213–22.

Liu, Y., Hsiao, W. C. L., Li, Q. *et al.* (1995). Transformation of China's rural health care financing. *Social Science and Medicine*, 41(8), 1085–93.

Liu, Y., Hu, S., Fu, W. *et al.* (1996). Is community financing necessary and feasible for rural China? *Health Policy*, 38(3), 155–71.

Mathiyazhagan, K. (1998). Willingness to pay for rural health insurance through community participation in India. *Health Planning and Management*, 13(1), 47–67.

Mbugua, J. K, Bloom, G. H., and Segall, M. (1995). Impact of user charges on vulnerable groups: the case of Kibwezi in rural Kenya. *Social Science and Medicine*, **41**, 829–36.

McPake, B. (1993). User charges for health services in developing countries: a review of the economic literature *Social Science and Medicine*, **36**(11), 1397–405.

McPake B, Hanson, K., and Mills, A. (1993). Community financing of health care in Africa: an evaluation of the Bamako Initiative. *Social Science and Medicine*, **36**(11), 1383–95.

Mills, A. (1991). Exempting the poor: the experience of Thailand. *Social Science and Medicine*, **33**(11), 1241–52.

Mwabu, G., Mwanzia, J., and Liambila, W. (1995). User charges in government health facilities in Kenya: effect on attendance and revenue. *Health Policy and Planning*, **10**(2), 164–70.

Normand, C. and Weber, A. (1994). *Social health insurance a guide book for planning*. WHO/ILO, Geneva.

Ogunbekuni, I. *et al.* (1996). Costs and financing of improvements in the quality of maternal health services through the Bamako Initiative in Nigeria. *Health Policy and Planning*, **11**(4), 369–84.

Peters, C. and Chao, S. (1998). The sector-wide approach in health. What is it? Where is it leading? *International Journal of Health Planning and Management*, **13**, 177–90.

Prest, A. R. (1985). *Public finance in developing countries*, 3rd edn. Wiedenfeld and Nicolson, London.

Ron, A., Abel-Smith, B., and Tamburi, G. (1990). *Health insurance in developing countries: the social security approach*. ILO, Geneva.

Russell, S. (1996). Ability to pay for health care: concepts and evidence. *Health Policy and Planning*, **11**(3),219–37.

Russell, S. and Gilson, L. (1997). User fee policies to promote health service access for the poor: a wolf in sheep's clothing? *International Journal of Health Services*, **27**(2), 359–79.

Russell, S. *et al.* (1995). Willingness and ability to pay for health care: a. selection of methods and issues. *Health Policy And Planning*, **10**(1), 94–101.

Sammon, A. M. (1996). An integrated approach to health care financing — the case of Chogoria Hospital. *Tropical Doctor*, **26**(4), 177–9.

Shaw, R. P. and Griffin, C. C. (1995). *Financing health care in sub-Saharan Africa through user fees and insurance*. World Bank, Washington, DC.

Stinson, W. (1984). Potential and limitations of community financing. *World Health Forum*, **5**, 123–5.

Thomason, J., Mulou, N. and Bass, C. (1994). User charges for rural health services in Papua New Guinea. *Social Science and Medicine*, **39**(8), 1105–15.

UNICEF (1988). The Bamako Initiative. Mimeograph, UNICEF, New York.

UNICEF (1995). *The Bamako Initiative: rebuilding health systems*. UNICEF, New York.

Viveros-Long, A. (1986). Changes in health financing: the Chilean experience. *Social Science and Medicine*, **22**, 379–85.

Waddington, C. and Enyimayew, K. A. (1989). A. price to pay: the impact of user charges in Ashanti-Akim District, Ghana. *International Journal of Health Planning and Management*, **4**, 17–47.

Walraven, G. (1996). Willingness to pay for district hospital services in rural Tanzania. *Health Policy and Planning*, **11**(4), 428–37.

World Bank (1987). *Financing health services in developing countries: an agenda for reform*. World Bank, Washington, DC.

World Bank (1993). *World Development Report 1993: Investing in Health*. Oxford University Press, Oxford.

World Health Forum (1994). *Round table discussion on inefficiency and wastage in the health sector*. WHO, Geneva.

Wouters, A. (1995). Improving quality through cost recovery in Niger. *Health Policy and Planning*, **10**(3), 257–70.

Xing-Yuan, G. and Sheng-Lan, T. (1995). Reform of the Chinese health care financing system. *Health Policy*, **32**(1–30), 181–191.

Xingyuan, G., Bloom, G., Sheng-Lan, T. *et al.* (1993). Financing health care in rural China: preliminary report of a nationwide study. *Social Science and Medicine*, **36**(4), 385–91.

Yang, B. (1995). The role of health insurance in the growth of the private sector. *International Journal of Health Planning and Management*, **11**(3), 203–16.

Yang, B. M. (1996). The role of health insurance in the growth of the private sector in Korea. *International Journal of Health Planning and Management*, **11**(3), 231–52.

6

Information for planning

Chapter 2 outlined the various stages of the planning spiral. Information is required at all these points in planning, although the type and indeed the accuracy necessary will vary at each stage. Planning is concerned with implementing decisions about change. In order to make, justify, and implement these decisions, information is needed. In the later chapters of this book detailed information requirements will be referred to as we examine the processes of each of these stages. This chapter sets the scene for this by examining a number of broad characteristics of information, and the various types of information and their sources. The following chapter then looks in more detail at the particular requirements of the first stage in any planning process, the situational analysis, when a broad information overview is required.

WHAT IS INFORMATION AND WHY DO WE NEED IT?

Before looking in any detail at information requirements and systems, some fundamental and interconnected preliminary points need to be made about the nature of information. The collection of information is viewed by some planners as a mechanical process involving statisticians, accountants, and record clerks, and as a rather tedious and marginal activity as far as the real work of planning is concerned. Such a view is not only unsustainable, but also foolish, if planning is to achieve its purpose of achieving necessary changes.

Information as the basis for planning

The first essential, though perhaps obvious, point to be made is that information is the lifeblood of the planning process. Without information it would be difficult to make any realistic decisions at all. We have argued that, to be successful, planning needs a combination of a 'rational' process and political analysis. Both of these strands need to be based on information.

The actual selection of information itself is, however, not a totally objective process. As we saw in Chapter 2, criteria are needed to select those aspects of a situation to be studied in more detail. These criteria are then translated into information needs. For example, concentration on the collection of information on particular groups in society (such as by class, gender, age, or area of residence) may imply interest in them as priority groups. Similarly, information about socio-economic or infrastructural factors (such as housing) suggests a particular view of health. Planners may look for specific information to enable them to pursue particular predetermined ends. The participants in the planning process all have their own preconceptions and values, which affect where they concentrate their attention.

There are a number of broad areas of health-related information which are generally accepted as prerequisites for planning, and these are discussed below.

Information as power

A second and connected point is that 'information is power'. Many readers will have experienced the situation where they are frustrated by opposition to a proposal coming from someone who claims to know the 'real situation' — to have better information. Such claims (however spurious), if presented convincingly, can be extremely powerful in a decision-making process. To put the same point more positively, a planner with a confident grasp of information is in a strong position to convince others of her/his case. No one involved in the planning process can afford to underestimate the importance of access to and familiarity with information.

Forms of information

The third point is that much of the information needed is not reducible to a statistical format. For example, the earlier chapters emphasized the need for a political perspective in planning. Information relating to this is rarely quantifiable, and as such may often not even be viewed as 'information'. It is important, however, not to confine one's view of information to what is already measured or easily measurable — what is sometimes known as *hard information*. *Soft information*, which may be impossible or difficult to quantify, is often ignored as being unscientific or difficult to deal with. Community views about health are a form of information that may be ignored by health professionals. Information about health workers' commitment or opposition to change may also be seen as being unmeasurable.

Some of this 'immeasurability' may of course reflect a historic lack of interest in such information. Within a PHC approach, the recognition of the importance of such information has led to the development of new innovative approaches to measurement. However, there will always be important information that is inherently unquantifiable, and would suffer from attempts at quantification. The elusive concept of 'political will' is one such example of an essential ingredient that cannot be quantified. Attempts to measure it, for example by counting the number of political statements made, may detract attention from the depth of commitment to a policy.

Lastly, we need to be aware of problems arising from what has been described as 'the measurable driving out the intangible'. This danger exists wherever soft information is given less explicit weight than hard information. We all give weight to certain values, and hence to corresponding soft information, but we are likely to do this implicitly rather than explicitly. This reduces the opportunity for recognition and debate about these differences. Later in this chapter we examine the potential dangers of reliance on computer-based information technology (IT) in relation to this particular area. Currently, IT is geared towards the analysis and presentation of quantifiable information. The adoption of IT-based management information systems (MIS) may carry with it the danger of an unwarrantable overemphasis on measurable information.

PARALYSIS BY ANALYSIS

Information is a necessary prerequisite for planning decisions, but it can also be used as an excuse for not planning. An all-too-frequent argument for not taking a difficult decision is the apparent lack of (sufficiently accurate) information. The phenomenon- of 'paralysis by analysis' may be the innocent result of a genuine desire for perfection, but it can also be used as a blocking device by an individual or group resisting change.

A balance needs to be sought; and a crude rule is to attempt to obtain only the minimum level of information needed *at that time* for the decision. Box 6.1 gives an example to explain this.

Box 6.1   Information as a blocking device

Two district planning teams separately carried out a situational analysis of their districts and discovered that 80% of the resources were concentrated on in- patient care provided at the district hospitals. These hospitals saw only 10% of the population. Both teams drew up plans to shift the balance of resource allocation gradually towards primary care facilities, by putting incremental growth resources into the primary sector and freezing, in real terms, the hospital sector's resources.

Hospital staff in both districts attempted to block this by asking the teams to define the ideal level of resource allocation for a balance between primary and secondary care. One team set about this task, and became immersed in gathering information to answer this question. The other team argued that given con- straints on the primary care sector's ability to absorb resources, the maximum growth rate for the primary care sector was 5% per annum. At this rate, the hospital would still be allocated 75% of resources after 5 years, which would still be regarded as out of balance. A definition of a balanced state' was seen as unnecessary and diversionary at that point in time. The second district started implementing their policy immediately.

ACCURACY OF INFORMATION

Before looking at types of information, it is important to recognize that information is rarely, if ever, completely accurate. Information provides a means of presenting a view about the real world. Such views can differ not only in terms of distortions or 'in- accuracies' but also, more fundamentally, as a result of genuinely different perceptions.

Box 6.2   Indicators

Indicators are variables that indicate or show a given situation, and thus can be used to measure change. There are two main types:

- *Shorthand*: indicator of something which one could in theory measure, but measuring which would be very costly. The use of community health workers per head of population could be seen as a shorthand measure of overall health service availability.
- *Proxy*: indicator of something which is, by its complex nature, inherently unmeasurable. For example, gross national product (GNP) per capita has been used as a proxy indicator of development.

There are both simple, single-measure indicators and composite indicators.

- *Simple* measures include infant mortality as a proxy measure of health status.
- *Composite* measures of health status include disability-free life expectancy.

The usefulness of indicators to 'indicate' the real nature of a situation is often assessed against the following criteria:

- *validity*: does the indicator actually measure what it is intended to?
- *reliability*: will the indicator provide the same information under differing conditions?
- *sensitivity*: does the indicator actually show changes in situation?
- *specificity*: does the indicator show changes in the situation as specified?

Examples of the above include:

- deaths under the age of 1 year in hospital are not a *valid* measure of infant mortality
- professional's qualitative judgement of disability within a community may not be *reliable*
- infant mortality may be a *sensitive* indicator of child health
- infant mortality will not be a *specific* indicator of measles, as a number of other factors may reduce infant mortality.

Information which is collected is rarely comprehensive, but is represented by indicators, of which there are two broad types, proxy and shorthand (see Box 6.2).

Much information collected depends heavily on both the skills of the 'collector' and how s/he 'views' or interprets reality. Box 6.3 gives an example to illustrate this.

Much medical information is even harder to obtain 'accurately'. Diagnosis is an art not a science, particularly where diagnostic aids are scarce.[1] For example, a lack of diagnostic tools may lead to every patient with high fever and blood in the stool being

---

[1] I am appreciative of help on this section from Marianne Lubben.

Box 6.3   Example of factors affecting accuracy of information

In carrying out a survey of a village population, one might imagine that obtaining the number and age-distribution of inhabitants would be fairly straightforward. However, various factors could affect the number recorded, such as:

- the definition of 'resident' (if a normal resident was not present at the time of the survey, should he or she be counted?)
- the level of motivation of the enumerator (would he or she bother to visit a home some distance from the main village?)
- enumerator training (do they ask the right questions to elicit accurate ages?).
- There may also be reasons why it is in the interest of the village (or indeed of the enumerator) to inflate or deflate figures — for example if a community tax is payable that is dependent on the size of the village.

---

diagnosed and treated for typhoid. A lack of knowledge can also lead to misdiagnosis — for example, the presence of a dark patch on the skin leading to a diagnosis of skin cancer, even when it is not. A lack of knowledge can also lead to a very high level of 'unknowns'. Furthermore, the way information is collected may itself force inaccuracy. Patients with TB and HIV may be registered as either. Most health information systems use the International Classification of Diseases as a basis for their diagnostic records. Such systems look for a single cause of death. For example, although in certain circumstances there may be no single cause of death (for example, measles in combination with malnutrition is often fatal), recording forms may require such single diagnoses. At a different level, hospital records may show the diagnosis on admission and not, more accurately, on discharge.

At a more fundamental level, the very concept of the cause of mortality or morbidity (and hence the information dependent on it) is not simple. In the above example, malnutrition and/or measles may at first sight be seen as the cause of death. However, at a second level, the real cause of death may be viewed as poverty. Hence the increasing attention being paid to social epidemiology, which by arguing for analysis of such broader social causation of disease challenges more narrow clinical epidemiological perspectives.

A further example of the complexity of information can be seen in feminist analytical perspectives which argue that gender issues have been ignored (Leslie 1989, Koblisky *et al.* 1993, Doyal 1995, Craft 1997, WHO 1998). A failure to incorporate such a perspective can lead in turn to an incomplete or inaccurate picture of the real situation. Ethnographic and participative forms of research (De Koning and Martin 1996) provide a very different and useful counterbalance to the more usual (and what has traditionally been seen as the more 'scientific') approach in the health service.

In many instances, therefore, 'accuracy' may also have both an interpretative and a political dimension, alongside the more obvious technical one. Even at the technical level there are important resource implications regarding levels of accuracy, which must be seen as a relative rather than an absolute characteristic. Different levels of accuracy are obtainable at different levels of cost, and these costs may not be solely financial. For example, time involved in collecting data may be used in other ways. It is important, in designing an information system, that we aim to obtain only the minimum level of accuracy required, in order to reduce the attendant costs of the information system. As one tries to refine information, the cost of collecting or analysing it increases. Trade-offs are therefore needed between the level of accuracy and the cost of obtaining it (see Figure 6.1).

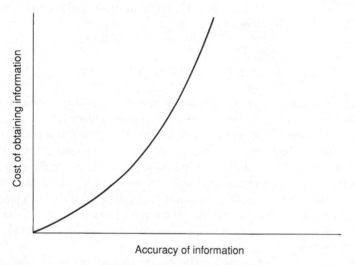

Accuracy of information

Fig. 6.1   Relationship between accuracy and cost of obtaining information in many situations

SPATIAL AND TIME CONSIDERATIONS

Information is often of most use when it can be compared, either on a time or a spatial basis. Projections of underlying trends are often important in planning. When comparisons are being used it is essential to ensure that the information is comparable (for example, does the term 'clinic' mean the same in both situations; does comparison of expenditure between years allow for inflation; does comparison of incidence rates between January and July make explicit seasonal variations; do international comparisons of personnel norms take account of different health service structures?).

As information systems become more sophisticated, the possibility of developing models for use in forecasting arises. Such techniques are already widely used in the demographic field to forecast future population in terms of its size and composition. Information on personnel employed within the health sector also lends itself easily to forecasting of future supply. The reliability of such forecasts depends of course on the realism of the underlying models and their inherent assumptions about relationships between variables. For this reason disease patterns are less easy to forecast, in part because of the difficulty of establishing the exact causal relationships. Econometric forecasting techniques are widely used at the macro-economic level, and are used in some health systems. Their data requirements are such, however, that they are unlikely to be used in health planning systems in less developed countries for some time. An example of their use can be seen in Carrin and Politi (1996).

One of the dangers of using such approaches is that the technocratic mystique of such models creates a barrier between the forecaster on the one hand, and other professionals and the community on the other hand. Given the emphasis that this book places on a broad participative approach to planning, it is important that such models should make explicit the assumptions behind them, and should look for means of making these generally accessible.

LEVEL OF AGGREGATION OF INFORMATION

In some situations, large aggregations of data may be necessary to ensure a sufficient data field to allow useful analysis. However, the greater the level of aggregation, the more distributional disparities are hidden. Table 6.1, setting out income distribution for various countries, highlights this aspect. Peru, with the highest overall income of the three, has the greatest income disparities between the highest- and lowest-earning groups, whereas Bangladesh, with the lowest per capita income, has the lowest ratio. Concentration solely on aggregated data of the first column would mask this important information on distribution. Aggregation may also mask important gender differences, where for example utilization of health services are not broken down by sex.

In general, plans relating to the distant future require a less detailed breakdown than those relating to the near future, where distributional differences are more difficult to redress. For example, a programme to build 20 clinics annually can refer to plans for 5 years' time at the national level, but would need to specify exact locations for the next year.

Table 6.1   Income distribution: selected countries (in $)

	GDP per capita 1988	Per capita disposable expenditure[a] for those in		
		20% lowest-earning group	20% highest-earning group	Ratio highest to lowest
Bangladesh	170	79	331	4 : 1
Ghana	400	130	892	7 : 1
Peru	1300	286	3374	12 : 1

Source: Adapted from World Bank (1990).
The table assumes similar household size in different income-groups. In reality this is unlikely. The *World Development Report* stresses that data should be treated with great caution, as the methodologies are not always strictly comparable.
[a] Income distribution figures relate to different years: Bangladesh 1981/2, Ghana 1987, Peru 1985.

TYPE OF INFORMATION

Different stages in the planning process require different types of information. Collecting, analysing, and presenting information all have attendant costs, yet much information is processed without any end-use. Not only is the processing of un-necessary information costly, but it may also lead to inaccuracies, as the staff involved see little purpose in their work. An efficient information system should routinely collect only that information for which there is a use, and the cost of which is outweighed by the benefits seen in improved decision-making. It is not always necessary, of course, for the health service *itself* to collect the data. Similar information may already be collected by other means, and this may provide an adequate low-cost substitute.

The next section examines broad types of information, and some of their indicators and characteristics. It is perhaps salutary first to remind ourselves of the saying:

The information you have is not what you want.

The information you want is not what you need.

The information you need is not what you can get.

It is all too common to find extremely active information systems providing informa-tion that does not match the requirements of the planners and managers; and it is an important part of the planning process to define its requirements carefully.

As we have seen, health planning is concerned with resolving the dilemma of scarcity of resources contrasted with unlimited needs, all within a socio-political context. Information can usefully be classified, therefore, into three types:

• information on the needs of specified populations

• information on resources and services

• information on the policy and political context.

These are discussed in turn. Before doing so, however, it is important to recognize the difference between the concepts of *inputs*, *outputs*, and *outcomes*, which are often loosely used, and yet which have very different implications for the type of measure eventually chosen. This is done in Box 6.4.

Indicators of need

The first type of information consists of indicators of the health and health needs of a specified population. Information is required which relates to demographic and socio-economic characteristics of this population. This is essential as a baseline against which health needs can be set. It is important that this information is not confined to traditional (albeit essential) demographic information, but also looks at wider indicators of poverty and of social justice, such as the status of different social groups.

Despite various attempts to get agreed indicators of health, there are still different approaches to the measurement of (ill) health. This, in part, results from differences

Box 6.4   Relationship between input, output, and outcome

Input indicators measure the resources that are used in the provision of services. These include personnel, finance, drugs, and buildings. Bringing these resources together leads to the provision of services. These are measured by output indicators, such as outpatient attendances, number of vaccinations given, bed-days, or pit latrines constructed.

Output indicators give no idea of the effect on health itself, and many argue that a further set of true health indicators which measure the change in health status are the crucial ones for the setting of priorities. These latter are known as *outcome* indicators and include the number of lives saved or extended, children protected (by for example immunization), or life years saved.

Example of input	Example of output	Example of outcome
Personnel	Outpatient attendances	Live years extended
Finance	In-patient days	Disability Adjusted Life Years saved

between concepts, and hence indicators, of health status, health needs, and health-care needs. *Health status* reflects a positive or absolute state. *Health needs* are the inverse, and reflect service requirements. These are often wrongly used interchangeably, and may become confused. Chapter 3 discussed different understandings of the concept of health. There are various ways in which a shift away from a narrow organic definition, using single disease measures, towards a wider more holistic view, has been attempted.

The simplest measures of (ill) health are those that measure the level (incidence and prevalence) of disease in an individual or community. Such measures correspond to a narrow definition of health. Although such information is important for planning, there is increasing recognition that overreliance on such indicators may be counterproductive.

Information about disease incidence by itself is not particularly valuable. Information as to its effects is also needed. Box 6.5 gives as an example a spectrum of alternative ways of viewing the disease polio. These range from simple measures of incidence rates to composite measures that bring together the number of deaths and the level of disability. The most recent is the DALY (Disability Adjusted Life Year), which is advocated by the World Bank (1993)as a means of measuring the overall Burden of Disease of a country.

Such measures still focus on the physiological aspects of ill health. A broader understanding of health is needed, to include not only measures of mental well-being, but also social and economic indicators. Contrast for example the health of two children, both 'disease-free', of whom one lives in a slum and the other is the child of a senior civil servant. The first is less healthy not only because of the undisputed effects of poverty on the child's physiological state, but also because the quality of life

Box 6.5 Possible health measures of polio	
Disease incidence	New cases of polio per 1000 population
Disease prevalence	Total cases of polio per 1000 population
Mortality rates	Deaths from polio per 1000 population
Life years lost	Aggregation of years of life lost as a result of polio
Disabilities	Number of disabled polio survivors
Physical Quality of Life Index	Measure of the functional quality of life for polio survivors
Disability Adjusted Life Year	Measure of the number of life years affected by polio and its disabling effects

itself is lower. This should be incorporated into any measurement of health. To be complete, profiles of a community's health need to incorporate not only traditional disease-based indicators, but social and economic indicators as well.

Even the broadest of the above measures of (ill) health, are determined by health workers and so still relate to a professional view of health. Our understanding of the health needs of a community is incomplete if we rely solely on medical data. Information on needs as perceived by the community is as important, although far harder to gather, analyse, and present. In part, this is because of the general problems of obtaining community views, referred to in Chapter 3. The heterogeneous nature of a community makes the notion of representation difficult. It is also particularly difficult in the area of health. The form in which health-care needs are perceived may differ between those who see needs in medical terms (such as measles), those who see them in health service terms (such as the need for a clinic), and those who see them in broader socio-political terms (such as income generation).

Resources and services

The second type of information concerns resources or inputs, and the services provided with these resources. Such information should relate to all health-related activities, and not only those of the health sector.

Resources
Information is required on the resources that currently provide inputs into services — personnel, buildings, equipment, supplies, and transport — and on those resources which will be available in the future. Planning and management both need access to information on the level, type, and distribution of these resources. Such information should not be restricted to the health sector alone, but should include any sector that has health-promoting potential. Underpinning these are the sources of these resources — financial resources and community in-kind resources.

One indicator for resources commonly used is that of money. As a common denominator it is very attractive. However, it suggests greater flexibility than is likely to be the case, certainly in the short term. Resources (although often expressed in a budget format) are usually committed to particular resource areas, and in particular personnel. Hence information about resources should be broken down as far as possible into the actual physical resources themselves. However, forecasts into the future may more easily use finance as a proxy for resources. Although in the short term resources are rarely substitutable (for example, drugs cannot be turned into vehicles; doctors cannot be transformed into nurses), the further one plans ahead, the greater flexibility there is to shift resources from one usage to another. This flexibility is represented then by the use of financial estimates.

Information on sources of finance is also important, and carries implications for the sustainability and flexibility of its use. For example, funding from donors is likely to be tied to particular uses, and may only be guaranteed for a certain period.

Chapter 13 stresses the need for information about personnel across all sectors as the basis for human resource planning. Similarly, Chapter 11 argues that financial information is crucial to the planning (and management) process.

Services
Accurate across-the-board information on service provision is, strangely enough, often unavailable. In particular, information on health-related services provided outside the health sector may be minimal. This situation contrasts with often quite elaborate systems of recording morbidity and mortality, usually at hospitals. Yet collection of service information is not technically difficult, and may be done easily either on a regular return basis or through sampling.

There is a relationship between resources and services analogous to that between finance and resources. In the short term it is difficult to shift the resource allocations which underly patterns of service provision (from, for example, hospitals to primary care services). This is due to the unsuitability of some resources for some services. For example, hospital buildings cannot be dismantled and recreated as a series of clinics; and theatre nurses may not make good primary care workers. Resistance to such shifts are also difficult to overcome in the short term. In the medium term, however, change becomes easier, with the possibility of shifts in the capital building programme and in training. In medium- to long-term projections there is more flexibility.

Information on service provision, where available, is often misleading.

- Firstly, the definition of a particular service may be unclear, or poorly specified. To describe an area as having 50 clinics may mask wide variations, either in terms of the services provided at the clinics, or of their frequency. Operational definitions of different facilities and services are an important starting point.

- Secondly, information may be confined to services in the government sector. However, as Chapter 4 has argued, significant health-care may be provided outside the government sector, either by the voluntary sector, or by private practitioners practising either allopathic or traditional forms of medicine.

- Thirdly, information on services will be incomplete without some measure of utilization. Information as to the coverage of health-care is frequently provided without complementary information on utilization. A health service may 'cover' 60% of the population, but if only 20% use it, this needs to be known.

Policy and political context

The third broad category of information relates to the policy and political environment. Planners do not operate within a vacuum, but start from existing political structures and policy. Information on this context is an essential part of the planning process. Some of this is possible to quantify, but much of it will be 'soft' information of the kind described earlier. Techniques such as stakeholder analysis and political mapping (see for example, Reich 1994) may be used to obtain a structured view of this context.

Table 6.2 sets out the different stages in the planning spiral, and gives the main categories of information required for each.

INFORMATION SYSTEMS

The preceding part of the chapter has discussed in general terms a number of characteristics of information. We turn now to the information systems themselves that provide this basic requirement of planning. We first examine methods of collecting information, and then discuss the need for feedback within information-collection systems, and issues of the analysis and presentation of information. Lastly we will introduce issues of system management.

Methods of collecting information

There is a variety of methods of collecting information. The choice of method for any type of information will depend, *inter alia*, on the level of accuracy required. One general introductory comment needs stressing. Methods of collecting information are frequently biased. For example, data collected on low birth-weight at hospital deliveries will be biased towards hospital users. As such, it is unlikely to be representative of the majority who deliver outside the hospital.

The main methods of collecting information are outlined below. Further readings are suggested at the end of the chapter for the reader wishing to become further acquainted with the different approaches and techniques.

Surveys
Surveys are episodic (though possibly regular) methods of assessing the wider situation by obtaining information from a selected, representative subgroup. They are useful for obtaining information that is not routinely required, is costly, or is not easy to collect regularly. The major difficulty in survey work is ensuring that the sample group is sufficiently representative for the purpose required. This depends

Table 6.2   Information requirements at different stages of planning

Planning stage	Information required
Situational analysis	General country characteristics
	Health status needs
	Health service availability
	Utilization of health-care and reasons for differences
	Other sector services
	Political context
	Resources present and projected
Priority-setting	National goals:
	• health
	• broader
	Community views on priorities
	Health-worker views on priorities
Option appraisal	Possible alternative options
	Appraisal information:
	• effectiveness
	• efficiency
	• equity
	• acceptability
	• feasibility
	• resource availability
Programming	Option chosen
	Budgetary information
	Resources
Implementation	Monitoring information at capital implementation stage
	• input provision/constraints
	• changes from plan information
	Management information at service provision stage
	• utilization of service
	• cost
	• constraints
Evaluation	As for appraisal and situational analysis

both on the method of selection and on the size of the sample. Examples of the use of surveys within the health sector include:

• health surveys, both medical and community-based

• knowledge, attitude, and practice (KAP) studies

• 'opinion polls' about services or needs

• health service utilization surveys

• personnel surveys for human resource planning

• financial and expenditure surveys.

A relatively recent development within the health sector is the use of rapid appraisals as a method of obtaining information for planning using, in particular, informed opinion; see for example *International Journal of Epidemiology* (1989), Kielmann *et al.* (1991), Chambers (1992), Nordberg *et al.* (1993). Participatory rapid appraisals provide a means of obtaining a picture of a community's needs within a short period of time.

The census can be considered as a special case of a survey in which the whole population is included. Censuses are generally conducted every 10 years, and provide a useful set of benchmark information, particularly on demographic data.

Governments may have survey units which carry out regular surveying on behalf of ministries. This can be a very efficient way of surveying. An example of this is a household survey, which collects wide-ranging information through surveys of a sample of households. Health ministries are often able to include specific questions in such surveys.

Surveys may be carried out by direct personal contact, selective record examination, telephone contact, or postal questionnaire. There are disadvantages and advantages to each of these methods for any particular purpose. Telephone surveys, for example, are easy to conduct, but can only provide information on a sub-group (those with a 'phone), and are therefore unlikely to be representative of the community as a whole. One particular approach within the health sector is that of sentinel reporting, in which designated 'sentinel' centres report fully on certain diseases.

Vital registration
Not all countries have a system of vital registration, whereby births and deaths are required to be registered by law. Where they do exist and operate accurately, they provide a valuable source of demographic information.

Treatment records
The most usual method of collecting information on health conditions within the health sector is from records kept as a result of services provided. This is an important source, but the biases inherent in it must be kept in mind. In particular, extrapolations from hospital-based records to the whole community need to be treated with great caution.

Notifiable disease returns
Many countries require particular returns from health professionals on certain communicable diseases for public health reasons. These can form a valuable source of information.

Management reports and returns
Routine returns from managers are often a neglected source of information for planning. The most obvious are financial returns, but personnel and supplies returns can also form an important source.

Informed opinion
'Soft' information may be obtained through meetings with individuals or groups (for example, in a community meeting). Although such meetings can be an important

source of information, their value is, of course, dependent on the representative credentials of the informants.

Information from other ministries, agencies, and institutions
Other agencies have information relating to their own activities. This is important in the context of a PHC approach. For example, the ministry responsible for community development may have information on housing conditions; the agriculture ministry may have information on population distribution. In addition, however, other agencies may have information relating to health service activities. Professional bodies are frequently an untapped source of information. For example, the register held by the national medical council can provide information on the composition of the medical profession.

Other sources
Other sources including international reports and journals and media reports may also be valuable. The World Wide Web is also increasingly becoming a useful source of information for those with Internet access. Examples of annual reports, and journals are listed in the References and Further Reading section at the end of this chapter. Web site examples are given on p. 22–23

Health systems research

Before looking at what is known as health systems research it is important to recognize that seeking and analysing information of different forms is all part of research activity. The terms health services research and operations research are also frequently used. Health systems research is the broadest of these terms. Certain activities are more specifically considered 'research', in part as a result of their one-off or specialist nature. There is an increasing awareness of the need to develop appropriate forms of research for the health system. Traditionally, the bulk of research in the health field has been of a clinical or epidemiological nature. This has widened, initially to a recognition of the need to look more broadly at the issues of health services, and most recently at health systems themselves; and a number of agencies have recently become interested in this area. Some have developed initiatives to strengthen health systems research, such as the International Health Policy Program and the Council for Health Research for Development. Some information requirements will only be answerable by specific research; in particular questions relating to the interactions between components of a system and 'what-if' questions will require such research. In planning terms, however, it is important both that such research is seen as meeting the information needs of the planning process and that the methodologies adopted are appropriate. These may include, therefore, more participatory and qualitative approaches to research than are traditional.

Analysis and presentation

Raw data is only of use after analysis and transformation into information.

- *Analysis* of information can occur at a variety of levels, from that of the original collector to that of a user at the central level. The decision as to which level of analysis occurs where depends partly on considerations of the cost involved and the skills required. However, wherever possible, analysis conducted as close as possible to the level of the data collector is likely to provide her/him with an interest in the information. This is likely to enhance motivation. It may also allow errors where a gross mismatch between the information and perceived reality exists to be detected sooner.

- *Presentation* of information is often neglected. There is no single correct way to present information. How it is presented will depend on its purpose and at whom it is aimed. It is essential to consider the target audience for the information (such as fellow planner, community, or politician) in determining the most appropriate means of presentation. For example, tables of detailed precise information on morbidity may be necessary for informing or persuading epidemiologists. The same information aimed at politicians may be better presented graphically. Box 6.6 provides an example of how the same information may be presented in very different ways.

Box 6.6   Different ways of presenting data

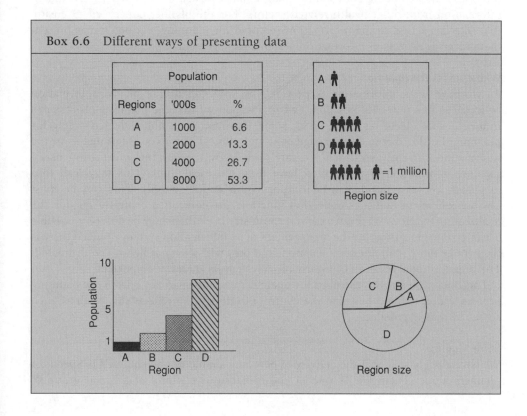

Feedback to data collectors

The technical accuracy of data depends largely on the skills and motivation of the data collectors. Many information systems suffer through insufficient attention being paid to this important aspect of an information system, on the automatic presumption that data are being collected properly. Information is often channelled in one direction only; or worse, raw data are collected at one place and analysed elsewhere, with no subsequent feedback on either the use to which they are being put or on the implications of the information.

There are a number of arguments for a feedback system. In particular the move towards decentralization and participative planning systems itself implies more information-sharing. Ideally, collectors should also be among the users of the information. Furthermore, feedback helps to motivate data collectors, and hence to maintain levels of accuracy.

Information systems management

From the preceding points, it is clear that the information which the planner uses will not be derived from one single information system. Traditionally emphasis within the health sector has been placed on health information systems, although increasingly interest is rightly being shown in management information systems (MIS) and in information from other health-related sectors. For the planner concerned to ensure that s/he has access to the information required for planning, various issues present themselves as aspects of information systems management.

Who controls the information?

As we have seen, information is power; s/he who can decide on the information collected is in a powerful position, and it is important that the planning process can influence such decisions. Of course, some information is not collected solely for planning, but for day-to-day management and clinical purposes. Decisions as to the information currently collected are rarely made by the current information users. Existing information systems often have long historical roots. This may lead to a mismatch between the demand for information and its supply. This can be most obvious where the statistics collection functions are controlled centrally, outside the health ministry. However, even within the ministry itself there may be different possible organizational locations for the management of its information systems. Indeed there is likely to be more than one such location, and they will often not be well co-ordinated. The organizational location of information systems is therefore important.

This book also stresses the need for openness and transparency within the planning process, and it is important that the control of information reflects this, with as open access to it as is possible.

Skills required

We have already seen that the activity of planning should not be confined to specialist planners alone. Their role is one of co-ordinating the efforts of a broad group of participants. The collection and analysis of information is an analogous case. Although a central core of information specialists is needed, it is both inevitable and desirable that a variety of groups are involved in the process.

The specialist skills required in developing an information system will reflect both the information to be collected and the system itself. Certain skills are required as a minimum — including epidemiological, social science, statistical, and computing skills — but it is also important that other perhaps less traditionally obvious skills are included in an efficient information system — including presentational skills. It is also important that a balance between types of skill is achieved. Too much emphasis on, for example, epidemiological skills will inevitably result in a bias in the system itself of the information collected towards medical data.

Lastly, within an information system, it is important that research skills are available. As we have seen, some information will be routinely available, but it may be necessary on occasions to develop research projects to answer particular questions. Even if research skills are not routinely available within an information system, there should be an understanding of the different approaches and the comparative advantages of various research methods. This will allow the commissioning of appropriate research, and the correct interpretation of its results.

Type of technology used

The use of computers in information systems is growing. There are various issues surrounding the technology chosen, including relative resource costs, maintenance capacity, and employment considerations. We have also briefly discussed the danger that computers can tend to overemphasize quantified information, with the consequent danger that less weight is given to qualitative information. The adage 'rubbish in — rubbish out' should also be remembered, as overreverent attitudes to computers can have the undesirable effect of attaching spurious legitimacy to their output.

SUMMARY

This chapter has introduced a number of issues in the area of information. Information is a critical component of the planning system, yet may be taken for granted. Information of different types and levels of accuracy is needed at different stages of planning. The collection, analysis, and use of information is not an objective process, but can very much depend on the attitudes and values of those who control it. The chapter has introduced a number of types of information and possible sources for information. The following chapter takes this further by looking at the information needs of the first stage in the planning process: the situational analysis.

INTRODUCTORY READING

The area of information, as we have seen, is extremely broad, and covers issues of what information should be collected, how, and by whom. It also involves issues of the type of technology and the methods of analysis and presentation employed. Lastly, its relationship to the broader management and planning function is also critical. No single text covers all of these aspects, and readers interested to pursue particular topics are referred to the readings listed below, whose focuses are self-explanatory.

EXERCISE 6

Spend 15 minutes writing down all the types of information which you can think of that is routinely collected in your own health system.
    Consider the following questions in relation to your own information systems:

- Is all the information collected used?

- What other information is needed that is not collected at present?

- How accurate does the information need to be?

- Who uses the information?

- What is the cost of providing the information?

- Is there feedback to the data collectors?

REFERENCES AND FURTHER READING

Abramson, J. H. (1988). *Making sense of data: self-instruction manual on the interpretation of epidemiological data*. Oxford University Press, Oxford.

Amonoo-Lartson, R., Ebrahim, G., Lovel, H., and Ranken, J. (1984). *District health care: challenges for planning, organisation and evaluation in developing countries*. Macmillan, London.

Andersson, N., Martinez, E., Cerrato, F., Morales, E., and Ledogar, R. (1989). The use of community-based data in health planning in Mexico and Central America. *Health Policy and Planning*, 4, 197–206.

Aubel, J. and Mansour, M. (1989). Qualitative community health research: a Tunisian example. *Health Policy and Planning*, 4, 244–56.

Barker, D. J. P. and Hall, A. J. (1991). *Practical Epidemiology*, 4th edn. Churchill Livingstone, London.

Berman, P. (1997). National health accounts in developing countries: appropriate methods and recent applications. *Journal of Health Economics*, 6, 11–30.

Bowling, A. (1997). *Research methods in health: investigating health and health services*. Open University Press, Buckingham.

Brownlee, A. (1991). *Health systems research training series, Vol. 1: Promoting health systems research as a management tool*. IDRC in collaboration with WHO, Ottawa.

Butcher, K. and Kievelitz, U. (1997). Planning with PRA: HIV and STD in a Nepalese mountain community. *Health Policy and Planning*, 12(3), 253–61.

Campos-Outcalt, D. and Vickers, P. (1988). For fuller utilisation of health data. *World Health Forum*, 9, 405–8.

Carrin, G. and Politi, C. (1996). *Exploring the health impact of economic growth, poverty reduction and public health expenditure*, Technical Paper 18, Macroeconomics, Health and Development Series, WHO, Geneva.

Cartwright, A. (1983). *Health surveys in practice and potential: a critical review of their scope and methods.* Kings Fund, London.

Casley, D. J. and Lury, D. A. (1987). *Data collection in developing countries,* 2nd edn. Clarendon Press, Oxford.

Chambers, R. (1992). *Rural appraisal: rapid, relaxed and participatory.* Discussion paper 311, Institute of Development Studies, Brighton.

Corrêa, S. (1994). *Population and reproductive rights: feminist perspectives from the South.* Zed Press, London.

Craft, N. (1997). Women's health is a global issue. *British Medical Journal,* 315, 7116, 1154–7.

De Koning, K. and Martin, M. (ed.) (1996). *Participatory research in action: issues and experiences.* Zed Press, London.

Doyal, L. (1995). *What makes women sick: gender and the political economy of health.* Macmillan, Basingstoke.

Eng, E., Glik, D., and Parker, K. (1990). Focus-group methods: effects on village-agency collaboration for child survival. *Health Policy and Planning,* 5, 67–76.

Garner, P., Thomason, J., and Donaldson, D. (1990). Quality assessment of health facilities in rural Papua New Guinea. *Health Policy and Planning,* 5, 49–59.

Griffiths, A. and Mills, M. (1983). Health sector financing and expenditure surveys. In *The economics of health in developing countries* (ed. K. Lee and A. Mills), pp. 43–63. Oxford University Press, Oxford.

International Journal of Epidemiology (1989). Supplement on rapid epidemiological assessment. 18, Suppl. 2.

Kadt, E. (1989). Making health policy management intersectoral: issues of information analysis and use in less developed countries. *Social Science and Medicine,* 29, 503–14.

Kielmann, A. A., Janovsky, K., and Annett, H. (1991). *Assessing district health needs, services and systems: protocols for rapid data collection and analysis.* AMREF, Nairobi; Macmillan.

Knox, E. G. (ed.) (1979). *Epidemiology in health care planning.* Oxford University Press, Oxford.

Koblisky, M. et al. (1993). *The health of women: a. global perspective.* Westview Press, Boulder, CO.

Kroeger A. et al. (1997). *The use of epidemiology in local health planning: a training manual.* Zed Press, London.

Leslie, J. (1989). Women's time: a factor in the use of child survival technologies? *Health Policy and Planning,* 6, 1–19.

Lippeveld, T., Sauerborn, R., and Sapirie, S. (1997). Health information systems — making them work. *World Health Forum,* 18(2), 176–84.

Newbrander, W. L. and Thomason, J. A. (1988). Computerising a national health system in Papua New Guinea. *Health Policy and Planning,* 3, 255–9.

Nichter, M. (1984). Project community diagnosis: participatory research as a first step towards community involvement in primary health care. *Social Science and Medicine,* 19, 237–52.

Nordberg, E. (1988). Household health surveys in developing countries: could more use be made of them in planning? *Health Policy and Planning,* 3, 32–9.

Nordberg, E., Oganga, H., Kazibwe, S. et al. (1993). Rapid assessment of an African district health system: test of a planning tool. *International Journal of Health Planning and Management,* 8(3), 219–33.

Nosseir, N. K., McCarthy, J., Gillespie, D., and Shaw, F. (1986). Using mini-surveys to evaluate community health programmes. *Health Policy and Planning,* 1, 67–74.

Opit, L. J. (1987). How should information on health care be generated and used? *World Health Forum,* 8, 409–17.

Reich, M. R. (1994). *Political mapping of health policy: a guide for managing the political dimensions of health policy.* Data for Decision Making Project, Harvard School of Public Health, Boston.

Ross, D. and Vaughan, J. P. (1984). *Health interview surveys in developing countries.* EPC Publication No. 4, Evaluation and Planning Centre, London School of Hygiene and Tropical Medicine.

Smith, D. L., Hansen, H., and Karim, M. S., (1989). Management information support for district health systems based on primary health care. *Information Technology for Development,* 4(4), 779–811.

Smith, G. S. (1989). Development of rapid epidemiologic assessment methods to evaluate health status and delivery of health services. *International Journal of Epidemiology,* 18, (Suppl. 2), S2–S15.

Solter, S. L, Hasibuan, A. A., and Yusuf, B. (1986). An epidemiological approach to health planning and problem solving in Indonesia. *Health Policy and Planning,* 1, 99–108.

UNICEF (1996). *State of the world's children 1996.* Oxford University Press, Oxford.

Vaughan, J. P and Morrow, R. H (1989). *Manual of epidemiology for district health management.* WHO, Geneva.

WHO (1988a). *Health systems research in action: case studies.* Programme on Health Systems Research and Development, Division of Strengthening of Health Services, WHO, Geneva.

WHO (1988b). Epidemiological and statistical methods for rapid health assessment. *WHO Statistics Quarterly* 44(3).

WHO (1998c). *Gender and Health:* Technical Paper, WHO, Geneva.

WHO (1993). *Guidelines for the development of health management information systems.* WHO. Manila.

WHO (1994). *Information support for new public health at district level.*Technical Report Series No 845, WHO, Geneva.

WHO (1996). *Catalogue of health indicators: a selection of important health indicators recommended by WHO programmes.* WHO, Geneva.

Williams, S. *et al.* (1994). *The Oxfam gender training manual.* Oxfam, Oxford.

Wilson, R.G, Echols, B. E., Bryant, J. H., and Abrantes, A. (eds) (1988). *Management information systems and microcomputers in Primary Health Care.* Aga Khan Foundation, Geneva.

World Bank (1990). *World Development Report.* Oxford University Press, New York.

World Bank (1993). *World Development Report. Investing in Health* Oxford University Press, New York.

Annual reports and journals

Human Development Report (UNDP/OUP annual publication)
The State of the World's Children (UNICEF/OUP annual publication)
United Nations Demographic Yearbook (UN annual publication)
United Nations Year Book (annual publications and sources of data)
World Development Report (World Bank/OUP annual publication)
World Health Statistics Annual (WHO annual publication)
World Health Statistics Quarterly (WHO quarterly publication).

Web sites

Chapter 1 gives a number of web sites which may provide sources of information.

7

Situational analysis

The last chapter discussed a number of general issues surrounding information and information management. As we have already seen, the first stage in the development of a plan, at whatever level — national, regional, district, or community — is to improve the understanding of the current situation. This chapter looks specifically at this initial planning stage.

The purpose of a situational analysis is to provide a broad basis of understanding. This is for two reasons. Firstly, it provides a common reference point for the rest of the planning process; and secondly, it provides the background for the selection of priority areas of concern for planning.

For many planners the situational analysis may seem an unnecessary activity, formalizing information that is often already well known. However, it is an important exercise. The very discipline of having to consider the background situation against which the plan has to be set may bring new insights. Furthermore, the act of planning needs to be made as public as possible, in order to assist in bringing other participants into the planning process. It is surprising how many health professionals operate within a narrow confined view of the health scene, often aware in great detail about their own field of work, but dismally ignorant of other perspectives, problems, and activities. The very process of carrying out a situational analysis can in itself be an educational process, for all planning participants.

Lastly, at a far more pragmatic level, the resultant document (and it is strongly advised that the analysis should be clearly documented) can serve at least two purposes beyond that of the immediate production of a plan. Firstly, it provides an invaluable form of feedback to health workers about the planning process, setting out the basis on which planning decisions are made. Secondly, such a document has important potential as a background document for the health sector, of the sort that outside consultants and donors frequently request and require. It is not a trivial point to recognize that the planning office is often (and correctly) seen as the focal point for such outside agencies. A significant amount of a planner's time can be spent in explaining the background of the health sector to such people. Although it would be unrealistic to think that even a good situational analysis can completely dispose of this activity, it certainly can reduce it to an acceptable level. We now turn to the content of a situational analysis.

As we have seen, a situational analysis outlines and assesses the current situation and projections in various broad areas. These are summarized in Box 7.1.

We will look at each of these in turn. While the emphasis will be on national-level planning, the principles and indeed categories of information are similar at regional, district, or even community level, although the variety and depth of information

---

Box 7.1   Key content of a situational analysis

Population characteristics

- demographic information
- religious, educational and cultural characteristics

Area characteristics and infrastructure

- geographical and topographical situation
- infrastructure
- socio-economic situation
- public and private sector structures

Policy and political environment

- overall national policies
- existing health policies
- political environment

Health needs

- medically perceived health needs
- community-perceived health needs

Services provided by and plans of the non-health sector health services

Health Services
- service facilities
- service utilization
- service gaps
- health service organizational arrangements

Resources

- financial resources
- personnel
- buildings, land, equipment, and vehicles
- other supplies

Efficiency, effectiveness, equity and quality of current services

---

required may be different. The categories chosen are, inevitably artificial and over-lapping, and could easily be classified differently.

POPULATION CHARACTERISTICS

The starting point of any analysis should be information about the people of the area under analysis and is here divided into different aspects.

Demographic information

Demographic information is necessary for a variety of reasons. Firstly, information is needed about the size and age- and sex-distribution, to provide a basis for estimates of service provision. Equally important is information about the rate of change of these indicators. High population growth rates not only create a strain on the overall provision of services, but lead to a predominantly young population, and hence a particular need for maternal and child services. By contrast, low or negative growth rates will lead to a higher proportion of elderly people in the population with different health needs. Baseline information is also important to help calculate the rates that need to be known when planning services, including the rates of morbidity, mortality, and service utilization.

Demographic information is also important in terms of the supply side of health-care. The health service is an extremely labour-intensive organization — often the largest single employer in a country — and therefore demographic changes can have important effects on the future supply of staff. In the UK health service, for example, major shortage of various categories of staff, such as nurses, are predicted partly as a result of the projected demographic profile.

The following list sets out the major population-information needs that a situational analysis should cover (in each case current and projected data are needed):

- absolute size and distribution of the population
- vital rates — birth, death, and fertility rates
- immigration and emigration rates
- overall population growth rate
- age and sex structure
- ethnicity.

Religious, educational, and cultural characteristics

These characteristics may have an important impact on health, and need to be analysed. For example, a recognition of a low educational level in women coupled with an undesirably high fertility rate may suggest the need for a literacy campaign, rather than just the provision of contraceptives. The main groups of information are:

- educational and literacy levels
- cultural or religious characteristics of any particular groups.

AREA CHARACTERISTICS AND INFRASTRUCTURE

In addition to information on the people, information is required about the physical and socio-eoconomic characteristics of the area under analysis and its infrastructure.

Geographical and topographical situation

This includes any particular characteristics that could affect health or health services, such as rivers or mountain ranges passable only at certain points or times; or climatic variations which have a direct bearing on health, for example rainy seasons that are related to malaria transmission.

Infrastructure

An understanding of the wider infrastructure is likely to influence the pattern of future health service provision. Knowledge of future road developments or resettlement schemes may affect the distribution of services. A high incidence of gastroenteritis, coupled with poor access to water, may suggest the need to emphasize the latter as a priority, rather than setting up services to provide oral rehydration treatment. Types of information could include:

- transport modes and routes

- communications

- water supplies and sanitation facilities

- utilities, including distribution of mains electricity.

Socio-economic situation

An important aspect of the analysis should be at the broad or macro level, with a description of the socio-economy. This important for two reasons.

- Firstly, the linkages between the economy, other sectors, and health, which we looked at in Chapter 3, imply the need to have a clear understanding of them. Changes in the pattern of housing or population settlement are likely to have important effects on the health of peri-urban communities, for example. A shift in the pattern of the economy from agriculture to manufacturing is likely to bring a different pattern of occupational ill health. Changes in the pattern of income distribution may affect the target groups for health-care. Numerous similar examples can be provided of the need to understand the current position and likely future changes in the factors affecting health.

- At the stage of planning, when options for interventions are being considered, an understanding of these causal factors may lead to very different health-promoting activities.

Public and private sector structures

Lastly, information is needed on the organizational characteristics and structure of the public and private sectors. Given the emphasis of this book on the role of the public sector, it is important that the situational analysis should set out clearly the overall position of the health sector within the public sector, including the relationships with central ministries such as finance and planning. Given current interest in both broad civil service reforms and more specific health sector reforms including for example any plans towards decentralization, this is of particular importance. Similarly the relationship between the private, NGO, and public sectors, and their relative roles, is important.

POLICY AND POLITICAL ENVIRONMENT

The next major category of information in the situational analysis concerns the less easily defined area relating to the wider policy and political (in its broadest sense) environment.

Overall national policies

This would include any stated national policies which go beyond the health sector. These may include broad development strategies, attitudes to the private or voluntary sector, economic policies, and policies related to self-sufficiency and to the role of women and minority groups.

Existing health policies

The situational analysis needs to refer to any existing health policies which need to be reflected in future plans. Planning at the regional and district level in particular will need to refer to national health policies.

Political environment

The next element of this section relates to the wider political environment. This section of a situational analysis, because of its potential sensitivity, may not be a public document. However, it is important that the wider context is recognized in the process of considering the current situation of the health sector. In particular, the concerns of various pressure groups influential in the health sector need to be considered: not necessarily done in order to comply with them, but rather in order to recognize potential opponents or supporters of eventual plan proposals.

HEALTH NEEDS

Information on health needs is a basic prerequisite for a plan. However, the issue of measuring health needs is a complex one, and is further discussed in Chapter 8. There are essentially two broad approaches, through medical indicators and through community perceptions of need. As we saw in Chapter 6, information on medically perceived need may come from a variety of sources, including community health surveys, and from records of health service contacts, as well as from the perceptions of health professionals.

Community perceptions of need are likely to be less easily available and less structured. However, such information may come from two sources:

• firstly, from surveys of the attitudes and views of community members as to their health needs

• secondly, indicators of community perceived need may be derived through existing community structures, such as village health or development committees, or indeed at the national level through democratic representative structures.

The pattern of ill health in most low income countries is well known, and one might think it unnecessary to repeat. However, there are clear differences between countries and within them between different areas. Furthermore, the fact that the pattern of service provision continues to fail to correspond to these needs suggests the continuing necessity to emphasize this disparity. The means of presentation of the information can help in this. For example, health problems can be grouped in presentation into those that are preventable in different ways (for example, through the provision of a water supply, or through immunization), and those that are not. This is required both for the present situation and for projections of future health needs.

Lastly, however, it is important to beware of the danger of paralysis by analysis discussed in Chapter 6. If it is known, for example, that malaria is a major health problem, lack of information on specific incidence rates where these are not available should not delay the development of anti-malaria activities. The main categories of health-need information are medically perceived health needs and community-perceived health needs.

• *Medically perceived health needs*

    – *morbidity rates*, including the incidence and prevalence by disease and by category of group affected (for example, age, sex, class, ethnicity, location (rural/urban/peri-urban))

    – *mortality rates*, including general population mortality rates, age-specific ones such as infant mortality, and disease and health need specific one such as TB mortality rates, and maternal mortality rates. Distributional analyses, as with morbidity rates, are also important

    – *disability rates*

    – *non-illness related needs*, including, for example, antenatal care and family planning.

• *Community-perceived health needs*. These are harder to define, particularly at the national level, and often expressed in terms of service deficiencies rather than 'health' indicators.

THE NON-HEALTH SECTOR: PLANS AND SERVICES PROVIDED

The next part of the situational analysis should give a brief description of the main services and future plans on those sectors which have a bearing on health, either negatively or positively. It is, however, important to sound a cautionary note here. It is all too easy to get immersed in long detailed descriptions of other sectoral developments which will never be read, and may well obscure issues. A good situational analysis should pick out salient points, and where necessary should refer the reader to other documents. Examples of the key sectors may include the following:

- education
- water and sanitation
- agriculture
- community development
- public works
- industrial and mining sectors.

HEALTH SERVICES

The second group of information on services relates to the health service itself. One might expect this category of data to be widely available and known within the health sector, but it is surprising how difficult it can be to find basic inventories of the facilities and service provision of the public sector, let alone other service providers.

Information is needed not solely relating to the public sector, but covering the various categories of health provider, including the private sector, employment-related health services, the non-government sector, and the traditional sector. The following sets out the principal minimum information needs:

Service facilities

- types and number of service facility, including:
  - community-based services
  - traditional practice
  - mobile services
  - clinics
  - health centres
  - district hospitals
  - referral hospitals
  - environmental service
- capacity of different facilities (for example, bed numbers)

- location of facilities
- ownership of facilities.

Service utilization

It is important that information is also provided on the level of utilization of services and by whom. Categories of information might include the following:

- hospital occupancy rates (where possible related to catchment areas — the population the facility is expected to serve)
- facility attendance rates (related to catchment areas)
- numbers of preventive activities performed, such as:
  - immunization rates
  - family planning accepters
  - drinking-water springs protected
  - pit latrines dug.

Service gaps

Service gaps that are known about need to be documented to include both current service gaps, such as areas not covered by basic facilities and likely future projected service gaps arising from population changes, new health needs, changed expectations, or changes in service standards.

Health service organizational arrangements

It is important that the analysis provides information on the current organizational arrangements of the health sector and any projected changes, such as decentralization of the public sector. In particular the degree of centralization of decision-making, opportunities for community participation in decision-making, and linkages between sectors, both within the overall pattern of health services (including the private, non-governmental, industrial, and traditional sectors) and with other health-related sectors need to be addressed. This is of particular importance during periods of changing organizational composition and relations, such as in countries pursuing policies of health sector reform.

RESOURCES

This refers to the resources currently deployed in the health sector and likely to be available in the future. The term 'resources', when used by economists and planners, refers not only to the finance available but also the real resources, including most importantly personnel, buildings, and equipment. While the levels of finance are crucial, it is easy to forget that finance by itself is of little use without the ability to use it to purchase real inputs or resources. These are discussed in greater detail in later chapters — in particular those relating to finance and human resources. However, the following basic information is suggested as important as a planning prerequisite.

Financial resources

The types of financial resource information required are:

- present and likely future capital and recurrent budget for the public sector services
- present and likely future expenditure in other parts of the health sector
- constraints on spending such as foreign exchange shortages
- projected inflation rates.

Information on the financial resources available to, and used by, the health sector and its different component parts is often not readily available but is important as a baseline against which to plan the allocation of future resources. It is important not only to have information about the total resource levels but also about their distribution within the sector and pattern of flow. Financing and expenditure surveys may be required to obtain information about the macro-level flows within the health sector; see for example Griffiths and Mills (1982), Mach and Abel-Smith (1983), Gilson (1987) and Gish (1987, 1988). More recently there has been growing interest in a technique of measuring the national health accounts; see for example Berman (1997). Figure 7.1 illustrates the complexity of flows within the health sector.

Personnel

- number of staff employed within the public sector, by major categories of staff
- number of staff employed in health fields outside the public sector
- projected output from training
- projected losses from the service
- projected transfers between the public and private health sectors; and
- current and projected gaps in staff.

Buildings, land, equipment, and vehicles

- type, age, location, ownership, and state of repair.

Other supplies

- constraints on the provision of other supplies, such as drugs.

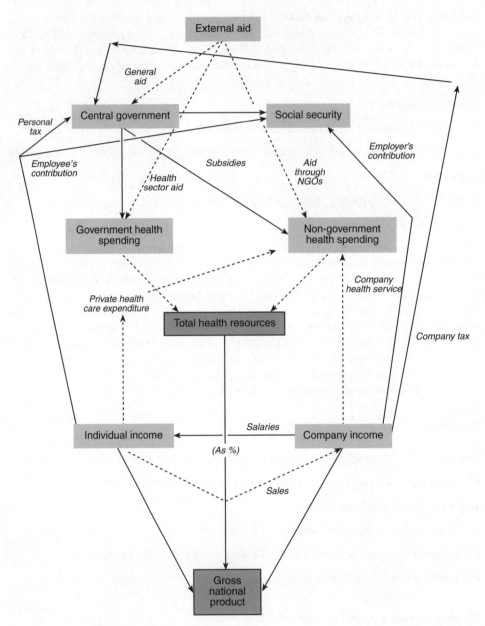

Fig. 7.1   Example of resource flows within the health sector

EFFICIENCY, EFFECTIVENESS, EQUITY, AND QUALITY OF CURRENT SERVICES

It is important that the situational analysis should provide some analysis of the efficiency and equity of the distribution of the various current services as a basis for the future plans. In this sense it is providing an evaluative function, which, as we saw in Chapter 2, is the lead in to a situational analysis within the planning spiral. Chapter 8 looks more closely at option appraisal and economic techniques of cost-effectiveness and cost–benefit analysis, and the details will be left till then. However, a good situational analysis will provide some indicators on the basic cost per activity, and, where possible, comparative data between facilities. Such information is important in assessing the current use of resources in different situations, and hence in planning future allocations. If, for example, a particular hospital is more expensive per patient than others for no particular reason, this would lead to a closer examination of the way the hospital was operating. Perhaps more important, however, is information comparing different types of facilities or services. For example, if it costs £10 per in-patient-day, compared to £0.50 to treat an outpatient, each in-patient-day implies the equivalent of 20 outpatient treatments. Although this does not imply that in-patient provision is unnecessary, it does suggest that a careful watch needs to be kept on the balance of resources going to different types of services. As part of this the effectiveness and quality of services need to be assessed.

Given, as we have seen, the importance of equity in PHC, it is also important that the situational analysis should explicitly examine and, where possible, provide information on the distribution of health-care resources between different population groups — including ethnic, locational, and class groupings. One simple indicator, if appropriate utilization and cost data exist, is an estimate of the resources in financial terms allocated or spent on different groups in comparison with their needs. Alternatively, information on the relative access of different groups to health facilities provides some indication of current distribution.

ANALYSIS OF THE SITUATION

As the term situational analysis implies, a description of the current situation is only part of this early and crucial part of the planning process. Although the preceding discussion has covered the major pieces of information required, it is important that a commentary on this should be provided as a backcloth to the selection of priorities and action. Such a commentary should attempt to match current and projected health needs with the present service provision, and to highlight likely gaps both in terms of services and particular resources. It should also comment on any particular salient aspects of the efficiency and equity of current health provision. It is also important to focus on interaction between the health service and other sectors, given the principles of PHC. Lastly, the commentary should, where necessary, address the appropriateness or otherwise of the current organizational arrangements for the health sector.

Examples of the major items which such a commentary might highlight for many developing countries are given in Box 7.2.

Box 7.2   Typical issues in a situational analysis

- High population growth rates
- High infant and childhood mortality
- Pattern of health problems which for the large part is preventable or treatable by primary care facilities, income generation, or better water supplies
- Poor prospects for future growth in resources for the health sector
- Inappropriate organizational structures of the health services, with highly centralized, bureaucratic structures and few mechanisms for community participation
- Lack of co-ordination between the public sector and other health services
- Inefficient allocation of resources between levels of facility, with hospital budgets absorbing the major and an increasing part of the resources
- Strong demand from middle-class urban elites for resources to be spent on high-technology medicine
- Major functional items of expenditure being drugs and personnel, both of which have above average inflation rates
- Low morale among health workers, and staff transfers between the public and private sectors
- Inequitable distribution of resources between population groups, and, in particular, the peri-urban and certain rural groups being particularly disadvantaged

---

WHO SHOULD CARRY OUT THE SITUATIONAL ANALYSIS?

It has been suggested earlier that there are a number of advantages in having a document setting out the results of the situational analysis. The task of drafting this document is likely to be the responsibility of the health planning body or secretariat at whatever level for which the analysis is being written. However, it is also important that the gathering and analysis of the information is seen as a broad-based activity involving not just health planners but three other groups as well:

- health professionals and service managers

- representatives of other sectors related to the health sector

- community representatives.

Involvement of these groups is important for two reasons: to ensure inclusion of their views, and as a preliminary step in garnering their support for the eventual plan.

SUMMARY

This chapter has set out the rationale for a formal situational analysis as a precursor to the development of a plan at any level within the health sector. It has suggested a number of components for such a situational analysis, and argued that broad participation in the process is important.

INTRODUCTORY READING

The specific areas on which information needs to be sought are covered in the reading for the previous chapter. However, the article by Abel-Smith and Leiserson (1980) provides a good example of a number of common resource issues facing many health sectors.

EXERCISE 7

Consider the different information requirements for a situational analysis outlined in Chapter 7, for a country known to you. What are the key features and sources of information required?

REFERENCES AND FURTHER READING

Abel-Smith, B. and Leiserson, A. (1980). Making the most of scarce resources. *World Health Forum*, 1, 145–52.

Arredondo, A. (1997). Costs and financial consequences of the changing epidemiological profile in Mexico. *Health Policy*, 42(1), 39–48.

Berman, P. (1997). National health accounts in developing countries: appropriate methods and recent applications *Health Economics*, 6(1), 11–30.

Gilson, L. (1987). Swaziland: health sector financing and expenditure. *Health Policy and Planning*, 2(1), 32–43.

Gish, O. (1987). Bias in health services: can expenditure data tell us who gets what? *Health Policy and Planning*, 2, 176–182.

Gish, O. (1988). More on health sector expenditure and what they can and cannot tell us. *Health Policy and Planning*, 3(1), 74–9.

Griffiths, A. and Mills, M. (1982). *Money for health*. Sandoz Institute, Geneva.

Griffiths, A. and Mills, M. (1983). Health sector financing and expenditure surveys. In *The economics of health in developing countries* (ed. K. Lee and A. Mills), pp. 43–63. Oxford University Press, Oxford.

Mach, E. P. and Abel-Smith, B. (1983). *Planning the finances of health sector.* WHO, Geneva.

Maier, B. *et al.* (1994). *Assessment of the district health system: using qualitative methods.* MacMillan, London.

Mills, A. (1990). The economics of hospitals in developing countries. Part 1: expenditure patterns. *Health Policy and Planning*, 5(2), 107–17.

Nyamwaya, D. *et al.* (1998). Socio-cultural information in support of local health planning: conclusions from a survey in rural Kenya. *International Journal of Health Planning and Management*, 13, 27–45.

Satia, J. K. *et al.* (1994). Micro-level planning using rapid assessment for primary health care services. *Health Policy and Planning*, 9(3), 318–30.

Vissandjee, B. *et al.* (1997). Utilisation of health services among rural women in Gujarat. *India Public Health*, 111(3), 135–48.

Wright, J. and Walley, J. (1998). Assessing health needs in developing countries. *British Medical Journal*, **316**, 1819–233.

8

Setting priorities

As we have seen, the fundamental rationale for planning is the inevitable shortfall between available resources and the competing uses to which those resources could be put. We turn now to discussion of issues relating to decisions as to the use of such resources should be made — in other words, on how priorities should be set. Chapter 1 suggested that there are two broad approaches to deciding how such limited resources are best allocated: a *demand-based market* mechanism or through a *needs-based planning* approach. Reliance on the market to determine health priorities was seen to be inappropriate with particular implications for equity. Within the context of this book it will be largely ignored in favour of the alternative needs-based allocative planning approach.

One major function of the planning process, therefore, is to determine these major needs, to devise suitable programmes for meeting them, and to allocate resources accordingly. There are not (and it can be argued, never will be) sufficient resources to meet all health needs. We need to decide which ones to focus on and which, therefore, have to be left. Of course, such decisions are not confined to countries with extreme resource shortages. Economic development will not remove the need for priority-setting, although the pattern may well alter. For example, even in the relatively well-resourced UK National Health Service today, there are waiting lists of patients untreated through lack of resources.

How such decisions are made has a major effect on the allocation itself. Different approaches and priority-setting mechanisms will lead to very different results. Techniques are neither objective, nor neutral, nor interchangeable. This chapter there-fore concentrates on the key questions of who should set priorities, and how. It also examines the complex issues of the factors underlying and attitudes towards priorities.

HEALTH AND NEED

We have already recognized that the ultimate aim of a health plan is to improve levels of health rather than health services — although the latter may, of course, be an important means to that end. At first sight, therefore, the process of setting priorities appears simple. We would expect planning to allocate resources to the areas of greatest need. If so, our priorities should be focused in the first instance on health needs rather than health service needs. Such priorities are often expressed in terms of a hierarchy of objectives starting with broad inclusive goals and gradually focusing on specific, measurable and time-bound targets. Box 8.1 explains the differences between these various terms, which are often confused.

Box 8.1   Goals, aims, objectives, and targets

Goals, aims, objectives, and targets are all ways of describing the desired direction of a service. They differ in terms of breadth and detail.

- **Goals** are broad statements. There is generally one goal for a service. The best-known has been '*Health for All by the Year 2000*'
- There are a number of **aims** relating to the goal. They are specific to particular health problems. One might be '*To raise the nutritional status of women and children.*'
- For each programme aim, there may be a number of **objectives** which are specified in measurable terms. An objective for the above aim might be '*To ensure that 95% of children under 5 are adequately nourished by the year 2010.*'
- For each objective, there may be various **targets** which specify various points on the way to the attainment of the objective. They are defined in relation to a point in time. For example, a target for the above objective might be '*To ensure that 75% of children under 5 are adequately nourished as pre-defined by the year 2000.*'

Health need is an elusive concept, loosely related to our understanding of the concept 'health', its inverse. The term 'need' is used widely, but with a variety of meanings. It can, for example, be interchanged with any of a number of phrases, including 'ought to have', 'must have', 'would like', 'will die without', or 'demand'. These phrases, although not identical in meaning, share two characteristics.

- Firstly, need refers to a lack of something — in this context, health. The measure for need, then, relates directly to the measurement of health.

- Secondly, need (like health) is not an absolute concept. There are gradations of need, and hence priorities among different needs. Less immediately apparent is the idea that need is a judgemental rather than a scientific concept. Perceptions of need will vary depending on the observer. This may be demonstrated through the simple exercise at the end of this chapter.

From within the context of the medical model, health needs have traditionally been viewed predominantly from an epidemiological perspective, with emphasis on mortality and morbidity. However, a number of criticisms can be levied against such a narrow view of health.

- Some of these criticisms relate to methodological issues. For example, as we saw in Chapter 6, morbidity and mortality data in many developing countries are often derived from information systems which are likely to give a biased picture of the overall health of the community. An example of this can be seen where hospital-based data on deaths are used as a proxy for overall mortality rates in a country where only a small proportion of deaths occur within a hospital. Such criticisms, although important, can be overcome with improved information systems.

• Secondly, medical concepts of need are less scientific than we might like to believe. Culyer (1985, p. 24) discusses an interesting experiment first reported in 1945. A number of children were screened by a group of doctors, who judged whether the children needed tonsillectomies (a popular form of treatment at the time): 45% were judged as in need. The children regarded as not in need were then seen by a further set of doctors, unaware of the earlier screening, who declared that 46% of this group were in need of a tonsillectomy. The experiment continued a third time with the residual 'clear' children being screened again — with a similar result! A number of interpretations can be put on this — perhaps the most plausible being that the doctors had a preconceived idea that in a sample of children they would expect to find a certain percentage of 'needy' children, and proceeded to diagnose a number of children as being in need. If the same experiment were repeated today it is conceivable that the same pattern would be detected, with one major difference: the level of tonsillectomies recommended would be lower, reflecting a further dimension in the nature of need. As the knowledge-base changes — in this case the medical understanding of tonsillitis — so do medical perceptions of need.

However, there are more fundamental concerns over the traditional epidemiological basis for determining priorities. Chapter 3 described the shift towards a broader concept of health. This broader understanding of health and rejection of a simple medical model of health, together with the related principle of community participation, has major implications for the process of priority-setting. It makes the measurement of need itself far more complex. It also raises questions about who should make such priority-setting decisions. Indeed, the debate around the appropriateness of a 'selective' approach to Primary Health Care (PHC) focuses to a large extent on these issues of priority and need determination.

NEED AS PERCEIVED BY THE COMMUNITY AND BY THE HEALTH PROFESSIONS

Who determines the need is clearly important. Increasingly the term 'perceived need' is used, in recognition that need is neither a scientific judgement nor the province of the medical profession alone. Figure 8.1 sets out diagrammatically the difference between the perceptions of the medical profession and those of the individual or community. While there are likely to be large areas of agreement between professionals and the community (*b* and *c*) in their judgements of need, there will be some differences. The area *a* represents need that professionals perceive, which is not viewed in the same way by communities. This might include some areas of preventive medicine. Areas *d* and *e* represent needs that may be perceived by a community, but not by the health professions. This might include some forms of traditional medicine, for example. The diagram also shows the relationship between (economic) demand and need. For economists the word 'demand' is reserved for the desire for a good or

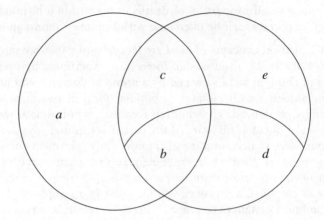

Professionally determined need = $a + b + c$
Needs as perceived by community or individual = $b + c + d + e$
Economic demand of the individual or community = $b + d$

Fig. 8.1   Perceptions of need

service (such as health-care) backed up by the ability to pay for it. On this basis only a proportion of community-perceived need can and will be translated into demand, because of income limitations. Indeed it is this difference between economic demand and need that underlies one of the arguments against the use of (demand-led) market mechanisms. Areas b and d together represent the needs for which the community would be prepared to pay (at current charges). This may include some needs not viewed as important by health professionals (d).

The diagram illustrates that, while there are likely to be large areas of agreement between health professionals and communities, there may also be differences. Figure 8.1 is oversimplistic in that it sees needs as absolute — as either being recognized or not. The situation is complicated by the fact that, as we have seen, need is not an absolute but a relative term. Some health problems may be considered to be more important by health professionals than by the community, and vice versa. Within the community itself there are also likely to be significant differences of opinion, arising from the heterogeneous nature of the community. Health professionals will also differ among themselves in their views about relative need. Perceptions of need will also vary over time. The origin of the differing weights given to need derives from differing perceptions of health; and it is to that that we now turn.

UNDERLYING PERCEPTIONS OF HEALTH

Groups in different positions within the health system (including different professional groupings, users, and more generally community members in different socio-economic and class contexts, as well as politicians) will have very different perceptions of health and its underlying importance. It is important to be aware of a number of possible dimensions to this which result in these different views. It would be inappropriate within the book to get immersed in discussion as to why health is generally regarded as high on the list of both individual and social desiderata. However, it is worth spending time considering some aspects of this, as it sheds light on why there may be differences in view as to priorities between different individuals and groups. Various themes are briefly introduced below.

Effects of ill health

Ill health is undesirable not in itself, but because of its effects on the individual or the wider community. There are various types of effects. These include:

• death

• pain and discomfort, either acute or chronic

• disability

• distress to the individual, family, and friends

• social effects

• economic effects on the individual, such as loss of earnings.

Different health problems will have varying combinations of these effects. For example, polio may result in disability and cholera in death; and chronic TB may lead to unemployment; alcoholism may have social effects.

A first underlying aspect to the setting of priorities, therefore, is attitudes towards the particular effects of different health problems. At first sight death may be viewed as the most serious consequence of a health problem, but priorities for community health also need to take account of the other effects. Indeed, in practice, health problems which result in death are not automatically accorded a higher priority than other health problems. As the health situation in countries improves and mortality rates drop, it becomes harder to decide whether to allocate resources to 'adding years to life' through focusing on life-threatening health problems, as opposed to focusing on the quality of life and adding 'life to years'.

Health as an investment or a consumption good

One aspect of the effects of ill health is influenced by whether we consider health as an investment or a consumption good. If individual health problems have varying effects on both the individual and society, this has implications for broad developmental policies towards health. As we have seen, over the last two decades development policies in many countries and donor agencies have shifted away from the early identification of development with growth in gross national product (GNP). Although health was not ignored in the development plans of countries taking such a view, the prime focus of development energy was targeted towards the productive sectors of industry, agriculture, and mining. Such strategies, although seeing health as an important aim of development, took the view that growth in the economy should be seen as the first priority as being the only way, in the long run, to achieve a better standard of living, including health. Economists and planners concerned with the immediate development of the health sector shifted their arguments for increased resources away from issues of social welfare towards a line of argument more consistent with that of the current development priorities. Health was talked of as an important factor in improving productivity. Investment in human resources was therefore seen as an important element of a growth-oriented development strategy. This view sees health as an *investment good*.

The apparent failure of such growth-focused strategies to ameliorate the position of the vast majority in developing countries led to a further shift in development thinking away from such a purely growth-oriented approach. Emphasis shifted towards the immediate rather than the long-term goals of development in terms of meeting the basic needs of the population. Health became an important contender for resources in its own right (rather than as a means towards growth). Such a view of health sees it as a *consumption good* — i.e. one valued in its own right. This shift towards basic needs, which largely took place in the 1970s, was cut short by both the world recession and the (related) rise of the New Right ideology in the West. The combination of these factors led to pressure on public sector approaches to social welfare, and confused and differing perceptions as to the importance of the health sector.

Which view of health is taken has enormous implications for priority-setting. The discussion is perhaps at its most stark in the area of economic appraisal, where the benefits of health need to be carefully stated. Under a consumption or social welfare view of health, issues such as equity are more likely to be seen as paramount. If we view health as an end in itself then we should not discriminate against different groups in terms of how we view their health needs on grounds other than the needs themselves. An investment view of health which sees health as a means to an end — better productivity and growth — would however deliberately favour one group (producers) against another. Under such a view one would see the health of the elderly, disabled, or unemployed as being of lower priority than that of the young, employed, fit adult. Yet ironically the health needs of the first group, almost by definition, are likely to be greater. Suggestions that one can combine the two approaches run counter to notions of equity, as they introduce the possibility of ranked health needs being distorted by considerations other than need.

The debate is not theoretical, but has real implications for policy. For example, it was argued in the early 1970s that the social insurance system predominant in Latin America, which was based on the industrial sectors, was inequitable. Such inequity in the short term was seen, however, as an inevitable and acceptable short-term consequence of the need to promote growth as a precursor to wider long-term health benefits (see Roemer 1971).

Target groups

A further perspective on priorities and perspectives on health can be seen in the concept of target groups. These may be groups which share a variety of characteristics such as age, location, or disease.

Perhaps the commonest target for priorities is that of particular disease-based groups. In particular, infectious diseases have often had a high priority — traceable back to the origins in many countries of public sector health services as a means of protecting civil servants, the army, and the burgeoning bourgeoisie. Vertical programmes set up in response to these concerns included those aimed at smallpox, malaria, TB, leprosy, and more recently AIDS. The use of disease groups fits in neatly with a medical model of health, and suffers from the corresponding deficiencies. The selective primary health-care approach examined earlier takes this view in comparing the characteristics of different diseases. The more recent Burden of Disease (BoD) approach (see World Bank 1993, Murray *et al.* (1994) using cost per Disability Adjusted Life Year (DALY) follows this medical model vertical tradition (Anand and Hansen 1997, Barker and Green 1996).

A second means of targeting groups can be seen in health-sector plans which have laid emphasis on particular population groups. The most commonly targeted groups are women and children. The rationale for emphasis on maternal and child health is not always clearly specified, but is assumed to be widely understood and accepted. It is, however, important to consider why such groups may be seen as priorities for health resources. There are at least three reasons why this may be the case, each with differing implications for future priorities.

- Firstly, the group may be seen to have the greatest needs in terms of demonstrated morbidity. Death rates for infants, for example, are generally far higher than for any group other than the very elderly; and maternal mortality may also be very high. Such a policy suggests that children and women are not being targeted in themselves, but rather as a result of the morbidity they face. Were their morbidity to be reduced, then the priority would shift to another group with higher morbidity.

- Secondly, the young may be regarded as of high priority because of the investment effect, with the young age groups forming the next generation of producers. Such a view has all the problems inherent in the investment approach to health noted above. One stark example is the possible priority that might be given to older surviving children over younger ones. Feminist analysis suggest that emphasis on women's health and maternal health-care may reflect only women's and children's roles in society as producers and reproducers.

- A third view suggests that children are given higher priority because they have a longer life expectancy than adults. Related to this might be some notion of fairness, suggesting that children who have not yet experienced 'life' are entitled to higher priority than elderly adults. An alternative rationale for this would be one of 'efficiency' in the resources being deployed to groups with higher potential life years to gain. In practice, of course, all these and other views become intermixed in the process.

Other target groups in health-care plans have often been inhabitants of rural areas — largely on the grounds that they have less access to health-care facilities and greater morbidity rates. More recently there has been recognition that 'ruralness' is not necessarily a good proxy for either access or morbidity. Within both rural and urban groups there may be wide variations. Attention has focused, in recent years, for example, increasingly on the position of the peri-urban dweller. Paradoxically, low income groups have not often been explicitly targeted, despite the well-known links between income and health.

The above examples of different target groups suggests that the choice of such groups is not simple, and often not dependent on explicit criteria.

Cost, ease, and effectiveness of intervention

All the above are concerned with the health effects of a particular problem. From the perspective of the planner, another important consideration is the ease and cost of intervention in the problem. A planner facing two health problems perceived as having similar health consequences, one of which is easier or cheaper to control, is likely — other things being equal — to choose that one into which to put resources. The overall health gain will be greater for the same resources. This is essentially the logic behind economic appraisal, which will be examined in more detail in Chapter 10. It is this aspect of a problem that leads to the fact that some life-threatening health problems which are not easily amenable to interventions are given lower priority than other non-fatal health problems which are relatively easy to deal with. For example, expensive radiotherapy treatment for certain cancers may not be seen as a priority in comparison with prevention of hookworm. In order to make such comparisons between cost and health gain, indicators of the latter are needed.

Simple outcome indicators such as the number of lives saved are easy to apply, but have a number of drawbacks.

• Firstly, they take no account of the age or indeed other health characteristics of the person affected by the health problem. Thus the life of a 3 year old and that of a 63 year old would be treated in the same way. Similarly, comparison between the treatment of two people for pneumonia, one of whom also has terminal untreatable cancer, would show no differences. To deal with this, alternative outcome indicators which incorporate the effects of other factors over and above the particular disease being treated, such as 'healthy days of life lost' or 'life yeas gained', have been developed.

• Secondly, both these indicators relate only to life-threatening health problems, yet health plans need also to deal with other types of health problems. Although simple indicators of morbidity, such as the number of cases of a new disease, can be used, and indeed are, their usefulness on their own is limited. Morbidity is difficult to compare not only with mortality, but also with other morbidity. How does one compare an episode of TB with leukaemia, measles, or an arm fracture? Yet if we are to make decisions about the allocation of resources between differing health needs based on indicators of health, we require a measure that allows direct comparison between them.

Attempts therefore have been made to devise more sophisticated measures of morbidity, such as the Physical Quality of Life Indicator (PQLI). In the US and UK more recent attempts have been made to develop even more sophisticated outcome measures, known as Quality Adjusted Life Years (QALYs; see Loomes and McKenzie (1989) for a discussion), which combine different types of measure of the effect of an intervention on a health problem, both measures in terms of life expectancy and measures in terms of the quality of the life expected. The outcome measure that is being promoted by the World Bank is the Disability Adjusted Life Year (DALY) which combines measures of life years gained and disability prevented (World Bank 1993, Murray *et al.* 1994).

Such composite indicators allow the comparison of different health problems in terms of their effects on these variables, and appear to be a step forward. However, they can be criticized on a number of counts. Firstly, they require sophisticated information systems, which currently do not exist in the health sector of most developing countries. Further, although goal-setting in terms of health problems constitutes the ideal, in practice individuals may find it hard to shift from thinking in terms of service objectives towards health objectives. This is particularly (and understandably) true of communities who may be more likely to frame their requirements in terms of services, rather than in terms of a reduction in particular diseases. Of more concern, however, is the criticism that although such outcome indicators may appear to be neutral measures of outcome, they actually mask subjective value judgements. For example, if we examine the difference between two measures — lives saved and length of life extended — the latter builds in a judgemental weighting towards diseases which affect younger people.

This concern is fundamental. Setting priorities is ultimately an exercise in judgement. Individual members of society will exercise that judgement in different ways depending, *inter alia*, on their perceptions of health. None of the 'sciences' involved in the planning field, including economics, sociology, or epidemiology, will have any better judgement of those priorities than the individual members of society, although they may, of course, be able to provide useful information upon which such judgements can be based.

WHO SHOULD SET PRIORITIES?

Within any priority-setting decision there are two broad processes which need to be conceptually disentangled.

- The first concerns the provision of information. This is an important function of the planning system, and in Chapter 7 we discussed the elements of a situational analysis which would form such a base for priority-setting. Although, as we have seen, communities should be important providers of information, there is also a clear role for health and other professionals in both the provision and the analysis of information.

- Secondly, there is the decision as to how health and health need is viewed. Preceding sections examined a number of possible different perspectives on health and health need. As we have seen, assessment of health needs and priorities is not a simple technical issue. Different individuals, professions, or groups will have different attitudes, and a critical decision relates to how such views are to be weighted. The philosophy of PHC suggests that such decisions should be made at the national level by society as a whole, and at the local level with the full involvement of the communities concerned. The difficulties in achieving this should not be underestimated, however. National level representation will depend on political structures. These vary between countries, from fully representative broad-based democratic structures to military dictatorships. At the local level, communities are rarely homogeneous, and have within them widely differing views. These views are affected by a variety of factors, including class, age, sex, and education, and how they are mediated is critical. Use of traditional power structures may be attractive, but may reinforce existing inequities. The setting-up of alternative structures, such as village health committees, requires careful consideration as to how representation is reached. The use of community health workers as an informal means of garnering opinion may, in view of their relationship with the rest of the health service, lead to biases in their information collection.

There are also questions as to the relationship between the political structures at the national level and those at the community level. Health services are often controlled by the central political structures, although in some countries decentralization policies are leading to local government increasingly playing an important role. Although it may be argued that the national political structure, if representative, can provide one means of participation, this is unlikely to meet the genuine requirements of a PHC approach. The role of the centre is rather to ensure that there is equity of resource availability between areas, maintenance of standards, and the provision of a framework for the determination of local needs. This needs to be done in a way that allows full participation by local communities in decisions which affect their health. The only constraint is that this should be done without negatively affecting the decisions of other communities or clashing with other national development policies.

Such an approach suggests different roles both for communities and for health professionals from those currently operating in many countries. Frequently, priorities are set on the basis of narrow morbidity information controlled by the health professionals, with little input from communities. Furthermore, such priority-setting is rarely done in an open, systematic fashion, which can be challenged. An essential function of the planning system, therefore, is the development of an open framework for setting priorities which allows communities a role and redefines the role of health professionals.

The above has focused on the two main groups with a claim to involvement in priority-setting: communities and health professionals. In practice, as we saw in Chapter 2, there are likely to be a number of other groups with a desire to influence priorities, each with more or less legitimacy. Examples of these include NGOs, trade unions, universities, and commercial companies. The political nature of planning that we have stressed makes their involvement inevitable. It is important that planners recognize this and ensure that the process is as open and transparent as possible, without giving undue access to any one group.

The other group that can, and in practice does, play a major role in determining priorities, is donor agencies. Through their control of external funds, such agencies can often impose their own set of priorities on a country. This is most likely to occur where there is a lack of a clear national framework; in such circumstances it is not only easy, but perhaps understandably tempting, for such agencies to attempt to fill the policy vacuum.

ESTABLISHING PRIORITIES WITHIN
A PLANNING FRAMEWORK

So far in this chapter we have looked at a number of issues and perspectives in the area of priority-setting without trying to suggest a particular approach. As has been stressed elsewhere in this book, none of these perspectives can be judged as 'correct', although some are likely to be closer to the philosophy of PHC than others. A planner, however, is left needing to use a framework to get priorities set and expressed in a form that allows for implementation. Some mechanism for establishing rankings is required. Such a framework needs to satisfy various criteria. In particular it needs to:

- achieve balanced participation between different groups and in particular communities and professionals

- encourage a multisectoral perspective

- achieve a balance between the centre and the periphery

- result in aims and objectives that are clear and feasible

- be an open and understandable system.

The rest of this chapter looks at a variety of methods and processes that can be used to assist in the making of such decisions about priorities. There is no 'correct' approach, and the process chosen in any particular country will depend on factors specific to that country, not the least important of which is the political framework.

The resource allocation process

The broad philosophy of PHC suggests that local decision-making involving communities should be encouraged as far as is possible and sustainable. Where such decentralization is possible, the decisions as to the precise pattern of health-care can be left to local decision-makers. In such circumstances central decisions as to the level of resources to be made available at the local level are necessary. This requires a resource allocation system, based on the principle of equity, that determines the broad levels of resources which each region or district will receive. This is discussed in Chapter 11.

Even where there is a highly decentralized system of planning, however, it is unlikely that the decentralized districts will have complete freedom in allocating resources. Firstly, guidance on broad policy will be provided from the central level. Secondly, it is likely that some services will be provided centrally; these might include training, specialist systems, and technical support, if not actual service provision, relating to particular diseases such as communicable diseases.

Decentralization of decision-making does not obviate the need to set priorities. Instead it alters the level at which these priorities are set. We will now look at various techniques used to set such priorities.

Economic appraisal

Chapter 10 looks in more detail at the techniques of economic appraisal. Such techniques (and in particular cost-effectiveness analysis and cost–benefit analysis) compare the resources needed for intervention with the outcome (or benefit) of such intervention. At first sight such techniques might appear to provide the answers to priority-setting questions, in that they bring together the issues of the cost of interventions and their impact on health problems. The World Bank approach of using estimates of the BoD, measured through DALYs, which compares the cost of interventions for different health problems to reduce the BoD is an important example of economic appraisal being used for this purpose (World Bank 1993, Murray *et al.* 1994).

In practice there are a number of problems with using economic appraisal techniques, which we explore later. See Green and Barker (1988) for a critique of economic appraisal techniques, and Barker and Green (1996) and Anand and Hansen (1997) for a discussion of the World Bank approach to setting priorities. The difficulties of comparing outcomes (necessary for cost-effectiveness analysis), let alone translating these outcomes into monetary values (as required in cost–benefit analysis) imply that currently the most important usage for economic appraisal is in comparing options to achieve the same objectives, rather than in setting priorities. Furthermore, economic appraisal techniques offer no escape from the need for the same subjective value judgements discussed earlier. In particular the techniques themselves offer no insights into why some health problems might be regarded as of greater importance than others. Economic appraisal techniques as currently practiced also have the danger of mystifying such decisions by making them appear very technical. As such they are unlikely to be immediately accessible to communities.

Economic appraisal techniques tend to follow a rather narrow medical model. Alternative approaches to looking at other factors which might affect priorities have also been tried; and these we will look at now.

Multivariable decision matrices

We saw earlier that there may be a variety of reasons why we might want to give priority to particular health problems. Various techniques exist that try to bring together such factors. Table 8.1 gives an example of one such.

Under this approach, various reasons for giving priority to a health problem were set. These included:

- size of the problem in terms of morbidity

- consequent suffering and disability

- effects of the problem on disruption to the family

- economic consequences of the problem

- likely demand from the public for the problem to be dealt with

- technical feasibility of a solution to the problem

- social consequences of the problem.

Professionals with expertise related to each of the variables were asked to rank which health problems they thought were most important *in terms of that variable alone.* For example, economists looked at the economic consequences of different problems, social workers at which problems caused the greatest family disruption, and epidemiologists at which problems had the greatest morbidity.

Table 8.1 was constructed, and showed the major health problems identified according to these criteria in the form of a matrix. At this point the process shifts from being a professional technical process to the more evaluative one of deciding between the importance of the different factors. This could be done in advance, with a decision being made as to the different weighting to be applied to each of the variables. Alternatively, the table is presented as background information to the 'political' decision-makers, who may be either at the community level or at the national level, depending on the level of decentralization. From this information a single list is derived for the major health problems.

Such an approach, although allowing for limited community input, is still professionally dominated in terms of the initial selection of problems. It could be broadened in a number of ways — in particular by setting other parameters, for example specific gender effects. One of its advantages, however, is that it does not rely on quantified indicators.

It is, of course, possible to incorporate the use of numerical rankings within the process. For example, diseases in each list could be given a number from 0 to 10 depending on their importance. Each variable could, in turn, be assigned a weighting (cost for example being seen as twice as significant as social consequences and thus given a weighting of 2). An overall priority list of diseases could then be obtained by adding the weighted numbers assigned to each disease. Although this is superficially attractive in that it gives an unequivocal answer, there is a clear danger that the process appears to be more objective and technical than it is, and that the nuances of priority-setting are glossed over.

Table 8.1   Ranking of disease groups by different factors

Priority ranking	In-patient morbidity	Family disruption	Economic* consequences	Public and potential demand	Technical feasibility of solution	Social consequences	Suffering and disability
1	Enteric diseases	Alcoholism	Alcoholism	Malaria	TB	Leprosy	Leprosy
2	Complication of pregnancy	Psychiatric disorders	TB	Complication of pregnancy	Measles	Alcoholism	Polio
3	Respiratory diseases	Skin disease, inc. leprosy	Bilharzia	Alcoholism	Polio	Sexually transmitted diseases	Eye disease
4	TB	TB	Trauma		Malnutrition	Psychiatric disorders	TB
5	Malnutrition	Sexually transmitted diseases	Polio		Water-borne diseases (inc. enteric)	TB	Trauma
6	Measles		Leprosy				
7	Skin diseases, inc. leprosy						

* Both in terms of cost of treatment, and loss of production
Source: Swaziland County Report for presentation to Nampula PHC Workshop, Nampula April 1980.

Decision-making processes

The two preceding approaches, economic appraisal and decision matrices, share a desire to develop a 'scientific' approach to setting priorities. Given that one of the criteria we have set for a planning framework is an open system, this is understandable. However, one of the major themes of this chapter has been that priority-setting is ultimately a process involving the application of different value judgements. Such quasi-scientific techniques may mask these important value judgements, and thus may, ironically, result in a less transparent system than was desired.

Although there are advances in the field of operational research which may bring 'soft' techniques that will assist in the making of such decisions, it would be unwise to assume that these will be easily available and applicable in the short term. It would also be wrong to assume that they will remove the fundamental need to reconcile in some way the different value judgements held both by different professionals and by different members of communities.

In the absence of easy scientific techniques one is forced back on broader approaches to decision-making. Two such approaches can be distinguished. The first involves a clear leadership role, where an individual is charged with the job, usually because of her/his position, of reaching a decision. S/he may consult colleagues and communities, using such techniques as those described above, but ultimately the final decision is seen to be theirs. The strength of their position will determine the degree to which they may vary from the majority view.

The second approach is based on a desire to reach a clear consensus of opinion, and is closer to the philosophy of PHC, though it may be a far more laborious process. Various techniques may be used to facilitate this process, but the end-result is that a group decision is reached which is seen to have been reached in an open and fair manner. In the Delphi technique (for an example see Rainhorn *et al.* 1994), a set of individuals are asked to give answers to questions (in this case related to priorities), and the answers are shared among the group. The same question is then asked a second time. As a result of the first sharing of answers, some individuals may shift their position. The process continues until a consensus is reached.

An interesting example of a process involving communities in priority-setting in an industrialized health-care system was that carried out in Oregon, USA (Crawshaw 1991, Dixon and Welch 1991, Honigsbaum *et al.* 1995).

PRIORITY-SETTING AND PHC

It is clear from the above that there are no easy answers to what is probably the most difficult stage of the planning process, yet the one given least attention. Different political, cultural, and health-care structures are likely to lead to different approaches. However, we will attempt to synthesize briefly some of the themes, and suggest the sort of priority-setting structure that would be consistent with the principles of PHC.

Such an approach would have four stages.

- The first stage would involve the production of a macro-situational analysis setting out the key information at the national level. The responsibility for the production of this document would be that of the national health planning unit, involving other sectors where necessary.

- The second stage would involve discussion by a national-level planning group, involving representatives of the major health-related sectors together with national-level political representatives. This group would be charged with producing, or bringing together where they already exist, broad guidelines as to:

  - broad (non-health-specific) national policies (such as gender policies; or putting emphasis on particular regions or on development strategies)
  - any specific national technical health-policy guidelines (such as towards immunization schedules)
  - resource allocation guidelines, taking account of equity principles.

- The third stage would involve the development of local-level situational analyses and priorities, by local-level health and other professionals and community representatives, with the assistance, where necessary, of the health planning unit. A group would be formed consisting of health professionals, other sector workers, and community representatives. The group would be set up in such a way that the community representative views were clearly protected; for example, by having a chairperson from the community. This group would be charged with:

  - reviewing the situational analysis, asking for further information where appropriate; and
  - setting feasible priorities for the area that are consistent with national policies and within the resource guidelines given from the centre.

- This group would be given a sufficient time-scale to meet to allow the members to consult their 'constituents' at various stages.

- The last stage would involve the review of these policies by the national health planning unit to ensure that they met the criteria set and were not inconsistent with other local area priorities. Sufficient time would be built into the process to allow the resolution of such divergences through dialogue.

SUMMARY

This chapter has explored a number of themes related to the process of setting priorities. It has argued that priority-setting is the most important part of the planning process, and yet is often not given sufficient attention. It has also argued that priority-setting involves a combination of technique and value judgement. Whose values are chosen is a critical decision; the philosophy of PHC suggests that communities should have a major role in the process. The chapter concluded by suggesting a number of criteria for the process of setting priorities, and gave an example of a process that would potentially satisfy these criteria.

INTRODUCTORY READING

Priority-setting (and its obverse, rationing) has become an important policy issues in the health-care systems of many industrialized countries and there is an increasing literature available focusing on this. Harrison (1995), Honigsbaum *et al.* (1995) Klein (1994, 1997), Shiell (1997) and Williams (1988) give a useful overview of the issues. Bowling (1996) and Doyal (1993) explore one critical aspect of this — the role of the public. The role of economic appraisal and in particular the use of QALYs is discussed by Loomes and McKenzie (1989) and Williams (1985). Recent interest in priority-setting in developing health systems has focused on the use of DALYs and the BoD through economic appraisal techniques with the *World Development Report* (World Bank 1993) and Murray *et al.* (1994). Critiques of this approach can be found in Barker and Green (1996), Anand and Hanson (1997), Cooper (1998) and Paalman *et al.* (1998). Some of this reflects the earlier debates (Walsh and Warren (1979), Unger and Killingsworth (1986) and Green and Barker (1986) around selective primary care of the early 1980s which are still relevant today.

EXERCISE 8

Ask each member of a group to rank the following in order of priority for medical attention:

- child with polio
- child with measles
- child with kwashiorkor
- unvaccinated child
- teenager with malaria
- unemployed single adult with glaucoma
- employed adult with TB
- elderly person with cancer.

1. Are the rankings of each respondent identical? If not, what are the differences and why?
2. What are the current priority areas for health action in your country?
3. Why do you think these are seen as priorities?
4. Are there health problems which are not currently viewed as a priority?
5. Why do you think this is the case?

REFERENCES AND FURTHER READING

Anand, S. and Hanson, K. (1997). Disability-Adjusted Life Years: a critical review. *Journal of Health Economics*, **16**, 685–702.

Barker, C. and Green, A. (1996). Opening the debate on DALYS. *Health Policy and Planning*, **11**(2), 179–83.

Bowling, A. (1996). Health care rationing: the public's debate. *British Medical Journal*, **312**, 670–4.

Braveman, P. and Tarimo, E. (1994). *Screening in primary health care: setting priorities with limited resources.* World Health Organization, Geneva.

Cooper, R. (1998). Disease burden in sub-Saharan Africa: what should we conclude in the absence of data? *Lancet*, **351**, 208–10.

Crawshaw, R. (1991). Oregon sets priorities in health care. *Bulletin of Medical Ethics*, **69**, 32–5.

Culyer, A. J. (1985). *Economics.* Blackwell, Oxford.

Dixon, J. and Welch, H. G. (1991). Priority-setting: lessons from Oregon. *Lancet*, **337**, 891–4.

Doyal L. (1993). The role of the public in health care rationing. *Critical Public Health*, **4**(1), 49–54.

Ghana Health Assessment Team (1981). A quantitative method of assessing the health impact of different diseases in less developed countries. *International Journal of Epidemiology*, **10**, 73–80.

Green, A. and Barker, C. (1988). Priority-setting and economic appraisal: whose priorities — the community or the economist? *Social Science and Medicine*, **26**, 919–29.

Harrison, S. (1995). A policy agenda for health care rationing. *British Medical Bulletin*, **51**(4), 885–99.

Honigsbaum, F. (1991). *Who shall live? Who shall die? Oregon's health financing proposals.* King's Fund, London.

Honigsbaum, F., Calltorp, J., Ham, C. *et al.* (1995). *Priority setting processes for health care in Oregon, USA; New Zealand; The Netherlands; Sweden and the United Kingdom.* Radcliffe Medical Press, Oxford.

Jamison, D. T., Mosley, W. H., Measham, A. R. *et al.* (1993). *Disease control priorities in developing countries.* Oxford Univrsity Press, New York.

Klein, R. (1994). Can we restrict the health care menu? *Health Policy*, **27**(2), 103–112.

Klein, R. (1997). The case against. *British Medical Journal*, **314**, 506–9.

Loomes, G. and McKenzie, L. (1989). The use of QALYs in health care decision-making. *Social Science and Medicine*, **28**, 299–308.

Lorenz, N. *et al.* (1996). The right objectives in health care planning. *World Health Forum*, **16**, 280–2.

Maxwell, R.J. (ed.) (1995). Rationing health care. *British Medical Bulletin*, **51**(4), 761–962.

Murray, C. J. L. *et al.* (1994). Cost-effectiveness analysis and policy choices: investing in health systems. *Bulletin of the World Health Organisation*, **72**(4), 663–74.

Paalman, M., Bekedam, H., Hawken, L. *et al.* (1998). A critical review of priority setting in the health sector: the methodology of the 1993 World Development Report. *Health Policy and Planning*, **13**(1), 13–31.

Rainhorn, J. D. *et al.* (1994). Priorities for pharmaceutical policies in developing countries: results of a Delphi survey. *Bulletin of WHO*, **72**(2),257–64.

Roemer, M. I. (1971). Social security for medical care: is it justified in developing countries? *International Journal of Health Services*, **1**, 354–61.

Shiell, A. (1997). Health outcomes are about choices and values: an economic perspective on the health outcomes movement. *Health Policy*, **39**(1), 5–15.

Stevens, A. and Gillam, S. (1998). Needs assessment: from theory to practice. *British Medical Journal*, **316**, 7142, 1448–52.

Unger, J.P. and Killingsworth, J.R. (1986). Selective primary health care: a critical review of methods and results. *Social Science and Medicine*, **22**(10), 1001–13.

Walsh, J. A. and Warren, K. S. (1979). Selective primary health care: an interim strategy for disease control in developing countries. *New England Journal of Medicine*, **301**, 1B, 967–94.

Williams, A. (1985). Economics of coronary artery bypass grafting. *British Medical Journal*, **291**, 326–9.

Williams, A. (1988). Priority-setting in public and private health care: a guide through the ideological jungle. *Journal of Health Economics*, 7, 173–83.

Wiseman, V. and Mooney, G. (1998). Burden of illness estimates for priority setting: a debate revisited. *Health Policy*, **43**, 243–51.

World Bank (1993). *World development report: investing in health.* World Bank/Oxford University Press, Oxford.

Zalot, G. N. and Lussing, F. J. (1983). A. process for establishing health care priorities. *Health Management Forum*, Winter, 4(4), 31–44.

9

Costs and costing

For many non-economists, it seems that a major preoccupation of economics is with cost calculations. One saying suggests 'economists are people who know the cost of everything but the value of nothing'. This rather unfair view of the discipline fails to recognize the more analytical side of economics, although an understanding of costs and costing is certainly one of the basic tools for economists and indeed for planners.

Chapter 1 argued that underpinning the rationale for planning is the reality of a scarcity of resources. In order to make informed planning choices between alternative and competing demands on these scarce resources, it is imperative that planners are aware of the resource requirements or costs of each alternative. This chapter examines different cost concepts, applications, and techniques.

WHAT IS MEANT BY COSTS?

Costs represent the resources given up in a particular situation in order to carry out an activity. For the sake of convenience and comparability they are usually expressed in terms of *money*. This should not obscure the fact that this money actually represents real resources used up. Costs are not the same as *prices*, which reflect a market rate of exchange. Some actions may have costs which have no price or market value, whereas others have market prices that do not reflect the real resource implications to society of an action.

As a result of the concept of scarcity, economists refer to the *opportunity costs* of an action. By this they mean the alternative actions (by implication the next best) that could have occurred if one had not gone ahead with the chosen action. For example, the opportunity cost of training one doctor might be the alternative of training two nurses.

Costing is the name given to the activity that estimates the costs of an action either in the future or in the past. There are three major points in the planning spiral at which costing is necessary — the option appraisal stage, budgeting, and evaluation. The principles of costing for appraisal and evaluation are similar; references to appraisal within this chapter can be read as references to evaluation as well.

The type and accuracy of the cost information required will vary depending upon how this information is to be used. This in turn depends on the particular planning activity being carried out. At the appraisal and evaluation stages (examined in more detail in Chapter 10), where programmes and projects are being assessed, either prospectively or retrospectively, it is important that the costs involved are well defined and sufficiently accurate. It is also important that within the public sector the real costs to society, and not just to the health sector, should be assessed. This is discussed further below.

Having decided, after an option appraisal, between alternative options (including the option of continuing existing programmes) it is important that the resources necessary to implement the chosen programme are available, in the right form, at the right place, and at the right time. Costs therefore need to be estimated also as a prerequisite to setting budgets.

WHOSE COSTS?

In determining the costs of any action, it is important to identify all the costs arising, and on whom they fall. Providing an antenatal service, for example, may incur costs for:

• the *health service*, for example, in the form of drugs or personnel

• the *individual*, in the form of charges, transport costs, or time away from home or work

• the *individual's employer or family*, in covering for her absence.

Planning in the public sector is a mechanism for determining the best option for a community as a whole. Indeed, this is what distinguishes it from the private sector, whose motivating force is profit for the organization's owners. As such, decisions by public sector planners determining the best option for society should try to take account of all the effects throughout society (not just the effects on the implementing health institution itself). This implies the need to take account of all costs of these alternative options, irrespective of on whom they fall. This contrasts starkly with a private sector concerned only with the resource implications for the institution providing the service, which would only look at its internal costs.

An example may clarify this. Box 9.1 sets out a hypothetical situation in which two alternatives for a new antenatal service are being considered — central and peripheral clinics. The assumption is that the quality of care and the utilization rates are similar (unlikely, but helpful for the example). Only the costs are different — relating in part to the effects of travel times falling on health personnel or on the user. In a proper assessment of such alternatives the differences in utilization and effectiveness of the service would also be taken into account, through techniques such as cost-effectiveness analysis (see Chapter 10). Here, however, the effectiveness and utilization are considered to be similar, in order to focus on the differences arising from the costs. Option A, the central provision alternative, faces lower health service costs than B, which involves staff travel time and transport. Option B involves lower costs to the users than A, as the closer location of clinics results in less travel time and travel costs.

If the assessment considered only costs to the health service (as for example in a private clinic), A would be chosen as the cheaper option. To society as a whole, however, option A is overall the more costly. Public sector appraisal seeking to minimize total social costs should therefore choose option B.

Box 9.1   Example of the effects of social costs

A new town is being planned. Health planners are considering alternative ways of providing antenatal care. Two options are available:

A centralized provision
B provision through outreach facilities at the periphery

The quality of care and expected utilization rates are assumed to be the same for both options.

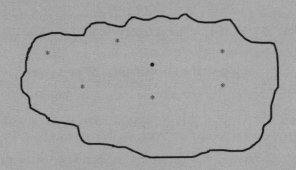

° central clinic (option A)
* peripheral clinics (option B)

Annual costs (£)

Options	Costs to health service	Costs to users	Total costs
A	60 000	40 000	100 000
B	70 000	10 000	800 000

Planners reading this, however, will recognize that such a comprehensive approach is rarely formally considered in cost exercises. This is for a variety of reasons.

- Firstly, there is a lack of awareness on the part of some planners of the importance of such wider cost assessments.

- Secondly, there is considerable difficulty in obtaining information on costs falling outside the health sector. Such data are rarely routinely available, and are often difficult to estimate.

- Lastly, and perhaps most important, an 'optimal solution' arising from a broadly costed appraisal may only be optimal if appropriate resource-transfer mechanisms exist. In the example above, option B is seemingly preferable; and yet in a situation of scarce resources this option, which requires greater spending by the health service, may be difficult for a hard-pressed manager to afford. It is only feasible if means can be found to transfer resources (which would have been used by the community for travel under option A) to the health service through some financing mechanism. If, for example, the community contributed an amount of £10 000, through a tax or fees, the health service would have the total necessary resources to provide option B, and yet overall the community would still be better off by £20 000.

The difficulty of achieving this means that costing in the public sector still tends in practice to concentrate on the costs to the institutions. Although understandable, this may result in decisions that are socially suboptimal. Planners undertaking option appraisals should therefore, at the least, make crude estimates of the likely implications of each alternative and, in particular, of any major differences between options.

The above example focused on costs falling on individuals or the community. A similar and perhaps more easily accepted principle exists for incorporating the effect of different options on other services, both within the health sector and outside. An option appraisal looking at alternatives for primary care services, for example, should incorporate any costs that may fall, as a result of the project, on referral services such as hospitals or laboratories, even if these are not directly covered by the primary care services budget. Furthermore, implications for other services not directly within the health sector (such as community development workers) should be included. Many problems in planning arise through the failure to recognize and incorporate such knock-on costs. Again, however, institutions may only be prepared to examine these wider consequences if compensatory transfer mechanisms exist.

To summarize, a public service such as a national health service which has the welfare of society as its aim should, as far as possible, in carrying out an appraisal of alternatives, consider all costs. A private health service, concerned to maximize profits is, in contrast, likely only to consider costs falling on itself, rather than on society. In practice the broad social approach is fraught with problems; but, as a minimum, planners should attempt to identify, and where possible make estimates of, the costs to agencies and individuals other than those directly involved in the project.

REAL OR MARKET PRICES?

A second broad distinction between the real and the market prices of costs needs to be made. Costs, as we have seen, are means of identifying the real resource implications of particular activities. The fact that for convenience we express them in the single common denominator of money should not obscure their basis in real resources. Some resources (air, for example) are not marketable, however valuable; and others, although bought and sold, may be exchanged at market prices which do not reflect the 'real' cost to society. Where the market price (that price at which a resource is actually bought or sold) fails to reflect the real resource implications to society, adjustments are needed during the appraisal stage for real incurred cost.

An example from outside the health sector may help to clarify this. Suppose a government subsidizes the price of fertilizer to bring it down from £1.00 to £0.75 per unit, in order to promote its use. The resultant market price (£0.75) under-estimates by £0.25 the overall real cost to society that the purchase of the fertilizer implies. Decisions in the public sector on agricultural projects which included such fertilizer should then cost the fertilizer at its real social cost (£1.00), rather than at the lower subsidized market price.

Large-scale development projects within the public sector frequently make such adjustments to market prices (known as shadow or accounting prices; see Curry (1987) for further discussion of shadow prices) when carrying out appraisals. Within the health sector, shadow pricing has been less widely employed, although it may be used in the case of large projects assessed by central planning ministries. The detailed application of shadow prices is complex and beyond the scope of this book; but some idea of the process may be helpful. The following shows its application in one area where market distortions have, in the past, frequently obscured the real social costs — that of the foreign exchange rate.

In some (though increasingly few) countries, the rate of exchange between domestic and foreign currency is fixed by the government at a rate higher than that at which it would settle if the market operated freely. Fixing the exchange rate in this way is done for macro-economic reasons. A higher exchange rate raises the price of exports and lowers the price of imports. However, through the supply-and-demand mechanism, this 'false' rate of exchange has the effect of encouraging a greater purchase of imports than the economy (and its overall availability of foreign exchange) can support. This is illustrated in Fig. 9.1.

As a result, strict controls, usually administered by the central bank, are imposed on the purchase of foreign currency (one side-effect of this is the frequent occurrence of an illegal market in foreign currency at rates above the official rate — and closer to the 'free market' rate). For the public sector, projects which involve the importation of goods, if costed at market prices, would underestimate the real effect of such imports on the economy. As a result, during the appraisal stage, such goods may be given a 'shadow price' to reflect this market distortion. Box 9.2 gives an example of how this operates.

Shadow pricing is only used during the appraisal stage. Once a project has been assessed and approved, the actual budget required to implement it is costed at the market price, and is that amount required to purchase the goods.

The above has set out the two major differences between costing for an appraisal and costing for budgeting. This is summarized in Table 9.1. In the example given in Box 9.2, option A is chosen on the basis of social costs, costed using shadow prices at £120 000; the budget required for the health service is £100 000, costed at market prices.

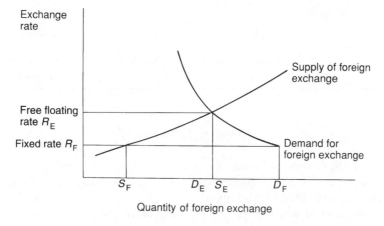

Fig. 9.1   Effect of Foreign exchange controls.
At equilibrium, free-floating position, where one unit of local currency = £1.00, demand and supply for foreign currency are equal at *DE*, *SE*. At the fixed rate of one unit = £1.50 (*RF*), the demand (*DF*) for foreign currency is greater than the supply (*SF*) available

---

Box 9. 2   Shadow pricing example

Two options are being considered, both with identical health outputs, the costs of which are shown in the table below. If market prices (i.e. the prices paid in local currency) are used during the appraisal, it suggests that option B should be chosen becasue of lower costs. However, applying shadow prices to imported items changes the relative real costs, and option A seems more attractive.

Note that the final budget required for the health service for option A is calculated in market prices as £100 000 (£10 000 + £90 000), and excludes community costs.

	Costs (£000) Market prices		Shadow prices[a]	
	A	B	A	B
Health service costs				
Imported goods (e.g. drugs)	10	40	15	60
Non-imported goods (e.g. labour[b])	90	50	90	50
Community costs				
Travel, time lost	15	15	15	15
Total (£000)	115	105	120	125

[a] A conversion factor of 1.5 is used, i.e. the local currency ios overvalued by 50%.
[b] Not shadow-priced in this example, although in practice it may be, to account for labour market distortions. The shadow wage rate is different from the shadow price used to correct for foreign currency distortions.

Table 9.1   Costing for what?

	Costs	Activity
Whose costs?	All agency and individual costs	Agency costs alone
How priced?	At real, nor market prices	At market price

COSTING METHODS

A number of short cuts are used in actually carrying out costing. However, the following sets out the basic approach to what may be called bottom-up costing. This requires the identification of all the resources required in the implementation of the activity; and of whether the costs are capital or recurrent (see below). These resources are then translated as far as is possible into money terms, using shadow prices for an appraisal costing where necessary. The steps are outlined in Fig 9.2, and are considered in more detail below.

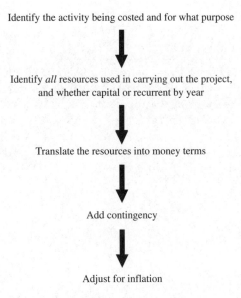

Identify the activity being costed and for what purpose

Identify *all* resources used in carrying out the project, and whether capital or recurrent by year

Translate the resources into money terms

Add contingency

Adjust for inflation

Fig. 9.2   Costing steps

Identify the activity

This first stage may sound so self-evident as to be unnecessary. However, it is surprising how many costings go astray through a failure adequately to specify the object of the costing. Take for example the 'costing of a health centre'. A variety of different interpretations of such a broad specification could be understood, including the following:

- some or all of the activities at the health centre

- other activities, not based at the health centre, but provided from it, such as outreach activities

- support activities not based at the health centre (for example, supervision, training, drug-supply systems, laboratory tests, administration)

- activities carried out from the health centre on behalf of other services, for example, supportive visits to health posts

- the cost to hospitals of referrals from the health centre.

Which of these is chosen will depend largely on the purpose of the costing.

Identify the resources

The second stage involves identifying the resources required to carry out the activity. For an immunization outreach programme, for example, this might include staff time, transport costs, subsistence or *per diem* payments, vaccines and syringes, cold chain equipment, preparatory publicity, immunization records, and staff training. In addition to these health service costs, there are likely to be costs related to the community. These broader social costs may, as we have seen, be harder to identify, but are likely to include:

- transport costs

- lost wages or production.

There may also be costs for other agencies which are similar in nature to those of the health service.

The identification of these resources is often helped by the use of a checklist. Table 9.2 provides one for health service items, which readers may wish to modify for their own purposes and use. For each item it is helpful to separate costs into *capital* (or development) costs and *recurrent* (or operating) costs. Capital costs are one-off costs, while recurrent costs continue to occur as part of the operation of the activity. Thus the construction costs of a building are regarded as capital, whereas the lighting in the building is recurrent.

On closer examination it is obvious that even 'capital' items such as buildings require replacement eventually, and the frequency of replacement is often important in the distinction, replacement at intervals of less than a year being regarded as recurrent. A further distinction may also be made as to the value of the item. Some small items of equipment (for example, stethoscopes) may well last for several years, yet be purchased from a recurrent equipment budget, partly because of the value of the item and partly because in any one year some, although not all, are being replaced.

In the end, there are no universal hard and fast rules as to categorization between

Table 9.2 Checklist for costing items

	Item	Capital	Recurrent
1	Buildings	Construction costs Land purchase[a]	Maintenance, small buildings, rent, rates, depreciation
2	Equipment and furnishings	Purchase of large new items	Maintenance, replacement, hire, depreciation, small equipment items
3	Transport and travel	New vehicles	Maintenance, replacement, fuel, hire[b]
4	Communications	Radio, telephone including installation	Maintenance, operating costs
5	Energy panels, connection to electric grid	Generator, solar fuels, electricity	Oil and other
6	Water, sanitation, waste disposal	Installation, building costs	Maintenance
7	Food equipment (see 2)	Kitchen	Food costs for staff/patients
8	Housekeeping	Equipment and buildings (see 1, 2)	Housekeeping supplies
9	Medical and laboratory supplies and equipment (1, 2)	Theatre, diagnostic, treatment, buildings	Reagents and drugs for out-patients, in-patients, clinics[c]
10	General administration	Computers, typewriter, desks (see 2)	Stationery, record system software and maintenance
11	Personnel	Initial training	Salaries and on-costs (pensions, statutory payments), refresher training
12	Consultancy services	For project preparation	For specialist services

This is an example of a checklist for use in a general health service situation. Specific situations or countries require adaptations.
[a] Square metre costs may be used to provide initial estimates of building costs.
[b] Unit costs for travel costs per kilometre can be easily calculated, and are a useful aid in estimation.
[c] Costs which are directly related to the number of patients can be estimated from a unit cost for one patient.

recurrent and capital budgets; different accounting and budgeting systems will have their own rules, which need to be followed. In order however to allow incorporation of capital costs into total annual costs, *depreciation* techniques are sometimes used. There are various approaches to depreciation which converts one-off capital costs into annual equivalents. Some take account of the real costs of capital in terms of interest rates; others are simpler and spread the capital cost over the expected number of years of life.

For each resource, whether capital or recurrent, the level required to carry out the activity is needed. This might include, for example, 6 hours' time from a registered nurse, 1000 BCG vaccines, and 400 km of four-wheel-drive travel. Even if accurate specifications are difficult, quantification is necessary, together with notes for future reference on how estimates were made (see below on accuracy). In some instances where a similar activity is already occurring this information can be established through existing records, observation, or discussion with staff — adjusting where necessary for any likely differences in level or type of resource.

Where an activity is completely new, the resources will need to be estimated from a description of the activity in the operational policy which describes the detailed functioning of the service. Clearly, if the activity is being costed in order that a decision as to its viability can be made, then detailed operational policies are unlikely to be available, and cruder estimates are necessary.

Translate into money terms

The third step involves expressing the resources identified in money terms. Whether shadow prices or market prices are used will depend both on the reason for the costing and, in particular, as we have seen, on whether the costing is for appraisal or budgeting. The sources of information for this stage will vary. Where good budget and accounting systems already exist this should provide much of the information. For example, information on the cost of personnel will be available from the wages office. The cost of drugs can be obtained from the chief pharmacist or the medical stores. In some cases commercial firms will need to be approached for estimates of specialist equipment costs. Building costs may be provided by the government building department or ministry, or by a private architect. At an appraisal stage this is likely to be done on the basis of average costs per square metre of building space. When budgets are being set there should be more precise information available from architects and quantity surveyors, based on prepared and costed drawings.

Add contingencies

Contingencies should be used to cover for the unexpected, rather than to cover for lazy costing. While it is worth including a contingency figure in the costing for budgets, it is important not to let this grow out of hand by adding contingencies at every stage. Contingencies may vary between 5% and 10% of the total sum, depending on the accuracy and certainty of the costing.

Inflation

Up to this stage costs have been expressed at present-day or current prices. Where an activity is to continue over a number of years, a figure to cover any possible price increases may be necessary. In budgeting, this is essential. In appraisals, whether incorporation of inflation is necessary will depend on any differential time-flow between projects and differential levels of inflation for different inputs within the projects. This situation is illustrated in Box 9.3.

Predictions of the likely future inflation rate usually can be obtained from central government offices, such as the finance ministry. However, their estimates are likely to

Box 9.3   Example of effects of differential inflation

Two projects are being costed — first using an average inflation rate of 10%, and then using item-specific inflation rates (drugs 8%, staff 11%, others 16%). For project A, the total costs are the same whichever approach is used, but the effects on individual items (important for budgeting) are different. For project B, because of its different cost profile, the resultant total is different.

Costs in £000

	A				B			
	Drugs	Staff	Other	Total	Drugs	Staff	Other	Total
Actual inflation	8%	11%	16%		8%	11%	16%	
Base costs	500	400	100	1000	300	600	100	1000
With inflation at 10% average	550	440	110	1100	330	660	110	1110
With differential inflation	540	444	116	1100	324	666	116	1106

be of general price inflation. Item-specific inflation (for example drugs versus salaries) will vary, and such detailed information may need to be estimated.

LEVELS OF ACCURACY AND SOURCES OF INFORMATION

The preceding paragraphs have set out the key steps involved in carrying out a costing. One issue raised was that of the accuracy required. In many situations the type of information needed either may not be easily available, or is only available in an accurate form at considerable cost. The trade-off between information accuracy and the cost of attaining such accuracy entails decisions in all areas of planning, and has already been discussed more generally in Chapter 6. It is easy to become trapped into chasing a detailed piece of information when the decision for which it was sought would not have been affected by it. Within the area of costing for appraisal decisions, it is often possible to dispose of certain options very quickly on the grounds of crude estimates of likely cost. This is made easier by the labour-intensive nature of much health-care, and the fact that personnel costs are usually relatively easy to estimate.

The planner should not shy away from the legitimate use of 'guesstimates' (informed guesses) at early stages of appraisals. During the actual appraisal of shortlisted alternatives greater accuracy is needed; but the area of costing where most accuracy is required is after the appraisal, when a budget needs to be set.

Related to the above are problems surrounding the sources of cost information.

Expenditure records kept within accounting systems may be the most obvious starting point, though these are often neither comprehensive nor well kept, in which case other sources need to be sought. Sometimes these are readily available. For example, as we have seen, cost information relating to labour costs can be readily obtained from personnel departments, or to medical supplies from the central stores or pharmacy. On other occasions, however (for example costs for new imported equipment), a large amount of effort may be needed to obtain such information. It is good practice to note down the sources of such information, and the level of confidence placed in these estimates.

UNIT COSTS

In order to avoid continually 'reinventing the wheel' it is useful to develop a series of unit costs. Such unit costs might reflect the cost of an outpatient attendance, a vaccination, 100 ambulance-kilometres, an in-patient day, or a nurse training. Box 9.4 shows how an average kilometre cost can be calculated. Although such unit costs are often invaluable as building-blocks at an early stage of appraisal, care needs to be taken in their use, as the exact unit cost of an activity will depend on the type and level of activity. For example, an out-patient attendance at a hospital with a doctor and laboratory facilities is not directly comparable with out-patient attendance at a health-post provided by a dispenser alone. Economies (and diseconomies) of scale also affect unit costs. A busy health centre may have lower unit costs than a quiet centre with the same facilities. This is further discussed below.

Box 9.4   Calculation of average kilometre cost

Suppose a four-wheel-drive vehicle.travels on average 20 000 km a year, with the costs as below.

Petrol is calculated on the basis of £0.8 per litre, and with a fuel consumption of 5 km per litre. Deprciation is.based on an initial cost of £15 000 for the vehicle, which is expected to last 3 years (interest charges not included) Annual maintenance is estimated as £1000.

Annual maintenance	:	£1000
Total amount petrol	:	£3200
Annual depreciation	:	£5000
Total annual costs	:	£9200

The average cost per kilometre under these assumptions would therefore be £0.46 [9200/20 000].

RECURRENT COST COEFFICIENTS

Attempts have been made to use a technique known as *cost coefficients* to assist in the estimation of recurrent costs. This approach estimates costs on the basis of a capital-to-recurrent cost ratio derived from experience of similar projects.

The technique is based on an assumption of a relatively fixed relationship between the capital costs of an activity and its resultant operating costs. Thus, if a hospital cost £5 million to build and costs £1 million to operate each year, the cost coefficient would be 0.20. On the basis of experience of existing activities, recurrent cost coefficients can be calculated to cover different categories of activities, for example district hospitals or health centres; recurrent costs of new activities can then be estimated on the basis of an examination of the appropriate capital costs.

Although potentially a more 'scientific' approach than 'guesstimating' and possibly useful at a early stage of option appraisal, the cost coefficient method is insufficiently accurate to be generally relied upon. It has a number of major drawbacks.

- Firstly, for small countries there may be an insufficient number of examples of the particular facility to obtain an accurate sample upon which to calculate the co-efficient. The temptation in such circumstances may be to aggregate 'similar' facilities to increase the sample — for example, to use an average figure for all hospitals; however, the different varieties of hospital are unlikely to have similar ratios.

- Secondly, recurrent cost coefficients may be 'imported' from other countries with different health or health service characteristics, leading to the use of inappropriate ratios.

- A third practical problem is that at the early stages of appraisal it may actually be easier to calculate recurrent costs than capital costs.

- The last difficulty, however, is perhaps the most serious one. It is that the approach has a built-in conservatism, in the shape of an assumption that the relationship between capital costs and recurrent costs will and should continue. Attempts to change the technology mix may, therefore, be hindered by such approaches.

COSTS RELATIONSHIPS

An understanding of various economic concepts in cost is important. Without these it is difficult, for example, to analyse whether a facility or a proposed activity is running, or is likely to operate, as efficiently as possible. The following sets out the basic relationships between different costs.

The total costs of any activity can be divided into its *fixed costs* and its *variable costs*. The fixed costs are those that remain constant within a range of activity, while the variable costs will alter with the activity level. In a training programme, for example, the costs of teaching staff and of office and classroom accommodation may not vary within a certain range, in contrast with the costs of books and of student accommodation. As more students join a programme, the *total* costs will increase, but the cost per student trained (the *average* or *unit* cost) will decrease, implying that the programme is becoming more efficient. After a certain point, however, additional teaching staff and classroom space will be needed, and the fixed costs will change, leading to a reduction in the level of efficiency. It is a task of planners and managers to identify such costs, and thereby to estimate the most efficient level of activity. Box 9.5 sets out the basic relationships between costs.

Box 9.5   Cost relationships

Total costs	=	**Fixed costs** (costs which remain constant in the short run)	+	**Variable costs** (cost which vary in the short run, depending on the activity level)
Average costs (average cost of carrying out one task)	=	Total cost/quantity of tasks	=	TC_n/Q_n
Marginal cost (cost of carrying out one *additional* unit)	=	$(TC_{n+1} - TC_n)/(Q_{n+1} - Q_n)$		

This box introduces a further concept — that of *marginal costs*. This is the cost at a particular level of activity of one further unit of activity. Thus if the level of student numbers was currently 20, the marginal cost would be the cost implications of adding a 21st student to the class. Marginal costs are essential tools in planning, as decisions are frequently made as to whether to increase levels of programme activity or not. In such instances, the average cost figures are misleading, as they contain the fixed cost element. Marginal costs, on the other hand, take account of the fact that fixed costs are already funded. Box 9.6 sets out examples of the relationship between average and marginal costs which illustrate their importance. A further example is given at the end of the chapter for practice.

In the example in Box 9.6, salaries are fixed costs, but petrol and vaccines are variable. In making the decision as to whether to expand or not, the marginal cost figure of £0.53 should be used. This represents the real cost of each additional vaccination. A decision is then needed as to whether the benefits of the extra vaccinations outweigh the cost of £0.53 (or, by implication, whether there is a better use of the money).

The example given in Box 9.7 demonstrates the relationship between fixed, variable, total, average, and marginal costs. Knowledge of the shape of such curves and the consequent implications can be extremely important. An example of this can be seen

Box 9.6   Marginal and average cost example

At present a mobile immunization team visits 20 schools a month to give 2000 immunizations. It is intended to increase this by going to 5 more schools. It is estimated that this will result in 500 more immunizations. The cost implications are in additional petrol and vaccines. What are the cost implications?

Cost per month	Present	Proposed
Salaries	£400	£400
Vaccines at £0.05 per vaccine	£100 (2000)	£125 (2500)
Petrol at £0.80 per km	£240 (300 km)	£480 (600 km)
Total	£740	£1005
Average cost per vaccination	£0.37	£0.40

The marginal cost per additional vaccination is £0.53. This is calculated by dividing the extra costs associated with increasing the programme (£265) by the extra vaccinations given (500).

in the issue of how long patients should be kept in hospital, illustrated in Box 9.8. For a further discussion of this, see Green (1990).

APPORTIONMENT OF JOINT COSTS

In many situations costs may be shared by more than one activity, in which case the question of how to apportion such costs arises. For example, a mobile immunization team may use rural clinics as bases for vacinations, and the costs of maintaining the building need to be allocated to both programmes.

One of the areas in which this is often important is in developing cost structures for hospitals. The breakdown of overall hospital costs into different activities is often complex yet necessary. It may for example be useful to know the cost per out-patient, or per in-patient-day. Costs of treating particular health problems or carrying out procedures such as X-rays or operations may also be needed for planning changes in services. Hospital budgets, however, rarely express allocations in these terms, with broader categories such as staff, or medical supplies, and disaggregation of these is necessary to obtain the costs of specific activities. Step-down costing techniques are often used in such situations, whereby costs are allocated initially to cost centres such as pharmacy or theatres, and then reallocated down to activities. A good example of this can be found in Mills (1990a).

Box 9.7 Relationship of costs in a 5–bedded hospital ward as a function of patient numbers

Costs per day

Number of patients	Fixed costs[a]	Variable costs[b]	Total costs[c]	Average costs[d]	Marginal costs[e]
1	20	10	30	30	30
2	20	15	35	17.5	5
3	20	20	40	13.3	5
4	20	35	55	13.8	15
5	20	55	75	15.0	20
6	30	78	108	18.0	33

[a] Includes maintenace, lighting, administrative time.
[b] Includes drugs, food, nurses' time.
[c] Fixed and variable costs added.
[d] Cost per patient-day.
[e] Cost of one more patient.

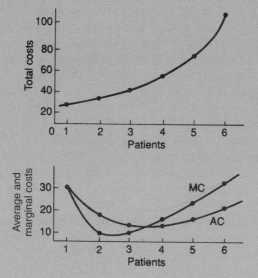

These figures illustrate the relationships graphically. The typical U-shaped arc of average costs shows both economies and diseconomies of scale. *Economies of scale* is a term used to explain the fact that, under certain circumstances, it is more efficient to operate at a higher level; *diseconomies of scale* implies the opposite.

Box 9.8   Cost implications of early discharge policy

A hospital manager is considering a policy to reduce the length of stay of hospital patients. The typical profile of a patient's stay is shown in the figure. Reduction in length of stay for patient A from, say, 8 days to 5 would save the hospital the shaded area (although of course it may raise the real cost to the patient, family or community of providing nursing care at home). Some of these costs to the hospital would be realizable immediately (for example, food costs); others would depend on the flexibility with which resources such as personnel could be redeployed or reduced. However, in the likely situation where there exists unmet demand for health-care, early discharge of patients is likely — other things being equal — to result in the immediate admission of a further patient. The patient (B) admitted would incur higher costs to the hospital than the saving made from the patient discharged early.

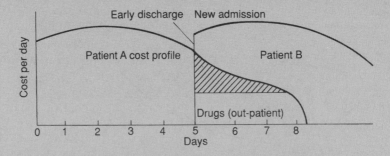

Cost profile of an in-patient, demonstrating the effect of a reduction in length of stay

Overall, the result would be that the *cost per patient* would reduce (a sign of efficiency), but the *overall cost* to the hospital associated with the additional patients would increase. The alternative of holding beds empty is inefficient; the other alternative of closing beds or wards may be difficult to implement and, in terms of the relationship between fixed and variable costs at a small ward size, may also be inefficient.

CASH-FLOW ANALYSIS

Cash-flow analysis shows the actual cash requirements at different stages in the implementation of a project, and is essential for budgeting purposes. Projects are often phased in, and may not immediately require *full* annual costs, because of the time taken to employ staff and to get the project geared up.

SUMMARY

Although this chapter has only scratched the surface of issues in the area of costing, it has introduced the rationale for the process. Costs represent resources given up. As such, they may not always be reflected by market prices — particularly when an appraisal or evaluation is being conducted. The chapter also suggested the need to consider, within the public sector, the effects of changes in health service activities on the community and other agencies. Various cost concepts, including marginal and average costs, have been introduced, and techniques and sources of information for costing have been outlined. We turn now, in the next chapter, to that stage of planning, option appraisal, which requires the integration of information cost with other information.

INTRODUCTORY READING

There are a number of general economics textbooks which provide an introduction to cost concepts. Culyer (1985) is one such, which includes a number of health-related examples. Creese and Parker (1994) and Hanson and Gilson (1996) provide excellent self-learning manuals for costing techniques. There are various articles which give examples of the application of costing. The Fiedler and Day article (1997) looks at costs in family planning; Pepperall *et al.* (1995) look at outpatient costs and quality of care; the Kasongo Project team (1984) gives a fairly simple approach to costing a primary health-care project. This should be contrasted with the more rigorous discussion in the Chabot and Waddington (1987) article. The book by Barnum and Kutzin (1993) and the articles by Mills (1990a, b, 1993) provide specific information on the costs of hospitals. The Berman (1986) article is a good example of the use of cost analysis in management.

EXERCISE 9: MARGINAL AND AVERAGE COST EXAMPLE

A hospital is considering the effect of increasing its throughput by increasing the occupancy-rate in a 10–bed surgical ward from 90% to 100%. At the current occupancy-level, 10 nurses are required. This will increase to 12 at the higher occupancy-level. Complete the table below, and consider the cost implications.

1. What is the average cost per patient at present and under the proposals?
2. What would the cost for each extra patient (the marginal cost) be?
3. Which should be used in determining whether to increase the throughput?

	Present	Proposed
Average length of stay	5 days	5 days
Occupancy rate	90%	100%
Turnover interval	–	–
Throughput	657	730
Costs (£)		
Lighting	10 000	
Staffing costs:		
Nurses at £8000 each		
Drugs at £50 per patient		
Surgical costs at £100 per patient		
Total costs		

REFERENCES AND FURTHER READING

Abel-Smith, B. and Creese, A. (1989). *recurrent costs in the health sector — problems and policy options in the three countries.* WHO, Geneva.

Barnum, H. and Kutzin, J. (1993). *Public hospitals in developing countries resource use cost and financing.* Johns Hopkins University Press, Baltimore, MD.

Berman, P. A. (1986). Cost analysis as a management tool for improving the efficiency of primary care: some examples from Java. *International Journal of Health Planning and Management*, 1, 275–88.

Bogg, L., Dong, H., Wang, K. *et al.* (1996). The cost of coverage: rural health insurance in China. *Health Policy and Planning*, 11(3), 238–252.

Chabot, J. and Waddington, C. (1987). Primary health care is not cheap: a case study from Guinea Bissau. *International Journal of Health Services*, 17, 387–409.

Creese, A. L. and Parker, D. (1994). *Cost analysis in Primary Health Care: a training manual for programme managers.* WHO, Geneva.

Culyer A. J. (1985). *Economics.* Blackwell, Oxford.

Curry, S. (1987). Introduction to shadow (or accounting) prices. *Project Appraisal*, 2(1), 64–6.

Fiedler, J. L. and Day, L. M. (1997). A cost analysis of family planning in Bangladesh. *International Journal of Health Planning and Management*, 12(4), 251–77.

Green, A. (1990). Health economics: are we being realistic about its value? *Health Policy and Planning*, 5, 274–9.

Hanson, K. and Gilson, L. (1996). *Cost, resource use and financing methodology for district health Services: a practical manual*, 2nd edn. Bamako Initiative technical report No. 34, UNICEF, New York.

Kasongo Project Team (1984). Primary Health Care for less than a dollar. *World Health Forum*, 5, 211–15.

Mills, A. (1990a). The economics of hospitals in developing countries: Part 1: expenditure patterns. *Health Policy and Planning*, 5, 107–17.

Mills, A. (1990b). The economics of hospitals in developing countries: Part 2: costs and sources of income. *Health Policy and Planning*, 5, 203–18.

Mills, A. *et al.* (1993). The cost of the district hospital: a. case study in Malawi. *Bulletin of The World Health Organization*, **71**, 329–39.

Pepperall, J, Garner, P., Rushby, J. *et al.* (1995). Hospital or health centre? A comparison of the costs and quality of urban outpatient services in Maseru, Lesotho. *International Journal of Health Planning and Management*, **10**(1), 59–71.

Philips, M. (1987). Why do costing?. *Health Policy and Planning*, **2**, 255–7.

Robertson, R. L. *et al.* (1984). Service volume and other factors affecting the cost of immunisation in The Gambia. *Bulletin of the World Health Organisation*, **62**, 729–36.

Waddington, C. and Thomas, M. (1988). Recurrent costs in the health sector of developing countries. *International Journal of Health Planning and Management*, **3**, 151–66.

WHO (1979). *Expanded programme on immunisation: costing guidelines*. WHO, Geneva.

Option appraisal and evaluation

This chapter deals with two closely related processes, option appraisal and evaluation. Option appraisal is the process of deciding between alternative approaches to reach an objective. It is carried out prior to the implementation of an activity. Evaluation refers to the process of assessing an activity while it is being carried out or on its completion. Many of the questions asked and the approaches followed are similar in each, and as such they are brought together in this chapter. The first part of the chapter deals with appraisal, and this is followed by a discussion of evaluation.

Chapter 8 discussed, in general terms, the role and difficulties of priority-setting within the health sector. Having set broad objectives, the next stage in the planning process involves deciding how these objectives are to be met. This is done through assessing the range of available alternatives, and is known as option appraisal. The options need not be confined to direct health service interventions, but given the current interest in health sector reform, such alternative options may be very wide — involving for example the contracting of services from other providers, or an increase in regulatory actions.

Economic appraisal techniques are regarded by many planners as one of the particular contributions that economics can make at the option appraisal stage. The increased squeeze on resources felt in recent years has provided the impetus for such economic techniques to be more widely promoted in health services, both as a result of increasing interest in looking at priorities in a more systematic fashion, and as a means of improving efficiency within existing programmes. The parameters behind an economic appraisal framework are those of scarcity of resources (the cost side) and competing needs (the benefit side). These are entirely consistent with the basis of planning. However, economic appraisal deals with only some of the aspects of decision-making. While providing a framework for setting out some of the factors important in making decisions, it can neglect other important variables. Many appraisals continue to remain narrowly economic, and fail to allow for other perspectives. Alternatively, they may present their results in such a way that decision-makers find it difficult to incorporate other perspectives.

Given the predominance generally accorded to economic aspects of appraisal, this chapter begins by describing economic appraisal techniques and analysing some of the issues raised by the uncritical use of such approaches. It then argues for the incorporation of other perspectives into an appraisal.

Although there has been a welcome shift away from the early days of health planning, when 'projects' were seen as the major means of implementing change, towards a recognition of the importance of looking at wider programme activities, the terminology and indeed attitudes associated with the narrower project-based approach often remain. Thus option appraisal may be encountered described in the literature as 'project appraisal'. Here we are using the term option appraisal to refer to the assessment of any set of activities, and not just of discrete projects. Fortunately, the appraisal techniques are similar.

ECONOMIC APPRAISAL TECHNIQUES

The basic principle of an economic appraisal is that it sets out a framework for comparing the resources (costs) used in a particular intervention with the expected outcome (benefits) resulting from it. It takes a view that generally those projects or programmes with the highest ratio between outcome (or benefits) and costs are the most appropriate to carry out. Essentially the process is analogous to any decision-making approach which compares the disadvantages (costs) and advantages (benefits) of alternatives.

There are three major techniques available, cost-benefit analysis (CBA), cost-effectiveness analysis (CEA), and cost-utility analysis (CUA). All three techniques compare the cost of an activity with its benefits. The difference between them is that in a CBA, benefits are valued in money terms, whereas in a CEA and CUA they are left as either simple (cost-effectiveness) or composite (cost-utility) outcomes. The implications of these differences will be discussed later. The techniques of appraisal for the private sector (often known as *discounted cash flow analysis* or *financial appraisal*) and the public sector are closely related, albeit with important differences.

- *Private sector appraisal* is predominantly concerned with maximizing the profits (the difference between revenue and costs) of the project. As such it is interested solely in the stream of internal financial costs and revenue (benefits) over time.

- *Public sector appraisal* follows the same principle of comparing benefits and costs over time. However, there are three major differences between a public sector and a private sector appraisal, reflecting the differences between the objectives of the public and the private sectors:

  - The benefits of public sector activities are not necessarily financial, and indeed are unlikely be so.
  - Effects falling on people or agencies outside the activity being appraised (known as *externalities*) should be considered alongside the direct effects.
  - Effects should be valued in terms of the real costs to the community, rather than purely financial costs.

These last two ideas were discussed in Chapter 9 in relation to costs.

Figure 10.1 sets out schematically the stages of an economic appraisal. In this chapter an introduction to the stages of an appraisal is given. However, for the reader interested in the detail of these methods, there are a number of articles and books concerned with economic appraisal. These are referred to at the end of the chapter. We now examine each of the stages of an appraisal in turn.

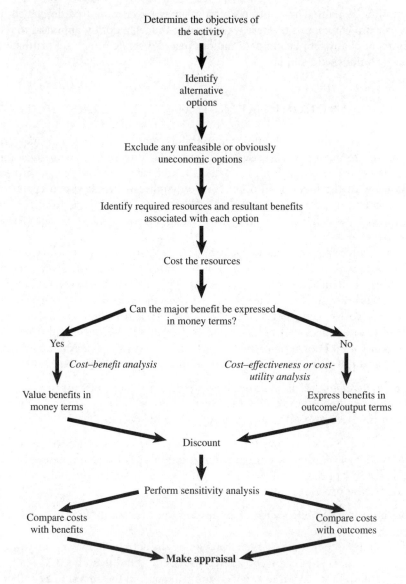

Fig. 10.1   Steps in the economic appraisal of an activity

Determine the objectives of the activity being appraised

The first stage of an appraisal involves determining the objectives of the activity being assessed. As we shall see, the choice of the decision criteria (and the indicators of these) used at the end of the process depends on the objectives of the activity. It is very important that these objectives are clearly spelt out. There may, for example, be distributional objectives, alongside more traditional health objectives. An Expanded

Programme of Immunization (EPI), for example, may aim not just to increase overall levels of immunization in a country by 20%, but also to reduce the gap between the best- and worst-covered regions of the country. These objectives should arise from the priority-setting process.

Identify alternative options

Having clearly identified the objectives that the activity would meet, the next stage requires the generation of alternative options for achieving this. Many economic appraisals are guilty of looking at one or two options in detail without first examining whether other alternatives exist to meet the specified objectives. It is helpful to try to draw up as comprehensive a list as possible initially, and then explicitly to exclude those which fail to meet defined criteria (see below). Canvassing of options from a wide variety of people (through brainstorming techniques, for example) is a useful way of generating a broad list of alternatives with which to start. It is also important to recognize that there is always the option of maintaining the status quo, i.e. of doing nothing. This is an option that can itself be appraised in its own right — essentially as an evaluation, as an alternative to any other proposals.

The most obvious means to achieve change is through options which focus on internal service interventions. Thus the government TB control programme may look towards the development of a DOTS (Directly Observed Treatment, Short Course) approach within the public sector as an option to tackling TB. However, it is also important to recognize that there may be approaches to achieving change which do not necessarily involve change in directly managed services. Thus in the TB example, options for consideration may include training of other sector workers, greater regulation of the private sector, or provision of free drugs to NGOs. Health Sector Reform (HSR) policies suggest the need to consider a much broader range of alternative options.

Exclude any unfeasible or obviously uneconomic options

It is unnecessary and a misuse of time and resources to try formally to conduct a full appraisal of every option. Criteria are therefore needed to weed out at an early stage any options which are non-starters, or are clearly less desirable than other contenders. The process of selecting options is an area which can be abused or manipulated. It is important therefore that planners are clear as to *why* they have made a decision not to consider further any particular options. Akehurst and Buxton (1985) give useful guidance as to criteria. They suggest four criteria that should apply in any situation:

- Any option which has very strong political support should be included. They argue that if this does not occur, such an option (even if very weak) must be carefully examined in order that, if rejected, the arguments for rejection are very robust.

- Any option that has a binding constraint that would make it unfeasible should be excluded.

- Any option that can be clearly improved on by another, in terms of its cost and benefits, should be excluded.

- Several options which are broadly similar should be represented by only one among them. If this particular option is seen as the best at a later stage, then those that it is 'representing' can be analysed further.

Identify the resources required to achieve each option and the benefits of each option

The next stage involves the identification of the costs and benefits associated with each of the remaining shortlisted options. At this stage it is necessary to decide how broad an approach is being adopted with regard to both the costs and the benefits.

Figure 10.2 shows diagrammatically the possible levels at which costs and benefits can be specified. An activity initiated at a departmental level may have effects at all these levels. As was argued in Chapter 9, a public sector analysis which aims to improve the welfare of society at large should ideally identify all of these effects, in order that the overall effect can be assessed. This, as we saw, contrasts with what happens in a private sector appraisal.

Ideally the effects considered should include all those changes directly attributable to the activity. In addition to the obvious direct costs and benefits (capital and recurrent costs and changes in health status) there may be various others, known as externalities. These may include hidden inputs and outputs, such as social costs to the community, training costs and benefits, environmental effects, or employment and linkage effects on the economy — for example, on the pharmaceutical industry.

In practice, appraisals within the health sector are often carried out from a narrower perspective. In part this is due to the methodological difficulties in identifying these wider effects and the scarcity of appropriate appraisal skills, and in part it is due to institutional introversion.

The choice of how broad a perspective is taken should depend on the objectives of the appraisal rather than on the availability of a methodology. Methodologies should be servants not masters. The perspective chosen can obviously affect the resultant

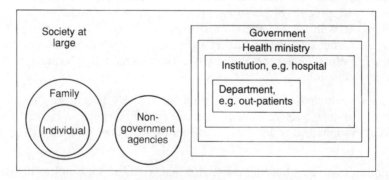

Fig. 10.2   Possible perspectives for economic appraisal

analysis, as we saw in Chapter 9 with the example of new antenatal services (see Box 9.1, p. 172).

Cost the resources required

The next step requires expressing the resources identified in money terms through costing techniques. Chapter 9 examined a number of issues in cost valuation. In particular, the two questions as to whose the costs are, and how they are valued, were discussed. It was suggested that ideally all costs should be included, whomever they affect, and whether they are financial or not. Furthermore, where market distortions are considered to mask the real costs to society, use of shadow or accounting prices is often advocated. Other costs (for example, the 'cost' of an injection includes the pain to the individual) may not, however, even have a price.

What type of analysis?

The next stage in the appraisal requires a decision as to whether a CBA or a CEA will be conducted. This decision depends largely on the type of benefits expected from the activity. Most programmes of activity (whether in the health sector or not) have multiple effects. Some of those which concern the health sector are shown in Table 10.1. Clearly some of these are linked. For example, productivity increases may occur as a result of changes in functional ability. How these different effects are valued depends in part on the weighting given to health as an investment or a consumption good, as was discussed in Chapter 8. Rarely, however, will an intervention result in only *one* of the above effects. There are three possible broad approaches in economic appraisal:

- *Full CBA.* Under CBA each of the benefits is valued in money terms in order that they can be aggregated to form a total benefit figure, which can then be compared with cost.

- *Full CEA or CUA.* Under CEA health-status outcomes are brought together to form a simple indicator of outcome, whereas under CUA composite indicators are used (see p. 197). Non-health benefits, such as productivity increases, cannot be included here.

Table 10.1 Health sector benefits

Reduction in morbidity
Reduction in pain, disability, or distress for the patient, family, or community
Reduction in functional ability
Improvement in quality of life
Reduction in mortality rates or increase in life expectancy
Increase in productivity (arising from above)
Reduction in future health or other service costs

- *Partial CBA, CEA, or CUA.* Much more common is the situation where some of the benefits are either valued or brought together as a single indicator, with other benefits being left 'outside' and not measured.

Which of these approaches is chosen will depend on the type of activity being assessed, appraisal objectives, and the availability of information. Of the three, the most powerful is the full CBA, for two reasons. By incorporating all benefits into a single measure (which neither CEA nor CUA does), it even allows activities with different forms of benefit to be compared. Furthermore, by using a monetary valuation of benefits they can be compared directly with costs. This gives answers not only to the question 'which alternative is better?', but also to the more difficult question 'is it worth doing?' In practice, CBA is rarely used in the health sector, because of the difficulties of valuation. Such analyses are particularly rare in developing countries, because of the information requirements.

CEA and CUA can rank approaches, but cannot answer the more absolute question as to whether any of them is actually worth carrying out. The reason why CBA can answer the latter question (which is based on value judgements) is because giving money values to health outcomes is itself assigning values. This is clearly the area which is most contentious, and to it we now turn.

Valuing benefits

Various methods exist to ascribe values to benefits. Behind them lies the concept of compensation. How much would society pay for the benefit, or need to be compensated for not obtaining the benefit? Perhaps the most difficult benefit to value is 'lives saved'. To put some value on this may be necessary in activities which are directly life-saving (as in the health sector), or which occur as spin-offs in projects (such as transport) where accidents may be increased or decreased. Various methods have been used by economists to impute values to life for this purpose (see Mooney 1977).

- Firstly, there is the *human capital* approach, which sees health as an investment (see Chapter 8 for further discussion of this approach). In this case the benefits of life are seen as being the losses or gains in productivity arising from the loss or saving of a life as a result of an activity.

- Secondly, the socially implied or *public behavioural* valuation approach imputes values as placed by society on life by analysing previous public decisions.

- Lastly, there is the approach which, through looking at the real or hypothetical behaviour of individuals, assesses the value they place on *reducing the risk of death*.

Discussion of the differences between and comparative advantages of each of these approaches can be found in the reading at the end of the chapter. It is important to recognize, however, that in each case a subjective judgement about the value placed on saving a life is being made by different groups. Thus economists may value life as a means to production; politicians may value life from a broader social perspective (often very inconsistently); and people may set a value on risks to their own lives as individuals rather than from a social perspective.

The preceding discussion has referred to the difficulty of placing a monetary value on the benefits of saving a life. Similar problems exist in trying to value the benefits of activities that result in improvements in the quality of life, decreases in pain, or any of the other effects set out in Table 10.1 on p. 195. Many readers will find the idea of valuing life in this way abhorrent; though it should be recognized that, given the fundamental dilemma facing a planner because of the scarcity of resources, in reality such valuations of the benefits of life-saving activities versus activities resulting in other effects are being made constantly, albeit implicitly. However, despite methodological advances, this valuative aspect of CBA is likely to present the greatest barrier to the adoption of such techniques.

In assessing or designing CBA studies it is important to be very clear as to what the basis for the valuation is, and what values lie behind it.

Measuring outcome for CEA and CUA

CEA and CUA sidestep the issue of valuing benefits by leaving them in outcome terms. No monetary value is placed on them. This is methodologically much easier, though it has the major drawback of limiting the benefits to outcomes, and not including directly other types of benefits CEA and CUA look at not just the cost of a health service output, but at the impact of that output in terms of health status.

A good example of such a study is that conducted in Botswana by an economist and an epidemiologist (Gish and Walker 1977) to compare the cost-effectiveness of different ways of providing primary care, whether through fixed clinics, or from mobile clinics operating either by road or by air. The study calculated the cost of patient contacts at the different types of facility. On this measure the most efficient appeared to be the land-based mobile clinic at a cost of £0.63 for each patient seen, compared to £0.68 for the fixed clinic. However, this output measure gives no idea of how effective such a contact is, in health terms. The study therefore examined the types of health problems which would be seen. Some of these problems would not be effectively dealt with on an occasional basis such as provided by the mobile clinic (for example, treatment requiring daily injections). The study therefore calculated the cost per likely effective patient contact (an outcome measure), excluding these 'unsuccessful' visits as positive outcomes. The result of this is to increase the cost of the 'successful' patient contacts. As mobile clinics are more limited in their availability and thus have more 'unsuccessful' contacts, their cost rise more than those of fixed clinics. The comparative cost per likely effective patient contact at the mobile clinic is £5.87 compared to £0.75 for the fixed clinic. The latter now appears more cost-effective.

In order to carry out CEA and CUA, indicators of change in health status are needed. There are two broad types of indicator:

- *simple indicators*, which measure only one aspect of health (such as years of life)

- *composite indicators*, which combine two or more aspects of health (such as years of life and quality of life).

Examples of these are given in Table 10.2. The simplest are indicators such as lives saved, children immunized/protected, or life years gained; but more recently attempts have been made to incorporate the quality of life, and to construct composite indicators such as the Physical Quality of Life Index (PQLI) or Quality Adjusted Life Years (QALYs). The most recent addition is that proposed in the World Bank *World Development Report* (1993) which combines disability and life years — the Disability Adjusted Life Year (DALY) (see Chapter 8).

Table 10.2   Examples of indicators of outcome

Simple indicators	Composite outcome indicators
Lives extended (saved)	Disability Adjusted Life Years (DALYs)
Children immunized	Quality Adjusted Life Years (QALYs)
Contraceptive acceptors	Physical Quality of Life Index (PQLI)

The difference between CEA and CUA lies in the choice of outcome indicator. CEA uses simple indicators and CUA composite indicators. Although CEA is widely used, it is limited to comparison between health interventions with identical types of outcome. Thus it is not strictly correct to compare, directly, lives extended through renal dialysis with lives extended through kidney transplant, let alone with a cure for an infectious disease. The resultant quality of life may be very different. A composite indicator such as the DALY allows more direct comparison. However, such compositing requires value judgements as to the way in which quality of life is measured, and how it is weighted against life expectancy.

All forms of economic appraisal make various assumptions about the distribution of the benefits of an intervention. Typically they treat them as neutral, irrespective of the beneficiaries; however, it is possible (and would probably reflect the prevailing values of many societies) to give greater weight to activities benefiting some groups rather than others. This has been further discussed in Chapter 8.

Because of the difficulties involved in valuing benefits discussed above, CEA and CUA are the techniques more commonly employed within the health sector. It is also common to find 'cost-effectiveness' analyses which actually measure the cost per output rather than per outcome. This is frequently an understandable response to the difficulty of finding a single outcome measure that captures the complex nature of many health activities. Thus, for example, comparison of a hospital out-patient department with a health centre may look at cost per patient seen, because of the difficulty of comparing the multitude of outcomes arising from such visits. Such analyses may be useful indicators of efficiency, but are not strictly cost-effectiveness appraisals.

Discounting

Many projects have costs and benefits that occur over time in an irregular fashion. For example, the construction and equipping of a new hospital in the early stages of the project would incur large capital costs, followed by recurrent operational costs after the hospital opens. Gradually, as the hospital increases its activities, there will be an increase in benefits, in terms of health improvements. Appraisal of alternatives needs to deal with such time-patterns. To do so, economists use the concept of *discounting*, which simply reduces the value given to both costs and benefits the further in the future they occur. It is applied in a similar way to an interest rate or an inflation rate.

There are two related concepts underlying the discount rate:

- The idea that all resources could be used in alternative ways, so that there is what is called a *social opportunity cost* of capital.

- A recognition that society itself values differently costs and benefits which occur at different positions in time. This is known as *social time-preference*. It should be noted that this does not depend at all on the presence of inflation, which is a separate issue.

Thus, for example, given the choice between two otherwise identical interventions, the first saving 100 lives this year and the second 100 lives next year, it is likely that most people would choose the former. Conversely, consider two services which both save 100 lives next year and have identical overall financial costs. However, for the first service the costs would occur this year, and for the second service, next year. It is suggested that society would normally choose the latter (which delays the costs for a year).

Such a view of time clearly involves important value judgements. Discount rates are used to reflect these. The higher the discount value, the greater the weighting towards the present. It can, of course, be argued that planners should not value the future less than the present, but instead have a responsibility as guardians of future generations. Clearly choice of a discount rate may affect the 'result' of an appraisal. In practice, the discount rate is usually provided centrally within a government. One use of discounting involves illustrating, the sensitivity of an activity to time, by the use of several discount rates,.

Once a cost or benefit has been discounted, this is known as its present value. The formula for applying a discount rate is:

Present value of $A = A/(1 + r)^i$

where r is the discount rate and i the year being discounted.

Box 10.1 gives an example of the use of discounting in a CEA.

Sensitivity analysis

A sensitivity analysis calculates the effect of changes in the value of one variable on the overall result of the appraisal; in other words, it shows the sensitivity of the appraisal to that variable. Sensitivity analysis should be undertaken wherever there is an element of doubt about variables within the appraisal. These doubts might be about discount rates, costs, outcomes, or indeed value judgements.

An example of a sensitivity analysis is given in Box 10.2. Where sensitivity analyses

Box 10.1   Discount example

Three alternative options for an immunization programme — A, B and C — are being appraised. The costs of each programme are the same. There are, however, differences in the number and time distribution of children immunized, as shown below.

Option	Children immunized (present value)				Discount rate (%)
	Year 1	Year 2	Year 3	Total	
A	40	100	170	310	0
B	100	100	105	305	0
C	140	100	60	300	0
A	40	95	153	288	5
B	100	95	95	290	5
C	140	95	54	289	5
A	40	86	124	250	10
B	100	86	77	262	10
C	140	86	44	269	10

The table shows that the choice of discount rate affects which option is deemed preferable (indicated in bold).

Box 10.2   Sensitivity analysis example

The current strategy (A) for immunization is through existing static health centres. The estimate of the level of protection provided is well known. A new approach (mobile services) is being considered and there is some uncertainty over how well the cold chain will work and hence the level of protection to be provided. Two alternative assumptions about the level of protection (B_1 and B_2) are made to determine the sensitivity of the appraisal to this.

Option	Assumption over level of protection provided by vaccination	Cost $	Children vaccinated	Children protected	Cost per child protected $
A	90%	150 000	700 000	630 000	0.24
B_1	60%	250 000	1 500 000	900 000	0.28
B_2	80%	250 000	1 500 000	1 200 000	0.21

show different values to key assumptions, then further investigation is suggested, or a political decision needs to be taken on the choice of value judgement.

Compare costs and benefits, or cost-effectiveness ratios

The penultimate stage of an appraisal is the comparison between the costs of projects and their benefits or outcomes. Various ways exist in which these can be expressed, each showing the relationship between costs and outcomes, but with subtle differences and possibly different consequences.

CBA

For CBA, the three major methods are net present value (NPV), internal rate of return (IRR) and benefit to cost ratio (BCR).

- The *NPV* for the project is calculated by summing the present values of all the costs and benefits. Projects are only worth doing on economic grounds if the NPV is greater than zero (i.e. the present value of costs is less than that of the benefits). Where there is more than one such project then the project with the highest NPV would be chosen:

$$NPV = \sum_{i=0}^{i=n} \frac{(B_i - C_i)}{(1 + r)^i}$$

where r is the discount rate, B_i is benefits in year i, C_i is costs in year i, and n is number of years.

- The *IRR* is the discount rate r for which the net present value is zero. Essentially this shows the rate of return for a project Comparison of different activities would lead to the choice of the one with the highest IRR.

- The *BCR* methods (gross and net) essentially divide the benefits by the costs, discounted where appropriate. If the resultant ratio is greater than 1 in the case of the gross BCR or than zero in the case of the net BCR (i.e. the benefits are greater than the costs), then the project is seemingly worth doing. Again, the higher the ratio the 'better' the project.

$$\text{Gross BCR} = \frac{\sum \text{benefits}}{\sum \text{costs}}$$

$$\text{Net BCR} = \frac{\sum (\text{benefits} - \text{costs})}{\sum \text{costs}}$$

Generally the three methods will lead to the same result, although occasionally they will differ. The major inconsistencies occur either as a result of the method of categorization of the benefits and costs or as a result of the size of the activity being appraised.

- *Effect of categorizing some costs as benefits.* Some projects specify averted (negative) costs, as one of the benefits. This can be misleading, with resultant inconsistencies between the BCR and the NPV (the latter being unaffected by how averted costs are treated).

- *Size of the project.* The NPV method favours projects with the greatest excess of benefits over costs. However, this depends in part on the scale of the project. The BCR is useful in comparing the benefits achieved per unit of cost, regardless of the size (see example in Box 10.3). There is no 'correct' decision criterion and the safest approach is to calculate using more than one, and then consider, where there are differences, what the reasons are.

Box 10.3　Example of effects of size

Two projects are being appraised, each providing similar primary care services. The projects are, however, of a different scale, with project A being much larger than project B. As a result the NPV of project B is smaller than that of project A because of its size, although the BCR favours B.

Project A:	Costs ($)	1000
	Benefits ($)	2000
	NPV ($)	1000
	BCR	2
Project B:	Costs ($)	200
	Benefits ($)	600
	NPV ($)	400
	BCR	3

CEA and CUA

For CEA and CUA, direct comparison of cost with outcomes is made; intervention with its lowest cost per outcome would normally be preferred under an economic appraisal.

Make appraisal

The last stage of an appraisal is the decision itself as to the relative or absolute worth of an activity. As we have seen, CEA can provide information only on the former question, whereas CBA provides it on both. CBA can only do this because it builds judgements of relative worth into the valuation of benefits (which is an integral part of the technique). The economic indicators which were outlined above are:

- *CBA*

  - highest NPV (at least greater than zero)
  - highest IRR (at least greater than the discount rate)
  - highest gross BCR (at least greater than 1)
  - highest net BCR (at least greater than 0).

- *CEA and CUA*

  - lowest cost per outcome.

OPTION APPRAISAL AND ECONOMIC APPRAISAL

Up to this point we have looked solely at economic appraisal. Such techniques may provide a useful framework for appraisal, but their narrow application can lead to a failure to consider wider issues. An appraisal needs to take account of other factors besides those covered by the two main criteria of economic appraisals — cost and outcomes. There may be other effects arising from an activity which are inconsistent with health service objectives but which would not show up under a narrow economic appraisal. Economic appraisal deals with the relationship between input (resources) and outcomes (benefits); it does not deal with the process of getting from input to output. Option appraisals need to do this. Consideration needs to be given to whether, for example, the project takes account of principles such as participation and service integration. The 'means' of the project may be as important as its 'end'. Thus a project that achieved its objectives in narrow health terms, but at the same time had negative effects on the social structure of a community, might well be rejected.

The usefulness of economic appraisal is as a means of laying out in a clear and methodical manner the issues surrounding any decision in order that the decision-maker can then apply value judgements on the basis of the best possible information. It is an aid to decision-making, rather than the means of decision-making. As we have seen in Chapter 8, it is important to recognize that an economic appraisal does not diminish the need for such value judgements.

A good option appraisal should:

- present both the quantified and non-quantified costs and benefits together as equal partners

- explicitly recognize and incorporate the need for economic and other perspectives

- recognize the resource and financial implications of a project

- explicitly examine the technical feasibility of a project

- explicitly consider the process effects of the project

- set out information on the methodology used

- perform where necessary sensitivity analyses

- set out key assumptions, and in particular make any implicit value judgements explicit.

Unfortunately such model appraisals are rare. A checklist for economic appraisal is given in Table 10.3. The technocratic nature of many appraisals tend to blur value judgements, and to concentrate on the measurable rather than the unmeasurable; a condition described by Blades *et al.* (1987, p. 471) as quantophrenia — the quantified driving out the important. It also often fails to recognize the need for other perspectives, including sociological ones, on the effects of projects.

We now look at some of these other criteria that need to be employed within an option appraisal, alongside the economic ones. Many of these are not amenable to quantification; yet it is important that they are given due weight alongside the quantified indicators of the economic aspects of the appraisal.

Table 10.3　Checklist for economic appraisals

---

1. Is the appraisal for priority-setting, appraisal of options, or evaluation?
2. Are the objectives of the intervention being appraised clearly identified?
3. Is it a CEA or CUA appraisal, or a CBA? Is this choice appropriate?
4. If a CEA or CUA, what outcome indicators are used? Are they appropriate?
5. Which options were identified? Were any important ones omitted?
6. Were all the resources identified?
7. Were the costings that were used appropriate?
8. Is a discount rate used? Is it appropriate?
9. Was a sensitivity analysis used? If not, should it have been?
10. Was the appraisal decision appropriate?
11. Were there other option appraisal criteria that should have been applied?
12. What value judgements were used? Were they explicit? Did you agree with them?
13. What were the main conclusions of the study? Given the preceding, do you agree with them?

Technical, administrative, and legal feasibility

An important necessary condition for the success of an activity is its technical feasibility. Will it actually operate as expected and intended? Activities may pass the economic appraisal criteria, but fail on technical grounds. Some of these technical grounds will relate in particular to the assumed linkages between the activity and the health status changes, i.e. to the epidemiological causality assumed. Related to this are the legal and administrative (or organizational) requirements that may constrain an activity. For example, an appraisal of a proposal to set up a new health cadre needs to consider whether the current health legislation is adequate, or whether legal changes are needed.

Knock-on effects

Projects may be assessed purely in terms of their direct activities. However, frequently projects have wider knock-on effects that should be incorporated into the approach. For example, the construction of a health centre may lead to more demands on district hospital facilities through laboratory tests or referrals.

Financial and resource availability

It is perfectly possible for a project to be deemed 'worthy' following an economic appraisal, but still lack the finance or resources to carry it out. Many good projects are not implemented owing to a shortage of a key cadre or other resource, or simply because the finances are not available.

Long-term sustainability

Activities may be cost-effective in the short term, but unsustainable in the long term. Models of causality which may hold true in the short term may break down over time. Alternatively, the managerial or financial sustainability of a programme may prove impossible to maintain over time.

Acceptability

A programme may prove to be unacceptable to a community or to health workers. The acceptability of an activity is an important consideration in an appraisal, and is most likely to be examined where the appraisal team is as wide-ranging in its representation as possible. Where changes in clinical practice are part of the activity being appraised, this acceptability may depend on ethical considerations.

Social, economic, and political effects

Projects may have a number of effects on communities which are not quantifiable. For example, they may affect the traditional social or power structure of a community. There is a serious tendency for economic appraisals to depreciate the importance of, or even to ignore, such factors, because of the difficulty of measuring them; yet their importance may be very great. There may also be wider economic effects (on employment, for example) which need consideration.

Distributional and equity effects

All appraisals should consciously assess the effects of an activity on different groups and classes within society. In particular, concern for equity suggests that the distributional effects of a project should be appraised.

Gender effects

Related to the last point, but of particular concern within an appraisal, should be the differential gender effects of a project. Given the position of many women throughout the world it is essential that an appraisal should deliberately assess the relative effects of any new activity on women and men.

Environmental and ecological effects

Project appraisals have often been formally expected to look at the effects of activities on the environment. However, this has often been done with a rather narrow focus. Given the increasing concern over wider environmental issues, it is important that appraisals consciously examine wider effects in this area.

Other development objectives

There may be wider development objectives from outside the health sector which an appraisal should take account of. For example, a government may have an explicit aim of localizing posts within the public sector. This policy would then need incorporation into the appraisal.

Expansion from a pilot activity or project

Some activities are initially tested through the use of pilot projects, to see either whether the model of causality holds true, or whether the activities planned are feasible and actually have the intended effect. However, though such piloting can be extremely useful, there is always a possibility that what is feasible, affordable, acceptable, and cost-effective at the pilot level may not hold for a wider application. This needs careful and explicit consideration in the design of the pilot project.

FORMS AND CHECKLISTS

It is useful to develop a pro forma for carrying out an appraisal which sets out the specific questions that are regarded as necessary within a particular country context. Central government ministries, and in particular the ministry responsible for development planning, may have such formats that they require ministries to use, at least as far as projects seeking either local capital or donor funds are concerned. Chapter 12 gives an example of one such format.

OPTION APPRAISAL AND PROGRAMMING

At this point, it might be helpful to recapitulate where we have reached in the planning spiral. The first stage of planning, the situational analysis (carried out at different organizational levels) set the scene for developing the plan. On the basis of this, broad national areas of priority were agreed. Depending on this, resources would be allocated to different priority areas and organizational levels. These would then consider different means of achieving their own prioritized objectives, through assessing different options. At the end of this process, there should be, for each priority area, a preferred approach to meet each objective. These would then be developed into a programme for implementation. This is discussed in Chapter 12.

APPRAISAL AND EVALUATION

At the beginning of the chapter, attention was drawn to the similarity between appraisal and evaluation. Up to this point, we have concentrated on *appraisal*, which seeks to assess whether an activity should take place or not, prior to its implementation. *Evaluation* asks similar questions, but after the activity has commenced, or in some cases after it has finished. Like appraisal, evaluation seeks answers to the basic question as to whether an activity should have been embarked upon or not. However, evaluation is not just interested in yes or no answers to this question, but also 'why' answers, and whether modifications would improve the activity.

Many of the detailed questions asked in evaluations are similar to those of an appraisal. Similar issues arise regarding the process itself, such as who should conduct appraisals and evaluations. Indeed, the same narrow focus on economic techniques of which we have been critical in appraisal can also be found in economically-focused evaluations which ignore wider issues.

The remainder of this chapter examines a number of issues in the area of evaluation, building on the basic techniques of appraisal discussed in more detail in the earlier part of the chapter.

EVALUATION

Evaluations can be carried out after the completion of a project or activity. Such evaluations are known as *summative* evaluations. Alternatively, evaluations can be conducted while an activity is still being carried out. These are called *formative* evaluations. There are various reasons for carrying out evaluations, and it is important to clarify in advance exactly what the purpose of the evaluation is. Different evaluative objectives are likely to result in different methodologies. Possible reasons for conducting an evaluation include the following.

- At the most basic level an evaluation may be conducted to decide whether the activity was worth doing. In the case of formative evaluations, this might determine whether the activity should be continued or not.

- Where an activity has finished, a summative evaluation is likely to be carried out to determine whether it accomplished the objectives it set out to achieve. It might also be carried out to decide whether it should be extended elsewhere. This might in particular apply to the evaluation of pilot projects specifically carried out as a test for wider application.

- In addition to such black-and-white questions, an evaluation may look for answers as to whether modification of the activity might make (or have made) a difference to its performance.

- More subtly, an evaluation might be conducted to answer questions as to whether related activities should be carried out — i.e. to provide a means of appraisal of an as yet untested activity.

- Lastly, it must be recognized that evaluations may have political purposes. There may be internal political reasons to carry out an evaluation to justify spending on a contentious activity. In addition, donor agencies frequently require evaluations to ensure that aid money is spent in line with donor policies, and to justify expenditure to the taxpayer.

EVALUATION QUESTIONS

Depending on its purpose, there may be a number of questions that an evaluation attempts to answer and it is important that these are made explicit in advance. The choice of such questions will affect the methodology chosen. The following sets out the key questions that most evaluations will attempt to answer. These questions essentially look at whether an activity achieved its purpose, and, if not, why not. There are, of course, a number of reasons why an activity being evaluated may fail to achieve its objectives, and it is important to distinguish between these. It is helpful to consider the relationship outlined in Chapter 6, between inputs, outputs, and outcomes. Failures to achieve the objectives can occur at any of these levels. Inputs (resources) may fail to be procured; resources may be available, but not be transformed into the services or outputs required; services may be provided, but fail, for a variety of reasons, to result in the anticipated health outcomes.

Inputs

The first set of questions relates to whether in fact the inputs planned as a means of providing the services themselves were available, and if not why not.

- *Did the inputs (i.e. resources) planned arrive?* One reason for the failure of a project or activity may be that, for a variety of reasons, resources did not arrive as planned. This may be for financial reasons (inadequate finances were planned or made available at the appropriate time). Alternatively, it may be that, despite the availability of finance, the actual resources themselves were not available. For example, there may not have been the required skilled personnel.

- *Were they sufficient to provide the services planned?* Resources as planned may have been available. However, it may be that they were inadequate to carry out the services required.

- *Were the resources transformed into services?* Resources may have been available (and sufficient), but, perhaps through lack of adequate management, were not transformed into the requisite services. Symptoms might include staff employed, but not providing services through a lack of adequate direction.

Outputs

The second set of questions is concerned with whether the services actually were provided in the form planned, and, if not, why not.

- *Were the services provided appropriate, relevant, and adequate?* Services may have been provided, but not have been appropriate, relevant or adequate for the task required. In particular, evaluations need to look at questions (similar to those of appraisal) of:

  - service quantity
  - service quality
  - efficiency of services
  - acceptability to the community and the provider
  - socio-economic effects
  - distributional effects
  - gender effects
  - technical difficulties.

Outcome effects
The last and most important group of questions relates to the outcome from the activity being evaluated.

- *What are or were the objectives of the activity being evaluated?* Perhaps the most fundamental question to determine is what the activity being evaluated was intended to achieve. It is against this benchmark that the activity's success or failure will largely be measured.

- *Were the objectives set achieved? If not, why not?* Following on from the above question is the key question as to whether the objectives set were actually achieved — i.e. whether it had the impact desired, and, if not, why not. Ideally the objectives would have been set in health-status terms, and the impact measured similarly.

- *Were any improvements observed, the direct result of the activity?* It is important that any improvements, such as in health status, detected are identified as being the direct result of the activity. An evaluation of a supplementary feeding programme which discovers an improvement in levels of nutritional status needs to ensure that they are the result of the programme, rather than, for example, the result of an increase in levels of income. This is essentially an epidemiological task, and requires a command of basic research skills.

Were there any other effects of the activity?
In addition to the planned effects of the activity, there may have been other effects which were not intended. These might have been health or other effects — such as socio-economic effects, or effects related to social structures or the position of women. It is important that such wider effects (whether positive or negative) are evaluated alongside the narrower health effects.

Design of evaluation methodology

The methodology for carrying out an evaluation can often be made out to be more complex than in practice it needs to be. The more complex a methodology becomes, however, the more closed it becomes. The design of an appropriate evaluation methodology can be seen as having four stages.

Stage 1
The first stage involves setting out clearly the questions that the evaluation needs to answer. These have been outlined, in general terms, above. To answer each of these questions, indicators are needed. Four types of information are likely to be required:

- *baseline information* to describe the situation prior to the activity

- *outcome information* to describe the situation after the activity

- *input information*, which describes the resources used in the programme

- *process information*, which describes the implementation process of the activity.

In addition to 'before and after' comparisons, it may be necessary to make comparisons between different areas, differentiating between areas where the evaluated activity has taken place and those where it has not. Where logframes (see p. 247) have been used in designing a project, these form a useful basis for evaluation.

Stage 2
The second stage involves determining measures for answering each of the questions. Sources of information for evaluation will depend on the indicators required. Some will be available in existing records (for example hospital statistics). Others may only be available through surveys (for example attitudes of communities or users of services to the provision of the service, or information obtained through social epidemiological surveys). Such information may be quantifiable or qualitative. As has been argued earlier in the book, it is essential that qualitative information is given due weight, and is not downgraded in importance by the presence of quantifiable indicators.

Stage 3
The third stage in the design of an evaluation is to determine how information relating to the indicators can be obtained. The sources of such information will vary but are essentially those discussed in Chapter 6.

Stage 4
The final stage involves deciding how, and, most importantly, by whom such information will be assessed.

Who should carry out an appraisal or evaluation?
There are two main issues that need to be considered in determining who carries out an appraisal or an evaluation; see Simmonds (1987) for a discussion of this. Firstly, what are the skills required; and secondly, is it advantageous or disadvantageous to have representation from people directly involved in the activity being assessed? There are three broad groups of possible evaluators:

- outsiders who are not directly in the service and who are considered to be impartial, but who will have less detailed knowledge of the activity (of course, as we have discussed elsewhere in the book, the concept of objectivity in such a context is spurious; however such people may bring particular skills to bear)

- service providers, who may be seen to be biased, but who have a good knowledge of an activity; and

- users of the service and community members.

The ideal is likely to involve a mix of the three groups. However, the balance will depend on the precise questions which a particular evaluation is intended to answer, as we pointed out above. To some degree the answer will also depend on attitudes to evaluation. Evaluation may (negatively) be considered as an 'examination' process, and thus be regarded defensively. It may also (more positively) be regarded as a learning process. In such cases the results of the evaluation should be fed into reformulation of the activity.

EVALUATIONS AND SITUATIONAL ANALYSIS

The concept of the planning spiral introduced in Chapter 2, suggests that the end-point of each cycle within the spiral is the evaluative function. Although formal evaluations are not required every year, and indeed at that frequency would be a costly and resource-diverting process, it should be recognized that the results of evaluations should provide an important input into the periodic revision of the situational analysis.

SUMMARY

This chapter has suggested that the techniques of appraisal of options prior to deciding on particular programmes or activities are closely related to those of evaluations of ongoing or completed activities or projects. The chapter has introduced economic techniques and suggested that they provide a useful framework for appraisal and evaluation. However, in the context of Primary Health Care, they require the addition of other perspectives which have also been discussed

INTRODUCTORY READING

Economic appraisal techniques are becoming more widely used within the health sector, and there are a number of sources of information on this. Drummond *et al.* (1987) provides a useful general introduction, though not aimed at developing countries in particular. Carrin's book (1984) is aimed at developing countries, but is less accessible. For a useful review of economic appraisal (set within the UK health service but providing a number of pertinent perspectives) see Blades *et al.* (1987). Green and Barker (1988) set out a critique of the narrow use of economic appraisal techniques and Anand and Hanson (1997) and Barker and Green (1996) provide a critique of DALYs and their use in appraisal. There are various case studies of economic appraisal techniques in use, including Aikins (1998), Ashworth and Khanun (1997), Fox-Rushby and Foord (1996) Hughes and McGuire (1996). An example of a wider approach to options can be seen in Evans *et al.* (1997).

Wider techniques tend to be dealt with in connection with evaluation rather than appraisal, and as a result there few good texts that deal comprehensively with all aspects. For example WHO (1981) provides a fairly standard look at evaluation. Feuerstein (1986) takes a more participative approach. Gosling and Edwards (1995) provide a practical guide to monitoring and evaluation. Simmonds (1987) looks at the issue of who should carry out evaluations. For a more formal approach from a donor agency see Bridger and Winpenny (1987).

EXERCISE 10

1. A district in your country has identified malnutrition as a priority health problem. Write down as many possible interventions as you can think of which might improve the nutritional situation. Be as free-thinking as you can, and do not restrict yourself only to health-care interventions or interventions by the public sector.

    Choose three very different interventions and consider:

    (a) what information you would need to appraise them

    (b) where you would obtain the information

    (c) who you would involve in the process of the appraisal.

2. A district is currently aiming to meet national immunization guideline targets of 80% coverage. Within the district there are disparities between the performance of different dispensaries where the immunizations are conducted. As a health manager you are concerned at the low level of immunization coverage (30% of children overall). You consider two alternative ways of achieving the target: to make existing dispensaries more efficient or to start mobile immunization services.

    Design an appraisal that would assess the two options.

3. A health ministry has been training community health workers for a number of years. It sees no reason to change its training programme, but the international agency that funds the training is insisting that an evaluation should be conducted before it funds the next phase. The community health workers are selected by community leaders and given training by a team that rotates between provincial centres where the training is carried out. Design an evaluation for this purpose.

REFERENCES AND FURTHER READING

Aikins, M. (1998). The Gambian National Impregnated Bednet Programme: costs, consequences and net cost-effectiveness. *Social Science and Medicine*, 46(2), 181–91.

Akehurst, R. and Buxton, M. J. (1985.). *A. guide to better decision-making: Option appraisal in the NHS*. Folio No 8, Nuffield/York Portfolio. Nuffield Provincial Hospitals Trust, London.

Anand, S. and Hanson, K. (1997). Disability-Adjusted Life Years: a critical review. *Journal of Health Economics*, 16, 685–702.

Ashworth, A. and Khanum, S. (1997). Cost-effective treatment for severely malnourished children: what is the best approach? *Health Policy and Planning*, 12(2), 115–21.

Barker, C. and Green, A. (1996). Opening the debate on DALYs. *Health Policy and Planning*, 11(2), 179–83.

Barnum, H. (1987). Evaluating healthy days of life gained from health projects. *Social Science and Medicine*, 24, 833–42.

Blades, C. A., Culyer, A. J., and Walker, A. (1987). Health service efficiency: appraising the appraisers — a critical review of economic appraisal in practice. *Social Science and Medicine*, 25, 461–72.

Bridger, G. A. and Winpenny, J. T. (1987). *Planning development projects: a practical guide to the choice and appraisal of public sector investments* (2nd edn). HMSO, London.

Carrin, G. (1984). *Economic evaluation of health care in developing countries: theory and applications*. Croom Helm, London.

Drummond, M. F. et al. (1987). *Principles of economic appraisal in health care*. Oxford University Press, Oxford.

Drummond, M. F., O'Brien, B. J, and Stoddard, G. L. (1997). *Methods for the economic evaluation of health care programmes*, 2nd edn. Oxford University Press, Oxford.

Evans, D. B, Azene, G., and Kirigia, J. (1997). Should governments subsidize the use of insecticides: the use of insecticide-impregnated mosquito nets in Africa: implications of a cost-effective analysis. *Health Policy and Planning*, 12(2), 107–14.

Feuerstein, M.-T. (1986). *Partners in evaluation: evaluating development and community programmes with participants*. Macmillan, London.

Fox-Rushby, J., and Foord, F. (1996). Costs, effects and cost-effectiveness analysis of a mobile maternal health care service in West Kiang, The Gambia. *Health Policy*, 35, 123–43.

Gilson, L. et al. (1997). Cost-effectiveness of improved treatment services for sexually transmitted diseases in preventing HIV-1 infection in Mzanza Region, Tanzania. *Lancet*, 350, 1805–9.

Gish, O. and Walker, G. (1977). *Mobile health services*. Tri-Med, London.

Gosling, L. and Edwards, M. (1995). *Toolkits: a practical guide to assessment, monitoring review and evaluation*. Save the Children, London.

Green, A. and Barker, C. (1988). Priority-setting and economic appraisal: whose priorities — the community or the economist?. *Social Science and Medicine*, 26, 919–29.

Griffiths, A. (1988). Cost-effectiveness and cost-benefit analysis of health services: the methodology and its application. *Health Policy*, 9(3), 251–65.

Hughes, D. and McGuire, A. (1996). The cost-effectiveness of family planning service provision. *Journal of Public Health Medicine*, 18(2), 189–96.

Jefferson, T. Demicheli, V. (1994). Is vaccination against hepatitis B efficient? a review of world literature. *Health Economics*, 3(1), 25–37.

Loevinsohn, B. P. *et al.* (1997). Using cost-effectiveness analysis to evaluate targeting strategies: the case of vitamin A supplementation. *Health Policy and Planning*, 12(1), 29–37.

McGuire, A., Henderson, J., and Mooney, G. (1988). *The economics of health care: an introductory text*. Routledge and Kegan Paul, London.

Mills, A. (1985). Economic evaluation of health programmes in developing countries. *World Health Statistics Quarterly*, 38(4), 368–82.

Mooney, G. H. (1977). *The valuation of human life*. Macmillan, Basingstoke.

Robinson, R. (1993). Economic evaluation and health care: what does it mean?. *British Medical Journal*, 307, 6905, 670–3.

Rossi, P. H. and Freeman, H. E. (1989). *Evaluation — a systematic approach*. Sage, Newbury Park, CA.

Simmonds, S. (1987). Evaluation at the local level: the roles of outsiders and the community. *Health Policy and Planning*, 2(4), 309–22.

Vaughan, J. P., Walk, G., and Ross, D. (1984). Evaluation of primary health care: approaches, comments and criticisms. *Tropical Doctor*, 14, 56–60.

WHO (1981). *Health Programme evaluation: guiding principles*. Health for All Series No. 6, World Health Organization, Geneva.

World Bank (1993) *World Development Report*. World Bank/Oxford University Press, New York.

11

Resource allocation and budgeting

One of the most powerful stages of planning is that of the resource allocation and budgeting process. Budgeting and resource allocation are two sides of the same coin and are key steps in the overall financial management process which are set out in Table 11.1.

Resource allocation implies the distribution of resources, and in particular finance, from the centre to peripheral levels. It is generally used to refer to broad levels of aggregated financial resources. *Budgeting* implies the more detailed determination of precisely how these funds are to be used. Given the importance we have placed on planning as a process that leads to action, budgeting and resource allocation are major planning instruments.

Unfortunately, it is common for planners to restrict their involvement in this area to capital or development budgets, or at least to concentrate on them. Although development budgets may provide a major impetus for change in periods of growth, this is less true in the tight financial situation facing many health sectors. The inappropriate allocation pattern for resources, a common feature of many health systems described in Box 7.1 (p. 138), suggests the need for alternative reallocative strategies to shift resources and budgets to the areas of higher priority. Even where there is growth, it is still incumbent upon planners to concern themselves with recurrent as well as development budgets. As has been stressed frequently in this book, planning is only successful if it achieves any necessary change it identifies. Plans which identify inappropriate uses of funds, but fail to redirect them, are of little use.

This chapter first outlines the major types of budget. It then looks at the main approaches to budgeting and resource allocation, and lastly discusses financial management issues relevant to the planner. It does not consider the detailed costing of the components of particular budgets, as techniques for this have already been discussed in Chapter 9.

Table 11.1   Key processes in financial planning and management

Resource allocation
Budgeting
Drawing and disbursing
Accounting
Expenditure monitoring and control
Virement or reappropriation
Auditing (internal and external)

Table 11.2   Typical health ministry budget structure

	Hospital A	Hospital B	Clinics	Enviromental health	HQ	Total
Salaries	150	300	80	30	40	600
Transport	20	30	20	10	20	100
Medical supplies	50	110	30	10	0	200
Equipment	15	30	5	5	5	60
Maintenance	8	15	5	2	0	30
Others	2	3	0	0	5	10
Total	245	488	140	57	70	1000

DIFFERENT FORMS OF BUDGET

Institutional versus programme budgets

Any budget format has essentially two components — the budget holders and the budget items over which they have control. Table 11.2 sets out a typical budget of the form frequently used in the public sector.

To understand some of the characteristics of different types of budget it may help to examine one institution. Consider a hospital for example. A hospital may have a manager responsible for the overall budget, perhaps the medical superintendent or the hospital administrator. Below this level there may be subsidiary budget managers. There are two main ways in which such budgets can be constituted.

- Firstly, they may relate to types of resources, such as nursing personnel, drugs, or transport. Under such a system, managers of different services (for example, the operating theatres) are provided by the budget holders with resources such as staff or supplies, rather than controlling a budget themselves. Such an approach is relatively easily managed by senior professionals in particular specialist areas of resources, as, for example, by a transport manager (transport), a matron (nursing staff), or a hospital pharmacist (drugs).

- The second approach decentralizes budgets on a basis of activity rather than of resources. The out-patient department, for example, would have its own budget and budget holder, covering all resources. The role of the professional head, such as a matron, in such circumstances is to provide professional support to the department mental managers as required.

Thus the form of organizational structure affects, and is affected by, the financial mechanisms. A structure that gives budget control over hospital nurses to the hospital matron weakens the power of individual departmental managers, who have to negotiate with the matron for nursing changes. Alternatively, strong departmental structures reduce the power of the professional heads, such as the matron.

The rationale for having managers (and hence budget managers) responsible for areas of activity is compelling. The aim of any health service is to achieve set programme objectives in terms of change in health status. Plans therefore need to be set in such programme terms, and backed up by relevant service budgets. Resources such as staff, supplies, or transport are the tools which the service managers have at their disposal to achieve these objectives in terms of health status, and hence of service. Such resources are only a means to an end, and not an end in themselves.

Many systems in fact combine the two approaches, with departmental managers having some discretionary budget, but with central control over major items such as staff. A third organizational model is possible, and this combines the two approaches by having departmental budgets which 'buy in' services such as nursing or pharmaceuticals from other managers. Under such circumstances, both the departmental and the resource managers have budgets. Such structures require a sophisticated and information-hungry system.

At the wider, health service level there has been interest in the concepts of *programme budgets*. Programme budgeting (related to Planning Programme Budgeting Systems — PPBS) attempts to relate resources (as inputs) to programme objectives (as outputs). Thus, for example, a mother-and-child health (MCH) programme budget would include all the resources related to MCH, irrespective of the part of the organization in which they were used. The rationale for this is that, in planning terms, it allows monitoring of the input–output relationship.

Tables 11.3 and 11.4 reanalyse Table 11.2 (a budget set in institutional terms) to show activities by programme. The programmes selected here, mother-and-child health/family planning (MCH/FP), communicable disease control, curative care, and headquarters support, are illustrative. Any set of programmes could be chosen, depending on the objectives and hence the programmes of the service. Table 11.3 shows the programmes by organizational location, and Table 11.4 by type of line-item expenditure.

Functional or line items can be seen, therefore, as describing the nature of the expenditure. Institutional budgets are based on where activities take place. Programme budgeting is concerned with the overall purpose. WHO's Managerial Process for National Health Development (MPNHD; WHO 1984) stressed the adoption of programme budgets rather than functional budgets. However, the practicalities of using programme budgets as a management tool are often complex. Arrangements for management are often based either on a function or a line item basis (for example, a nurse manager may manage and control the budget of nurses involved in a variety of different programmes), or are institutionally based (as in hospitals or health centres). Management of programmes across institutions is extremely difficult. Programme 'budgets' are often therefore used not as budgets but as an analytical tool to monitor spending by objectives.

Capital and recurrent budgets

The distinction between capital and recurrent (known in some countries as revenue) budgets has already been discussed in Chapter 9. It is based on the difference between items of expenditure which can be considered as one-off, as opposed to those which are repeatable. However, while some items, such as building construction, can be

Table 11.3   Programme budget by organization

	MCH/FP	Communicable disease control	Curative care	HQ support	Total
Hospital A	40	30	175	0	245
Hospital B	28	10	450	0	488
Clinics	30	10	100	0	140
Environmental health	0	57	0	0	57
Headquarters[a]	0	0	0	70	70
Total	98	107	725	70	1000

[a]Headquarters support could be spread over direct programme activities.

Table 11.4   Programme budget by line item

	MCH/FP	Communicable disease control	Curative control	HQ support	Total
Salaries	64	61	435	40	600
Transport	10	25	45	20	100
Medical supplies	10	5	185	0	200
Equipment	5	10	40	5	60
Maintenance	8	5	17	–	30
Other	1	1	3	5	10
Total	98	107	725	70	1000

clearly seen as 'one-off', other items, such as training or furniture, are less obvious. Such items are also repeatable, but at longer intervals than, say, drugs. Indeed, even buildings eventually also require replacement! Capital expenditure can be 'translated' into annual recurrent expenditure through depreciation techniques (see p. 178) which are useful reminders to health planners of the opportunity cost of capital budgets which may otherwise appear as 'free' goods. Indeed in countries, where health sector reforms are encouraging greater partnership between the public and private sector through initiatives which harness private sector finance for the public sector in the form of loans or commercial arrangements (sometimes known as Private Finance Initiatives) the distinction between capital and recurrent costs may be less obvious through the interest payable on capital.

There are, however, at least two reasons for a capital budget. Firstly, the inclusion of such one-off payments within budgets that deal with ongoing expenditure would distort projections of long-term funding requirements and it is therefore easier to keep them separate. Secondly, one-off expenditures which provide benefits in more than one year may be funded in a different way (such as through loans or aid) from those providing immediate benefits to society.

One difficulty which has arisen from this distinction, however, is the misperception that capital budgets relate to planning, whereas recurrent budgets are seen as related to 'management'. The rationale for such a view is, at first sight, understandable, given that capital developments lead to changes in the future. However, a danger arises when this becomes translated into a view that capital improvements are the only vehicle for altering direction (the role of planning). This is not the case. Reallocation of resources between services (particularly in a period of low, nil, or even negative resource-growth) may be the only realistic way to obtain change. Planning *must*, therefore, be involved in the setting of recurrent budgets. Furthermore, as capital expenditure almost inevitably leads to future recurrent budget requirements, it is essential that the two budgets are considered together.

Unfortunately, it is still the case that development or capital budgets are seen as the responsibility of many planning departments, whereas recurrent budgets are seen as the province of an accounts department. If planning systems are to be effective, then these distinctions must be broken down, and the process of setting recurrent budgets must be fully integrated into the overall planning process. The use of rolling plans, discussed in more detail in Chapter 14, provides a means for this.

Cash-limited versus volume budgeting

Some budgetary systems are based on agreed volume indicators (such as the number of personnel), and supplementary budgets for unexpected price increases (such as wage rises) during the financial year are automatically approved. Increasingly, however, financial constraints have led to the adoption of *cash-limited budgets*. Here, a fixed budget is agreed and it is expected that it will be kept to, irrespective of any changes that occur during the year after the budget has been set, such as price increases. In such situations unanticipated changes either in prices (for example through inflation-ary pressure) or in the level of activity (for example through an epidemic) are expected to be contained by compensatory reduction elsewhere in the level of activity and expenditure (although supplementary budgets may be provided in exceptional circumstances). Such cash-limited budgets have forced managers to be far more conscious of the financial implications of alterations in services. Later in the chapter, financial management techniques which can assist managers in living within such budgets are discussed.

BUDGETING AND RESOURCE ALLOCATION APPROACHES

We turn now to the different ways in which budgets may be set. Each approach has different implications for planning.

Budgeting, resource allocation, and decentralization

One central issue concerns the optimal system of resource allocation or budgeting. As we saw in Chapter 3, the Health Sector Reform (HSR) policies being pursued in a number of countries frequently include an emphasis on decentralization with the shifting of decisions as to how resources are used to as low an administrative level as possible. This requires budgets to be set at lower levels within a broad ceiling set by the central level. This needs to be done within a clear framework of equity, thus ensuring that resources are allocated according to need, so a strong central role in accomplishing this is still needed. One solution to this apparent dilemma is to allocate resources in broad financial terms on the basis of the needs of the decentralized management areas, leaving the local managers to determine the detail of how such resources are used and hence budgeted.

With policies of decentralization, increasingly districts and regions are responsible for the detailed budgeting within given broad constraints, with the centre-to-periphery allocative decisions being based on population characteristics to reflect need and equity, such as population, age, sex, social class, mortality, or morbidity. Resources are allocated to lower administrative levels, such as districts, with budgets being retained at the centre for particular activities. Figure 11.1 sets out diagrammatically the elements of such a resource allocation system. The components of such a potential formula are:

- health needs of a specified population

- differential costs of providing different services

- differential costs in different areas

- costs associated with non-service delivery such as teaching costs

- use by patients in one area of services in another (cross-boundary flows).

The most contentious of these criteria is the first (assessment of need) with potential measures of need being a combination of:

- size of population

- age and sex ratios

- direct measures of morbidity

- mortality measures (such as standardized mortality rates — see Box 11.1 — as overall proxy for different levels of health need

- indicators of deprivation (to reflect both potentially higher levels of relationship between morbidity and mortality and higher health-care costs).

In many instances (such as UK RAWP — see below), need has been split into different components such as acute care, maternity, chronic and psychiatric each with different proxy measures. Issues have centred around:

- whether mortality is a good proxy for morbidity

- whether measuring deprivation indices leads to double counting of need

- whether morbidity measures are influenced by accessibility to services

- weighting given to different aspects

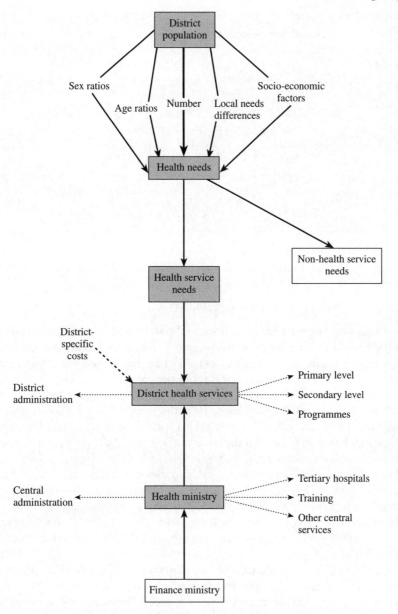

Fig. 11.1   Model for the allocation of resources

Box 11.1   Example of condition-specific standardized mortality ratios for an age group

Standardized mortality ratios (SMR) are a technique used to show the relative level of a health problem within an area, which shows the mortality rate in comparison with the national average, taken as 100.

	Region 1	Region 2	Total
Population (000s)	40	60	100
Actual deaths	10	20	30
Mortality rate	25%	33%	30%
Expected deaths	$0.3 \times 40 = 12$	$0.3 \times 60 = 18$	
SMR	$(10/12) \times 100 = 83$	$(20/18) \times 100 = 111$	

- whether the actual funding based on components of need are translated into equivalent services at the local level

- which services should be centrally provided.

A crude version of such a resource allocation system would distribute funds on the basis of the population size alone. However, such an approach takes no account of the particular health needs of one region over another, and a weighting system may be required which allows the allocative process to take account of such differences. Such systems may provide weightings for the elderly or the young, or for above-average incidence of particular health problems. How the weightings are chosen is of course extremely important, and will reflect central priorities and views on need. One method uses weightings between factors on the basis of the effect of the particular factor on the national costs of service provision. For example, if it costs more to provide care for under-fives, then this would be reflected in the under-five weighting. Box 11.2 gives an illustration of how such a system might operate. There are a number of judgements underlying such a process, including, for example, an assumption that current methods of service provision (and hence relative costs) are the most appropriate. For many countries such cost information is not available, however, and much cruder weightings are used.

Box 11.2 shows a crude weighted resource allocation model, based on age groupings and relative costs of care. The differences in population composition have no overall effect when no weightings are given to each age group. However, when weightings are given the different demographic composition leads to a change in allocation. Such a model could be made more sophisticated by developing the allocative groupings (for example to include particular disease groups), by indication of need (such as mortality), and by a further population weighting to reflect the different administrative costs associated with higher populations. The UK NHS allocative system developed in the 1970s, known as RAWP (Resource Allocation Working Party 1976), is an example of an allocative system which attempted to incorporate various indicators of need and

Box 11.2 Example of resource allocation weighted for age-specific costs

	0–4	5–25	25–60	60+	Total	% of total
Population (000s)						
Region 1	1100	2000	700	200	4000	40
Region 2	1400	3000	1500	100	6000	60
Total	2500	5000	2200	300	10000	
Equal per capita distribution of a total national budget of £10 million (£000s)						
Region 1	1100	2000	700	200	4000	40
Region 2	1400	3000	1500	100	6000	60
Total	2500	5000	2200	300	10000	
Relative cost of service provision[a]		2	0.6	7		
Allocation according to cost weighting						
Region 1	1879	1708	179	598	4364	44
Region 2	2391	2562	384	299	5636	56
Total	4270	4270	564	897	10000	
Total weighted costs	10000	10000	1320	2100	23420	

[a]This does not represent the actual cost but the relative ratio between different age-cohorts as illustrated in Fig 5.1, p. 96.
Allocation to each age band
= (population of each age band × relative cost of age band × total national population)/(sum of total of each national age group × relative cost)

which subsequent systems have refined. Under RAWP, health regions were allocated annual overall budgets from central government, based on a formula which aimed to reflect their different health-care needs. It was, however, recognized early on in the development of the RAWP process that (for historical reasons) there were severe divergences between current provisions and those suggested by the needs-based formula. An immediate shift towards regularizing this was seen as politically and managerially unfeasible, and a policy of allocating to regions in a way that reduced the gap over the medium term was instituted.

Resource allocation formulae have tended to concentrate on recurrent allocation costs. Capital allocations need to take account of the existing capital stock.

A shift towards an allocative system based on explicit criteria brings with it a number of issues around the implementation of such formulae. These include the following:

• *Speed of implementation*. This can be important and is related in part to the absorptive capacity of underfunded areas and the ability to reduce funding of 'overresourced' areas. The political strength of different areas is likely to have an important impact on the feasibility of shifting resources in real terms between areas. When such shifts occur at a time of overall growth of funding for the sector, then the shifts may be relative rather than absolute and as such there may be less resistance from 'losing areas. Segall (1983) in his study of the Zimbabwean health sector argued a similar point when suggesting that while it was both possible and desirable to shift resources from the city-based hospital sector to rural health-care facilities, this was best achieved through the use of differential growth rates for the different sectors over time.

- *Local revenue generation*. The second concern relates to alternative sources of funding for a district, such as from local revenue generation. Where this occurs, the principle of equity suggests that the potential for local generation of resources should be taken account of within the formula, though this may reduce the incentive to raise funds.

- *Information systems*. One of the major constraints on the development of needs-based allocative systems is the existence of adequate and widely accepted information. In some countries it may be necessary to start with very basic allocative formulae based on population before the development of more sophisticated formulae. Even basic population data may not available, or accepted by particular population groups. For example, the 1998 census in Pakistan was disrupted by demonstrations by regional groups which were concerned about the way in which the census was being carried out and the potential implications for resources for their areas.

- *Perverse incentives*. It is important the system does not lead to perverse incentives. We have seen above an example of this in connection with local revenue generation. Other potential problems include the linking of funding to (poor) health status as a proxy for need.

- *Cost shunting*. Lastly, the development of such allocative formulae may lead to attempts by health authorities in one region to shift costs to another region, by for example, encouraging the use of services in a neighbouring region. Though formulae may be able to account for this by incorporating measures of cross-boundary flows, these require information which may not be easily available.

Historical incrementalist budgeting

The most widespread approach to budgeting is the incrementalist approach, which allocates overall resources on the basis of the previous year's budget (possibly adjusted by estimates of expenditure). Alternative approaches are illustrated in Table 11.5. Table 11.5 A shows the current budget and Table 11.5 (B-D) the effects of alternative approaches. The crudest form of such budgeting is one where any growth in the overall resources (or cuts) is applied equally across the board. Table 11.5(B) gives an example of such a budgetary system.

Table 11.5 Examples of incrementalist budgeting

		Hospital	Clinic	Other	Total
A	Current year budget	7000	1500	1500	10 000
	Distribution (%)	70.0	15.0	15.0	100.0
B	With equal growth rate of: (%)	5.0	5.0	5.0	5.0
	Next year budget	7350	1575	1575	10 500
	Distribution (%)	70.0	15.0	15.0	100.0
C	With growth rates of: (%)	0.0	33.0	0.0	5.0
	Next year budget	7000	2000	1500	10 500
	Distribution (%)	67.0	19.0	14.0	100.0
D	With growth rates of: (%)	2.8	16.7	3.0	5.0
	Next year budget	7200	1750	1550	10 500
	Distribution (%)	68.6	16.7	14.8	100.0

Such an approach strictly maintains the status quo, with the proportion of the total budget assigned to each institution or activity remaining the same. It allows for no possible shifting in priority between different activities, and assumes that past budget shares not only were appropriate, but will remain so. This is too crude an approach to be widely used.

An alternative, allowing more scope for change, entails distributing the incremental growth in resources not equally, but among priority services. This is exemplified in Table 11.5(C), where all the overall increase in resources is allocated to the clinic programme. Such an approach is attractive, in that it allows for a shift in the proportion of the total budget given to any one budget holder. At the same time, by not cutting any absolute budget, it reduces resistance to the shift from the (relative) losers, in this case the hospital.

In practice, of course, it is unlikely that a shift of all incremental growth towards priority areas is possible. Pressure to increase budgets from all quarters is more likely to result in reduced differential growth rates. Such a scenario is exemplified in Table 11.5(D). This can be seen to be analogous to incremental planning. It conserves the status quo, and thus is both non-threatening and easy to administer, but offers little opportunity for radical change.

Capital-led allocations

One widely used variation on the above (often used in conjunction with it) views the major means of change to recurrent budgets as arising from approved capital development projects. Under such an approach, a project is approved in terms of both its capital and recurrent costs. The additional recurrent budget requirements are then added at the appropriate time to the budget. While this approach at least ensures that capital developments are provided with the necessary running costs (which is not, unfortunately, always the case) it has the danger of weighting change toward activities involving capital, such as construction or project-based activities.

Zero-based budgeting

At the other end of the scale lies zero-based budgeting. If historical incrementalism is analogous to incrementalist forms of planning, zero-based budgeting corresponds to a comprehensive rational approach. Under such a system, originally promulgated in the USA as a means of ensuring continuous reassessment of priorities, no budget is regarded as assured. Every year, each budget holder is required to justify the whole of her/his budget submission against stated objectives through the use of performance indicators. Failure to provide adequate justification can result in a reduction in budget size. Such an approach clearly allows far more opportunity for radical change. However, it also requires a large amount of information, and is administratively very costly. It can also be very destabilizing and demoralizing for staff, uncertain whether their position is secure from year to year. For these last reasons it is also the approach that is most likely to encounter strong opposition.

A modified version of zero-based budgeting requires managers to justify their budgets at the margin. Managers set out the effects on the objectives of their services of both an increase and a decrease of, say, 5% in their budget. The activities possible through an increase of 5% are regarded as the next highest priority for the service. Those which would be cut with a reduction in budget of 5% are assumed to be the lowest-priority services. These effects can then be compared between different services. Where the benefits of providing additional resources to one activity are seen to outweigh the disadvantages of a comparable reduction in another service, budget alterations will be made. Such an approach embodies some of the potential benefits of the zero-based budgeting approach as a means of obtaining allocative shifts, but in a more feasible manner. It can potentially be a powerful tool, provided clear monitoring of the budget is possible. If such monitoring is not carried out, the way is open to managers to manipulate the situation by suggesting that the effects of budget cuts would be more serious than would actually be the case!

THE BUDGETING PROCESS

Annual budgeting can be seen as the final stage of the planning spiral prior to implementation. A long-term strategic plan sets the context for shorter and more immediate 3–5-year plans, and annual budgeted action programmes. Planning and budgeting should therefore be seen as two ends of the same spectrum. In practice the process of budgeting is unfortunately often separated from that of planning, thus removing from planning a major tool with which to influence resource allocations, and hence to effect change. The rolling plan (see p. 289–90) provides a mechanism to bring annual budgeting and longer-term planning together.

It is not uncommon to find the process of budgeting being seen as the responsibility of an accounts section. Such a situation often results in either incrementalist across-the-board increases (or cuts), or priorities based on an accounts department's perspectives. This might lead to an undue emphasis on expenditure levels, rather than on the activities themselves and on priorities. Although financial information provided by such a department is essential for the budgeting process, it is important that organizational mechanisms should be devised which provide policy direction (based on plans) to the formulation of budgets. Budget committees constituted of accounts staff, planning staff, and policy-makers are one means of providing such a mechanism.

The details of how budgeting occurs vary in different countries. In particular, the role of central government ministries in relation to service ministries such as the health ministry will differ, reflecting in part the degree of decentralization within the government structure itself. As we saw in Chapter 3, there are various models of decentralization; each of these will lead to different budgeting processes. The following refers to a system of functional deconcentration. The central government functions of personnel management (including establishment control), financial control, and planning are normally brought together through the budgeting process. At the next level, the resource allocation and budgeting process within the ministry and its health services will vary, depending largely on the degree of decentralization.

Review of previous year

The first stage of a budgeting process should involve a review of the previous year, as part of the ongoing monitoring role of planning. This should occur at all levels of the service, and can be seen as part of the revision of the situational analysis. Within the specific context of budgeting, the review should consider the levels of expenditure by different services against the service targets set within the plan and against the indicators of achievement of these targets.

As this review inevitably takes place before the end of the financial year, estimates of likely expenditure in the current year, together with actual expenditure figures for the preceding year, should be set against the respective budgets, and against the service objectives stated in the plan.

The degree to which such objectives are both explicit and quantified depends largely on how well formulated the plan is. This again highlights the close inter-dependence between planning and budgeting. Questions which need to be asked include the following:

- Is the current year's expenditure likely to exceed or to fall short of what was budgeted? If so, why?

- Are the objectives of the service currently being met? If not, is this related to levels of budget, outside constraints, or poor management?

Review service objectives and targets

The concept of a rolling plan allows annual reviews of objectives and targets to affirm or amend them. During this process changes in emphasis may be placed on different areas of the service, as a result of either a change in external circumstances or priorities, or of experience of actual service provision.

Central government resource guidance

At a relatively early stage in the process, the central government ministries should provide guidance on the likely level of the budget for the ministry as a whole, together with any particular constraints on its use. In addition to financial regulations, there may be personnel or planning requirements. For example, there may be a requirement that only a certain amount should be budgeted for personnel costs, as a means of establishment control. Where such estimates of likely budget levels are not provided early enough in the budget cycle, the ministry will need to make its own estimates.

Ideally, information should also be provided on likely inflation rates in the following year, and how these are to be budgeted for. Where they are not available, estimates would again be needed. On the basis of the overall likely resource levels, the health ministry should determine the different regional or district allocations, as was outlined earlier.

Discussions and negotiations between different levels

The next stage in the process involves negotiation over the level of individual budgets with the managers of different services. Such discussions may take many forms, this diversity in part reflecting the differences between a bottom-up and a top-down approach, and depending on the budget-setting approach adopted. Negotiations should, however, focus on the review process described above. Usually there are intermediary levels of management (such as regional authorities); then the negotiations with district service managers are likely to be handled by these authorities, basing themselves on the regional allocation estimates of their own total budget, which is itself provided by the ministry through the application of an allocative formula.

The negotiations should, as far as possible, be based on proposals by managers for their services that are in line with the plan and will allow fulfillment of their service objectives. As such there are likely to be four elements to the proposals:

- a description of service changes (for example an extension of a mobile vaccination service) and their expected effects on plan targets

- any personnel implications (for example, the need to employ an additional nurse)

- recurrent budget implications

- development or capital budget implications.

In this way, the budget process, is tied in closely with the planning process. It is important to encourage service managers to recognize that change can occur not only through the provision of additional resources, but also through redeployment of existing resources. The budget process provides an ideal opportunity for explicit consideration of such possibilities.

Set draft budget

Following the discussions with service managers and provisional agreement on their budget proposals, the ministry (or where applicable, the regions) should be in a position to draft an overall budget close to the central government guidelines. In some countries a central resource guideline is taken as firm, and draft ministry budgets cannot exceed this. Elsewhere, there is room for manoeuvre, and ministry budgets which slightly exceed the guidelines may be accepted as the basis for discussion. Indeed the discussions which occur at this level are analogous to those carried out at lower levels within the service ministry staff.

Final budget set by central government

The last stage of the process involves the final approval of the budget by central government, and by the political level of government (for example the cabinet, president, or parliament). This approval then provides the authority for budget holders to commit expenditure according to the budget set.

Box 11.3 sets out a possible timetable for these stages. The exact process and timetable will clearly depend on the structure of the health sector and its form of decentralization It is important to note that the whole process, if it is to allow participation by service managers (and for them to consult their own staff and communities), can take at least six months; more if there are intermediate management levels such as provinces and regions.

FINANCIAL MANAGEMENT AND ACCOUNTING

Monitoring

Once budgets are set, monitoring systems are required to provide managers with information throughout the financial year as to the current situation and the likely end-of-year position (out-turn). Though such monitoring is primarily a management function, it has important implications for planning. If such monitoring leads to action, within the year, which deviates from an agreed plan, then it is important that planners are aware of this. The accuracy of such monitoring will depend on both an understanding of the *budget profile*, i.e. how one expects the budget to be spent over the year, and the *accounting system*, which provides information on how much has been *spent* or *committed* to expenditure. Three main accounting systems exist: cash accounting, accrual accounting, and commitment accounting, depending upon the point at which a decision to spend is reflected in the accounts.

Budget management statements such as that shown in Box 11.4 provide one means of monitoring expenditure. Such statements allow comparison of the expenditure (real or committed) at the end of each month with expected expenditure. The simplest form of such statements is based on an assumption that the budget will be equally spread and spent over the 12 months of the year. Thus, for example, by the end of the

Box 11.3   Annual budget cycle

Month	Activity
1	Financial year begins.
5	Health ministry receives provisional allocation for following year from central government, together with any special constraints or conditions.
6	Health ministry issues broad resource allocation guidance to regions[a] on the basis of provisional allocation.
7	Regions issue broad allocations to districts on similar basis.
8	Budget holders develop and return proposals showing: • review of service targets in line with plan • estimated expenditure for previous year • estimated expenditure out-turn for current year • reasons for under/overspending • budget proposals for following year, costed and showing how they will meet planned service targets.
8	Budgets totalled and reconciled at regional level and then at health ministry.
9	Adjustments made • to reflect national policy • to reconcile with other budget proposals • to reflect constraints • to reconcile with central government allocations.
9	Discussions with central government.
10	Adjustments with service managers.
11	Informal approval.
12	Government approves budget.
1	Budgets issued to budget holders.

* Where an organizational structure does not include regions or provinces, adjustments will be needed.

third month 25% of the annual budget should have been spent. In reality such 'straight line' spending is unlikely, for a variety of reasons. For example:

• economies of scale in purchasing may lead to above-average spending at the beginning of the year

• delays in recruitment over new posts may cause underspending on personnel

• equipment items are often indivisible, and purchased by the expenditure of a single large lump sum.

Box 11.4 Monthly financial management monitoring

The table below shows a monthly management statement after 3 months of the year. The budget-to-date column shows what might be expected to have been spent one quarter of the way through the year. It is assumed here that spending will be equal each month (which is unlikely); more sophisticated estimates could be made. The variance columns show the relative (not actual) over or underspending.

Item	Budget	Expenditure to date	Budget to date	Variance (+ under, − over)		Projected year-end Expenditure	Variance
	£000	£000	£000	£000	%	£000	%
Personnel	120	10[a]	30	+20	+66	40	+66
Drugs	80	40[b]	20	−20	−100	160	−100
Transport	40	20[c]	10	−10	−100	80	−100
Utilities	12	1[d]	3	+2	+66	4	+66
	252	71	63	−8	−13	284	−13

Possible reasons for variance
[a] Recruitment slow with new posts at beginning of year.
[b] Early stock-taking.
[c] Overspend due to petrol price increase.
[d] Water company strike: no bill received.

Where such patterns are known and predictable, more sophisticated profiles of likely expenditure can be built into the monitoring process — particularly where computer-based financial management systems are being used. Where such systems are not available, accurate, or appropriate, then manual systems based on the knowledge of the budget holders as to their likely spending patterns can provide good substitutes.

Systems of monitoring are essential means of detecting deviation from the budget early enough that remedial action can be taken to ensure not only that the budget is not exceeded, but that such action is taken in a measured way, consistent with the objectives of the service plans. Where recognition of potential overspending does not occur until late in the financial year, the remedial options are often extremely limited, and may lead to unplanned and undesirable shifts from the service objectives.

Financial monitoring may detect two variations from the set budget — a likely over or underspent out-turn. Such variations are likely to be the result of:

- poor initial estimation
- initial misallocation between budget items
- unplanned change in volume of activity
- unexpected change in prices
- change in efficiency levels.

In situations where a cash-limited manager is likely to be heading for an over-expenditure of her/his budget there are a number of actions that s/he can take. Which is most appropriate will depend on the reasons for the overexpenditure, and the consequences of the action on the plan objectives. It is therefore important to be clear as to the cause of the deviation, as this may lead to different responses from managers, and planners may react in different ways. For example a change in activity level may have been unavoidable (if it came about, for example, as a result of an epidemic). By contrast, the inefficient use of resources should be discouraged through budgetary mechanisms. An ideal financial management and budget system should aim to discourage both inefficiency and unplanned changes in activity level. It should also not encourage end-of-year 'spending-up', a common phenomenon when budget residues cannot be carried forward or budgets are related to the previous year's expenditure.

Corrective financial actions

The options open to a manager facing over or underexpenditure can be summarized as:

- virement
- a request for supplementary funds
- improvements in efficiency

- a reduction in activity levels

- a reduction in the quality of service.

Each of these is outlined briefly below.

Virement
Virement is the process of transferring funds from one budget line to another. Where the likely overexpenditure is only in one item, and is compensated for by an under-spending in another item, then a transfer of funds from one line item (such as transport) to another (such as drugs) may be possible. Financial control systems usually have restrictions on the ability of a budget manager to make such virements between certain items.

Request for supplementary funds
A second option is to seek additional funding. This may under certain circumstances be possible in the form of a supplementary vote of funds from the next level up in the health service (the region or ministry for example), or from central government. The possibilities of this and the appropriateness of such action will depend both on the availability of funds, either through a contingency budget or through underspending elsewhere, and on the cause of the overspending. Unanticipated increases in the levels of activity (for example through an emergency) may be seen as a reasonable cause for supplementary funding.

Efficiency improvements
The most attractive option for dealing with potential overexpenditure is an increase in efficiency, allowing the same level of service activity to be provided, at the same quality, for less resources. Striving for improved efficiency should, of course, be a concern of all managers at all times, and not just in situations of potential overspend. Possible techniques which may help to identify areas of inefficiency include economic appraisal techniques, or, even more simply, an examination of cost structures. Efficiency may, in general, be improved in three ways.

- by achieving the same ends by a completely different approach

- by looking for areas where economies of scale can be achieved, perhaps by sharing resources such as transport

- by negotiating a reduction in the price of inputs, such as drugs.

It should be noted, though, that often efficiency improvements take some time to filter through into budgets, and thus may not provide an easy solution to short-term over-expenditure problems. There are also efficiency traps which can lure the unsuspecting manager into worse situations. Chapter 9 gave an example of this in Box 9.8 (p. 186). As we saw there, a reduction in hospital stay may lead to greater efficiency in terms of individual patient cost, but may, in certain circumstances, lead to greater overall expenditure. It is worth remarking that undue attention spent on attempting to improve efficiency (which may, in the short run at least, have diminishing marginal returns for the effort invested — there is a limit to the efficiency savings available at any given time) may be counterproductive, and may divert attention away from more important managerial and planning issues. There is always an opportunity cost attached to a manager's time.

Reduction in activity levels
A fourth option involves reducing the levels of service activity, which, in contrast with the previous option, may lead to budget savings, but possibly also to lower levels of efficiency, where the activity level drops below the lowest point on the average-cost curve (see Box 9.7 on p. 185) for an example). Reduction of activity is rarely easy managerially, as there is likely to be understandable resistance to it from health professionals and the community. It may, however, be preferable to other options, or the only option available.

Reduction in the quality of service
The penultimate option involves the possibility of deliberately reducing the quality of a service. Again this is understandably unpopular; but it may be preferable to a reduction in service levels. The 'quality' of services may be lowered through, for example, a reduction in nursing care, or in the quality of food. It is obviously important in carrying out such a strategy that the quality of care does not drop to the point where service efficacy is lowered, endangering service objectives.

Line item control
The last three options have all dealt with alternatives ways of reducing expenditure. In many situations this may be the only realistic option open to a cash-limited budget manager. An alternative approach, commonly followed, starts with the existing line item budgets (such as transport or drugs) and looks for savings in these. Such an approach is a useful way of involving other functional managers. However, it is important to recognize that this and the previous approaches are closely linked. Any change in such line items will always result in a change in either the efficiency, the quality, or the levels of activity of services. Similarly, any change in efficiency, quality, or quantity can only be realized through changes in the actual budget lines.

SUMMARY

This chapter has introduced a number of issues in budgeting and resource allocation. The most appropriate form of budgeting and resource allocation will depend in large part on the organizational structure of the health service, and in particular on its degree of decentralization. We have stressed that budgeting is an integral part of effective planning, being the means to achieve resources and hence action. Planners who fail to get involved in the budgeting process are handicapped from the beginning.

INTRODUCTORY READING

There are few recent comprehensive texts on this area related to the health sector of developing countries. WHO (1984) provides an introduction to the techniques of programme budgeting. Brambleby (1995), Pole (1974) and Mooney (1984) give a good introduction to the issues around programme budgets as planning tools. Both of the Segall articles are important with one (1991) looking at the use of recurrent budget planning and the other (1983) more specifically at Zimbabwe. Chae *et al.* (1989) is a case study of the relationship between resource allocation and planning in Papua New Guinea, and Mahapatra and Berman (1995) look at resource allocation for hospitals. The original report of the UK National Health Service resource allocation process by the Resource Allocation Working Party (1976) remains a good detailed study of the mechanics of a broad allocative process; Judge and Mays (1994), Mays (1987), Carr-Hill and Sheldon (1992), and Sheldon *et al.* (1993) discuss issues in the RAWP formula including wider measures of need than those originally built into the RAWP formula. Rigden's (1983) text on budgeting and financial management in the UK National Health Service, though not aimed at developing countries, provides a practical introduction to these issues. Nirel and Gross (1997) and Green (1992) look at practical budgeting issues at the primary and district level.

EXERCISE 11

1. How are resources allocated within your country from the Ministry of Health to lower administrative levels (e.g. regions and districts)?
2. How are the budgets for individual parts of the health service decided?
3. To what degree does the above process incorporate equity?
4. What is the relationship between the planning and budgeting process?

REFERENCES AND FURTHER READING

Abel-Smith, B. and Creese, A. (1989). *Recurrent costs in the health sector — problems and policy options in three countries.* WHO, Geneva; USAID, Washington.
Berman, P., Ormond, B. A., and Gani, G. (1987). Treatment use and expenditure on curative care in rural Indonesia. *Health Policy and Planning*, 2, 289–300.
Brambleby, P. (1995). A survivor's guide to programme budgeting. *Health Policy*, 33(2), 127–45.
Caiden, N. and Wildavsky, A. (1974). *Planning and budgeting in poor countries.* Wiley, New York.
Carr-Hill, R. and Sheldon, T. (1992). Rationality and the use of formulae in the allocation of resources to health care. *Journal of Public Health Medicine*, 14(2), 117–26.
Chae, Y. M., Newbrander, W. C., and Thomason, J. A. (1989). Application of goal programming to improve resource allocation for health services in Papua New Guinea. *International Journal of Health Planning and Management*, 4, 81–95.
Chu, D. (1992). Global budgeting of hospitals in Hong Kong. *Social Science and Medicine*, 35(7), 857–68.

Cowen, M. E. *et al.* (1996). A guide for planning community-oriented health care: the health sector resource allocation model. *Medical Care*, **34**(3), 264–79.

Dean, P. (1986). Programme and performance budgeting in Malaysia. *Public Administration and Development*, **6**, 267–86.

Green, A. (1992a). Financial management in times of severe resource constraints: the role of the district manager. *Tropical Doctor*, **24**, 7–10.

Green, A. (1992b). Managing district finances. *Tropical Doctor*, **24**, 3–5.

Judge, K. and Mays, N. (1994). Allocating resources for health and social care in England. *British Medical Journal*, **308**, 1363–6.

Mahapatra, P. and Berman, P. (1995). Resource allocation for public hospitals in Andhra Pradesh India. *Health Policy and Planning*, **10**, 129–39.

Mays, N. (1987). Measuring need in the national health service resource allocation formula: standardised mortality ratios or social deprivation. *Public Administration*, **65**, 45–60.

Mooney, G. (1984). Programme budgeting: an aid to planning and priority setting in health care. *Effective Health Care*, **2**, 65–8.

Newbrander, W. C. (1987). Papua New Guinea's expenditure on hospitals: policy and practice since independence. *Health Policy and Planning*, **2**, 227–35.

Nirel, N. and Gross, R. (1997). Challenges in implementing a budget-holding programme for primary care clinics. *Health Policy and Planning*, **12**(2), 146–60.

Omolehinwa, E. (1989). PPBS in Nigeria: its origin, progress and problems. *Public Administration and Development*, **9**, 395–404.

Pole, J. D. (1974). Programme, priorities and budgets. *British Journal of Preventive and Social Medicine*, **28**, 191–5.

Resource Allocation Working Party (1976). *Sharing resources for health in England*. DHSS, London.

Richardson, R. and Waddington, C. (1996). Allocating resources: community involvement is not easy. *International Journal of Health Planning and Management*, **11**(4), 307–15.

Rigden, M. S. (1983). *Health service finance and accounting*. Heinemann, London.

Segall, M. (1983). Planning and politics of resource allocation for primary health care: promotion of a meaningful national health policy. *Social Science and Medicine*, **17**, 1947–60.

Segall, M. (1991). Health sector planning led by management of recurrent expenditure: an agenda for action research. *International Journal of Health Planning and Management*, **6**(1), 37–75.

Sheldon, T. A. *et al.* (1993). Weighting in the dark: resource allocation in the new NHS. *British Medical Journal*, **306**, 835–9.

Waddington, C. *et al.* (1990). Financial information at district level: experiences from five countries. *Health Policy and Planning*, **4**(3), 207–18.

WHO (1984). *Programme budgeting as part of the managerial process for national health development (MPNHD). Guiding principles*. World Health Organization, Geneva.

Wickings, I., Coles, J., Flux, R., and Howard, L. (1983). Review of clinical budgeting and costing experiments. *British Medical Journal*, **286**, 575–8.

12

Programmes, projects, implementation, and monitoring

Following the option appraisal stage discussed in Chapter 10, the next stage in the planning spiral is *programming*. This involves translating the results of the priority-setting process and option appraisals into a set of workable programmes of activity that form the basis of the plan, including the budget and staffing requirements discussed in Chapter 11 and 13.

This chapter outlines first some of the issues faced in programming, and in particular the relationship between programmes and projects and donors. It then looks at the record on the implementation of plans and how it can be improved.

PROGRAMMES AND PROJECTS

The end-point of a priority-setting process is a set of agreed objectives the plan should achieve. The option appraisal stage examines alternative ways of achieving these objectives. Sometimes this will result in a continuation of existing programmes of activity, possibly modified; sometimes new programmes will be needed. Not all activity will be directly managed by the organization within which the planning unit operates (such as the health ministry); for example, the ministry may contract with NGOs to provide services. Furthermore, as we have seen, not all activity will fall directly within the health (service) sector.

Plans may therefore cover a variety of forms of initiatives, each aiming to provide change within the health sector. They may incorporate a range of policy tools within them, including incentives to other sectors and other health agencies. Chapter 4 outlined a number of these. Each initiative is likely to require funding either:

- to provide directly (changed) service provision

- to contract services from other agencies

- to develop mechanisms to persuade or require other agencies to change their behaviour (e.g. incentive structures, or regulatory requirements).

Capital funding is often, though not always, required to achieve such change. Equally important, however, are the required changes in the recurrent budget that will allow the ongoing funding of the service once any capital items such as buildings or equipment have been put in place. Such initiatives must be consistent with the likely availability of resources — in particular, human and financial. For each initiative, therefore, the following documentation is required:

- the objectives which the programme is expected to meet

- how these objectives will be met (i.e. the services required)

- the resource implications of the programmes, and how these will be met

- other implications, such as legislative and organizational

- the timetable for meeting the objectives

- any likely risks involved or constraints.

Such a document forms the basis of that part of a more general plan document that sets out the intended activities of the organization. It lays the responsibility for effecting change in ongoing service delivery on the planning function, irrespective of whether there are capital inputs or not.

It is important, however, to remind ourselves of shifts of emphasis which have been occurring between *projects* and *programmes* as instruments for planning change. The early days of health planning introduced many of the planning approaches of the industrial and agricultural sector, including the idea of discrete project-based planning. Projects were viewed as one-off activities, usually funded under a capital budget. These were the precursor to a set of different service activities. Examples of such projects might include construction projects, the purchase of vehicles, training, or a revolving drug fund. This, coupled with the fact that many initiatives were either in the area of buildings or vertically controlled services, lent weight to a project-based philosophy of planning. Changes to existing service patterns were often viewed as resulting from discrete, capital-led, interventions — and this, in many countries, reinforced the idea of a planner being responsible purely for the capital budget and its related 'projects'. Planning was mistakenly identified with the implementation of *projects*, rather than with the implementation of *change*.

The recognition of the need to integrate services and to emphasize horizontal linkages, together with the tightening of resources in the 1970s and 1980s, led to a shift away from capital-led projects to a philosophy of 'programmes'. WHO's Managerial Process for National Health Development (MPNHD), for example, emphasized 'programming' as a key activity in planning. Such an approach is consistent with a theme of this book that planning is concerned with effecting necessary change at all levels, and not purely with the change through incremental service add-ons that is characteristic of a project-dominated process. However, although increasingly development of sustained services, through programmes rather than projects, is seen as more consistent with the philosophy of Primary Health Care (PHC), many donors still consider aid as best provided in the form of discrete projects.

In addition to any presumed desire to support the health-promoting activities of a country, donors have other concerns about the way their funds are used.

- They are concerned to ensure that funds that they provide are used in ways consistent with their own priorities.

- They are frequently also concerned to support activities which have identifiable results in the short to medium term, often for political reasons in their own countries. Linked to this, and to a concern not to encourage activities which are not sustainable in the long term, is a general interest in capital rather than mainstream recurrent budget support.

• They are concerned to ensure that proper financial control is exercised.

• Lastly, they are often anxious to ensure that, once an activity has been identified for support, and approval for provision of donor funds has been reached, disbursement of these funds occurs in line with the agreed timetable.

All of these reasons suggest that, from the donor's perspective at least, discrete project activities may be the most desirable and monitorable form of aid. Countries therefore still rely on projects as a major means both of attracting foreign aid and of determining the allocation of incremental funds to activities. The use of projects within defined programme areas has many advantages, particularly those connected with the development and monitoring of new activity, but difficulties arise (as discussed further in Chapter 14) when a project is defined by a donor agency in a way which crosses over existing programme boundaries, and essentially sets up new organizational structures within the health sector. Examples of such projects which are currently popular include family health projects or population projects. Although they may lead to the prompt disbursement of funds for those particular projects themselves (though even this may be doubtful, given the difficulties of managing such a broad-based approach), they may also adversely affect the ability of other programmes to implement their own projects. These implementation difficulties are discussed later in this chapter.

Recently there has been however, developing interest in broader Sector Wide Approaches (see p. 110) to donor support to the health sector. Though there is still little experience with them, they potentially offer a means of reducing the transactions costs associated with multiple donor activity with specific projects.

It would be naive to suggest that most planners at present have the power to alter donors' attitudes to project-based funding. Such changes are only likely to occur at the political level. However, encouragement to locate projects organizationally within the confines of existing programmes, rather than setting up new structures, may be more feasible.

IMPLEMENTATION

The penultimate stage in the planning spiral outlined in Chapter 2 is *implementation*. By this point in the planning process, agreement has been reached on the overall objectives and, through the option appraisal, on the approach which the plan will follow. Unfortunately, the record on the implementation of plans is generally poor. Indeed, it can be argued that the failure to implement plans successfully has been the major contributor to cynicism in some quarters about the whole activity of planning. There is some justification for this. Given the emphasis which we have placed in this book on planning ensuring that necessary changes occur, plans which remain as ideas or as documents are of little use. Insufficient attention has often been given to this element of planning.

As we saw in Chapter 10, in the discussion of evaluation, a failure to attain set health objectives can be attributable to one or both of two broad causes.

- It can amount to a failure to achieve the health objectives set, despite the provision of the intended inputs and the attainment of the service delivery targets. This type of failure is not strictly an implementation failure, but instead a failure to analyse correctly the relationship between the service provision and the health targets at the appraisal stage.

- The second cause of the non-attainment of targets can be traced to a failure to provide the services themselves in the form planned. It is this aspect of implementation upon which we shall focus in the rest of this chapter.

As we shall see, many of these problems can be attributed to design-failure at an earlier stage in the process, such as a failure to estimate the available levels of resources accurately. Some are directly the result of poor detailed programming, in the shape of not ensuring that resources are well specified in terms of type and quantity. This chapter will then introduce techniques for improving the success rate in the implementation of the programmes and projects which follow on from the option appraisal.

CAUSES OF POOR IMPLEMENTATION

A number of factors can be identified as possible causes of poor implementation. Poor implementation here is being taken to mean either delayed implementation, non-implementation, or implementation in a form different from that planned. Factors leading to such poor implementation include:

- changes in priorities or policies from those originally agreed

- a resistance to the changes inherent in the plan, either from within the health service or from outside

- a lack of the necessary resources which are required to implement the plan, whether these missing resources are financial or real (such as trained staff)

- imprecisely specified details of the project or programme to be executed

- a lack of the appropriate organizational structure or the appropriate managerial skills necessary.

There is of course a degree of interdependence between these, but it is helpful to try to separate them out, conceptually at least. Before we look briefly at each of them, a preliminary comment is worth making. A number of the factors liable to delay the implementation of a plan should have been recognized and addressed during the plan design stage. Indeed, failures of implementation can frequently be traced to inadequate earlier planning, rather than to incompetence on the part of those charged with implementing the plan. Figure 12.1 sets out diagrammatically how these possible failures may be traceable back to inadequate design.

Change in policies or priorities

The cause of the non-implementation of a previously agreed plan can frequently be traced to a change in policy or a shift in priorities. Where this is due to genuine reassessment by all parties, then it should not be a cause for concern, given that the

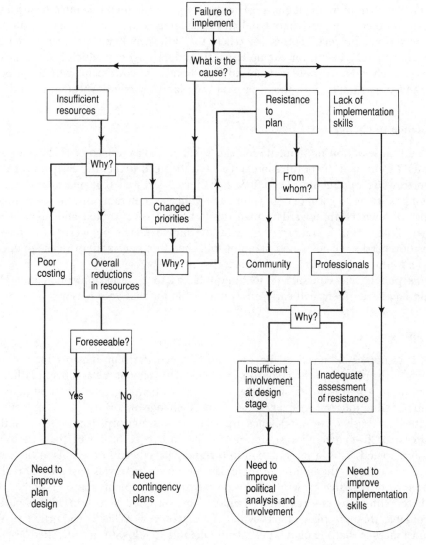

Fig. 12.1 Causes of failure of implementation

role of a plan is to further the adoption of agreed policies. This book has stressed that the concept of the planning spiral must not be taken too literally. It should not therefore be viewed as rigidly chronological. Flexibility is required, and there may be very good reasons for policies to be changed even at a late stage in the development of a plan. It is important, however, that the implications of such changes for planners should be clearly recognized. Delayed implementation of the (new) plan must be seen in such circumstances as likely. Attempting to reorient a plan in a very short time-frame can lead to disastrous effects, and planners need to point this out clearly to policy-makers.

On the other hand, when the change in policy is less the result of a deliberate change in priorities than of an inadequate earlier policy analysis, then this must be attributed to a failure to consider alternative policies adequately at the priority-setting stage.

More serious, however, is the case where the shift in policy is external rather than internal. This may occur, for example, within a donor agency which has changed its policies. Such changed policies may now no longer be consistent with those of the plan, and in particular with those parts of the plan they were expected to fund.

Resistance to change

A second cause of non-implementation can be identified as resistance to the plan itself. Chapter 2 examined the politics of change, and the need to identify early on the likely supporters and opponents of a policy. It has been stressed that one of the skills of planning is trying to garner support for such policies, preferably through engendering feelings of 'ownership' towards a plan through early involvement and identification with it. Where this is not possible then alternative means of overcoming possible opposition need devising. Good planning will therefore have anticipated such opposition, and either overcome it or absorbed it.

Some policies, of course, are so unpopular as to be non-implementable. These should have been identified early on as unfeasible for that very reason.

Lack of resources

Plans may not be achieved owing to a gap between the requirements for resources implicit in the plans and the resources available. This may occur as a result either of a reduction in the resources available or of costs being greater than anticipated. Resource reductions may occur either from a change in priorities (either internal priorities or those of donors) since the plan was drawn up, leading to a shift of resources, or from overall resource levels that prove to be lower than those that were anticipated. This latter situation in turn may have been foreseeable at the design stage. For example, the failure to implement because a plan was based on unrealistic projections of resource growth is a design rather than implementation issue.

Where extraneous unforeseeable circumstances have led to a shortfall it is perhaps unavoidable that the plan targets will not be achieved. What is important in such circumstances is that the plan is sufficiently flexible to allow for a controlled response to the resource gap.

Where the resource gap is due to poor costing or an inadequate assessment of the demand for services, then poor design again appears to be the cause.

Lack of programme specificity

A further cause of poor implementation can be traced to a failure to ensure that the various components of the programme or project being planned are well specified. A failure to quantify particular resources accurately, or to identify when the resources are required, can often lead to major delays or unplanned changes in the type of service provided.

Lack of appropriate managerial skills or structure

The last major cause of non-implementation can be traced back to a lack of managerial skills or inadequate organizational structure. Successful implementation of plans needs more than just acceptable policies, and adequate resources; it also requires managerial skills and an organizational framework within which these can operate.

IMPROVING THE RECORD ON IMPLEMENTATION

The preceding discussion suggests three types of poor implementation:

- unavoidable, through, for example, genuine policy changes or unforeseeable extraneous circumstances
- related to failures at earlier parts of the planning cycle
- related to failures at the programming and implementation stage.

The remainder of this chapter looks more closely at how the record can be improved through techniques at the programming and implementation stages.

Improving the relationship between planning and service management

Most plans suggest changes in service delivery, and, in this sense, the real implementers of a plan are the service managers. Failure to involve them may lead to a rejection of the plan or to poor estimation of the resources required to carry it out. A number of difficulties in implementation are attributable to a failure to define a proper role for service-managers in the planning process. Figure 12.2 suggests an appropriate balance between planning as an activity and the implementation of changes in direction, level or type of services, and the eventual ongoing management of those services.

At the early, formative stages of a plan the major responsibility for planning rests with the planner. However, involvement of service managers will help to ensure commitment to the plan. As the plan becomes more detailed and specific services or projects are planned it becomes even more important that the managers who will eventually be responsible for running the service are involved, to ensure that the

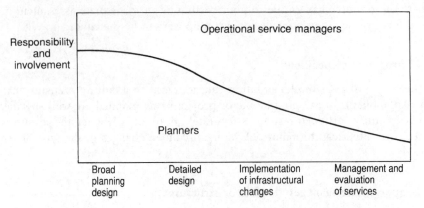

Fig. 12.2 Relationship between full-time planners and managers

service as planned is feasible. The people who will manage such services are those best placed to judge the resource and organizational requirements.

The next stage in the development of a new (or changed) service is the actual implementation of any necessary infrastructural changes. This may include construction of buildings, equipment purchases, or staff training. Again, in all these areas it is important to involve service managers and representatives of the professions who will operate the service. There are countless examples of badly designed buildings or inappropriate equipment that can be traced back to a failure to consult the future service providers.

The penultimate stage is the actual commencement and operation of the changed or new service. Responsibility now lies squarely with the service-manager, though in the early days close contact with the planner is desirable to overcome any unforeseen problems. The last stage relates to the point at which the services are operating normally, and the role of the planner at this stage is one of support and evaluation. Management theory that stresses the idea *of management by objectives* accords well with this approach, by ensuring that service-managers are constantly relating their activities to wider objectives.

The preceding may appear very obvious. It is remarkable, however, how often planners fail to co-ordinate with and involve the managers of the services — with resultant service deficiencies. Part of the reason for such co-ordination failures lies in the administrative processes and structures of planning, which are discussed in Chapter 14.

Ensuring a close and well-defined working relationship between planners and service managers is, however, not enough to ensure effective implementation even of a well-resourced plan with strong policy commitment. Implementation of changes involves the bringing together of resources of personnel, buildings, equipment, and supplies to the same place at the same time, and one of the major skills required here is an ability to co-ordinate the timing of such inputs. We referred to this process at the beginning of the book as *activity planning*, as distinguished from the broader, more strategic *allocative planning*.

The role of a planner at the programming and implementation stage is that of a co-ordinator of a team comprising members with very different sets of skills. Within this, one particular specialist activity is that of both co-ordinating, where necessary, architects and capital planners, and acting as a bridge between them and other members of the planning team. The responsibilities of the planner in this process are to ensure that:

- the inputs required for the service are well specified

- there is a clear and appropriate organizational and management structure

- those involved in the process understand both their general and their specific responsibilities

- a timetable for each activity is set and adhered to

- funding is secured and released on time

- the budget as set is adhered to

- monitoring of the activity occurs

- where relevant, there are clear links between the architect, the contractor, and equipment suppliers and the team (usually through the planner)

- links with other agencies, ministries, and the community are maintained.

Organizational and legislative framework

Some plans require legislative changes. There may also be a need for modification to the organizational framework of the health service. This is particularly the case with the current interest in Health Sector Reform (HSR) which, it has been suggested, should form an important part of health sector planning. Many plans lay emphasis on the physical resources required to implement change, and neglect these wider changes to the legislative and organizational framework. Responsibility for ensuring that this occurs lies with the planning function, though it may not itself have the requisite skills or authority to make the changes.

Documentation

Clear documentation is another way of improving implementation. Project or programme documents are formal documents outlining the precise nature of a new development activity. As such, they have three functions:

- to act as a checklist to ensure all aspects have been considered

- to provide documentation for the funding body's decision-making process[1]

---

[1] Each funding body is likely to have its own standard format. Such bodies include both external donor agencies and the central finance ministry. The health ministry itself may have such a standard format for approving new activities.

- to provide a document which can form the basis of the monitoring and eventually the evaluation of the activity.

Such documents are usually associated with projects, and particularly those which involve outside funding. It is important that the planning process also documents other major shifts in service provision, however, even where they do not involve capital budgets or external funding. These formal, usually standard-format, documents, are essentially used to seek authority and funds, and to ensure that no major obstacles exist. Allied to them are other working documents which are required to ensure that a project will both work and meet its objectives, from an operational point of view.

The relative timing of these two sets of documents will vary. Logically it may appear sensible to sort out operational details before applying for funding. However, it may be inefficient to go into great operational details until firm funding is secured. The issue is likely to be resolved by timing considerations specific to each country and its annual timetable.

It is important to note that submission of a project document (however well argued and presented) may be a necessary condition, but is not a sufficient condition for gaining support for a project. Any project which involves change of any kind will have its opponents. It is important that this is recognized in order that the case can be argued and support can be gained in the corridors as well as on paper. In many situations, in fact, the project document may serve only as a formal statement of a request which has already been informally canvassed and agreed.

The document's second function, however, that of acting as a checklist, can be an important tool for ensuring that the planner has considered all the possible difficulties which face the programme, and whether they will constrain the project unduly. These of course should have been examined at the appraisal stage, and include difficulties of the following nature:

- socio-cultural or ethical

- social, economic and political

- gender

- resource-based, including those of financial availability

- difficulties of sustainability

- difficulties of acceptability

- administrative and legal difficulties

- difficulties of scarcity of personnel

- technical difficulties

- ecological or environmental difficulties.

Chapter 10 examined these in more detail.

The third function of such documentation is as a means of monitoring the progress of an activity. As such a clear statement of the type and timing of inputs and activities is required. This aspect of planning, which was referred to at the beginning of the book as 'activity planning', is a crucial one in the process of implementation. Techniques for ensuring its success are discussed further below.

Box 12.1 provides an example of the information a project document may require.

It will be noted that the various issues raised above are covered in the different sections of the document. Some agencies use a *Logical Framework* approach as part of their overall project documentation; see Nancholas (1998) for a description of the logical framework approach. This requires the methodical identification of the hierarchical objectives and outputs of the programme and the inputs required to achieve them. What makes it different from a normal project document is that it also requires the identification of indicators to measure whether each of these have been achieved. It also requires, prior to the project, identification of any assumptions or risks upon which the objectives, outputs, and inputs rest. Failure to realize these assumptions would lead to a failure to meet these three levels of project success. Box 12.2 gives an example of a completed Logical Framework. It is a useful means of attempting to ensure that the various possible constraints to the implementation and success of a project are identified at the project design stage. It can also provide a mechanism for ensuring that a project team are in agreement as the specific aims, objectives and approaches of a project.

A second type of document which is invaluable is an operational policy for the service to be delivered. This is a document which lays out the detailed workings of the service. Box 12.3 gives an example of the content of an operational policy.

Timetabling of implementation

We have already suggested that many of the failures of implementation relate to a lack of co-ordination of the real resources (including personnel, equipment, and building) and a lack of realism about timing. Delays in project implementation are not only a problem in themselves, but may cause problems of cost overruns and frustrated expectations on the part of both staff and the community. Realistic timetabling is therefore essential as a means of accurate costing and maintenance of planning credibility. In order to minimize delays as a result of this, various managerial techniques exist. These are often given the generic name of *network analysis*. These techniques vary from crude flowcharts to the more sophisticated critical path analysis.

- A *flowchart* sets out, in order of occurrence, the various steps which need to be gone through, dividing where necessary where options occur and decisions have to be made. More than one activity can be occurring at the same time. Figure 12.3 sets out the main steps in a project, such as the construction and operation of a health centre, which has already been identified as part of a programme. While the exact sequence of events may vary for different projects, this shows the main steps for projects where building work is required. Where projects include no building work, the diagram can be amended suitably. Construction of such a flowchart with dates on it is a useful basis for the monitoring of a project.

Box 12.1   Example of the format of a project document

Summary:
Name of project
Budget number of project
Summary of project's objectives and scope
Summary of project costs

Details:
- Aims and objectives of project
- Quantifiable targets set
- Background documentation (consultancy reports, feasibility studies)
- Relationship with any national, including health, plans
- Description of the project
- Inputs required, quantified, and specified

  – personnel
  – other recurrent items
  – equipment
  – transport
  – buildings

- Costs by year by item, recurrent and capital. How costs were calculated
- Funding source

  – donor funds
  – loan
  – community
  – central government
  – redeployment of existing resources

- Arrangements for the activities of the project (where relevant) at the end of the funding period
- Any difficulties (other than financial) foreseen in procuring inputs.
- Any training requirements?
- If there is a building requirement, has a site been identified/procured?
- Legislative requirements
- Organizational and management arrangements
- Relationship with other ministries, agencies, communities?
- Any environmental or negative health effects?
- Timetable for implementation and critical points
- Process for monitoring and evaluation
- Flexibility to respond to change

Box 12.2   Example of a logical framework for a reproductive health programme
Source: Nancholas (1998) reprinted with permission

Vertical hierarchy of objectives	Objectively verifiable indicators (OVI)	Means of verification (MOV)	Assumptions
Goal: To improve reproductive health (RH) in Sambura Province	31 March 2001: Maternal mortality rate decreased by 20% Maternal morbidity rate reduced by 20% Infant mortality rate reduced by 15% Cases of STD/HIV/AIDS rduccd by 12% TFR[a] reduced by 4%	Provincial government health statistics Summative evaluation report	High morbidity, mortality and fertility rates are due to lack of knowledge and/or access to quality services Government and provincial government will endorse and support the programmes Funding will be approved and available Economic and political stability will prevail
Purpose: Increased use of RH services in Sambura Province	By 31 March 2001: Clinic attendance by women will increase by 30% Men attending men's clinics will increase by 15% Adolescent clinic attendance will increase by 60% Contraceptive prevalence rate will increase by 30% 60% of the rural population will report knowledge of and access to the CBD[b] and/of mobile RH program services	Programme monthly reports Clinic records for attendance, care given, and stocks used	The relevant people will be interested to listen to the broadcasts and more fully utilize the clinics Access to clinics and rural services will be much improved by the programme The services offered are acceptable and appropriate to the needs of the population
Outputs: 1 12 existing RH facilities upgraded and equipped, staffed and operational 2 Antenatal, postnatal, family planning, STD/HIV/AIDS, adolescent, men's and MCH services established and operational at each clinic	12 clinics upgraded, staffed and equipped by 30 September 1998 36 staff fully trained in the specialist services to be offered by 30 September 1999 All specialist clinic services available in each ccntre by 1 January 1999	Programme monthly reports Accountant's records Trainer's reports October 1999 Mid-term Review Recorded broadcasts Evaluation report	Equipment and supplies will be consistently available and logistically well organized Trained staff will serve the programme throughout its duration

[a] TFR = Total Fertility Rate
[b] CBD = Community Based Distribution

Box 12.2   *(continued)*

Vertical hierarchy of objectives	Objectively verifiable indicators (OVI)	Means of verification (MOV)	Assumptions
3 4 mobile clinic rural outreach services established and operational covering 80% of the province 4 CBD programme established in 4 areas 5 Monthly radio broadcasts organized for one year 6 End of programme evaluation report disseminated and revised continuation process established	4 mobile clinics for rural areas functional by 1 January 1999 8 CBD workers trained, equipped and programme established by 30 September 1998 12 monthly radio programmes, discussed, prepared and broadcast by 30 September 1998 Monitoring reports analysed to compile a summative programme evaluation report by 31 March 2001. Report disseminated to relevant stakeholders by end of March 2001		
Activities: 1.1 Secure funding and plans for RH facilities, appoint contractors 1.2 Ensure facilities upgraded to specifications 1.3 Order supplies and equipment for clinics 1.4 Arrange specialist refresher training for existing staff 1.5 Appoint new, qualified and experienced staff for programmes 2.1 Check that all services are provided and fully operational 2.2 Ensure radio broadcasts advertise these services 3.1 Arrange mobile outreach services with communities and staff	Inputs: Clinic upgrading rehabilitation programme (including staff salaries and training costs) $668 000 Mobile outreach services program $20 800 CBD program $30 353 Radio broadcast airtime $4 200 Monitoring/evaluation $5 000 Total: $728 353 NB. These costs are only approximate	Accountant's records	

Box 12.2 (*continued*)

Vertical hierarchy of objectives	Objectively verifiable indicators (OVI)	Means of verification (MOV)	Assumptions
4.1 Recruit and train CBD workers			
4.2 Prepare and implement CBD programme			
5.1 Prepare and organize monthly RH radio broadcasts for one year			
6.1 Set up fomative and monitoring processes. Monthly reporting systems for each programme			
6.2 Conduct overall evaluation, prepare, report and establish revised plans			

Box 12.3 Example of the content of an operational policy for a new health centre

- Objectives of the health-centre-based service
- Broad description of the services to be provided
- Detailed description of how the services will be organized (including, for example, outpatient flows between waiting, history-taking, diagnosis, dispensing, etc.)
- Resource implications — personnel, supplies, equipment, buildings
- Management arrangements
- Outline job descriptions for staff
- Relationships with other parts of the health service, other sectors, and the community.

- Figure 12.4 sets out a *bar chart* (sometimes known as a *Gantt chart*) for the same project, showing the order in which events have to occur, and their duration. Any change or delay in one of these activities may lead to a corresponding delay in subsequent activities. For example, a delay in arranging training may result in missing a course start-date, and ultimately to delay in starting the new service.

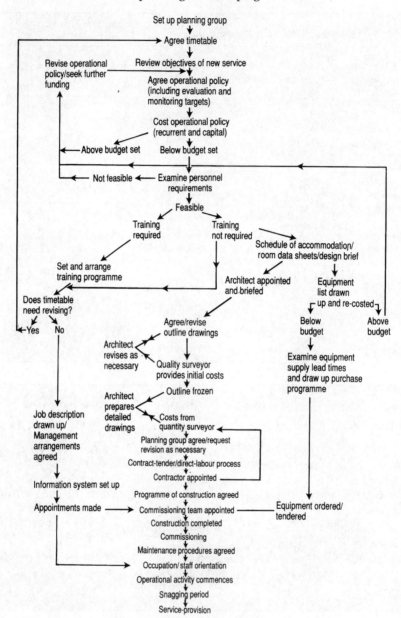

Fig. 12.3　Example of a flow chart for the implementation of a health centre project

Construction schedule

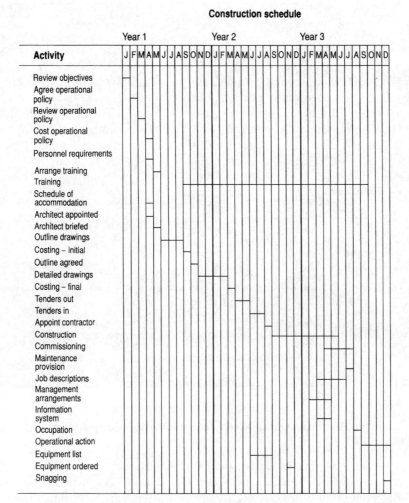

Fig. 12.4   Example of a bar chart for the implementation of a health centre project

- *Critical path analysis* uses the same basis but superimposes on it estimates of the time required to carry out each discrete component. The critical path is the path which provides the overall time constraints on the project. Delays may be possible in activities which do not fall on the critical path. Any delay in the critical activities will lead to an overall delay in implementation. Box 12.4 gives a simple illustrative example of a critical path analysis of a construction project, in which a number of activities can occur in parallel.

Critical path analysis is the most 'scientific' and precise of these techniques, but simple flowcharts in combination with an activity plan provide useful and adequate monitoring tools for most situations.

Box 12.4   Example of critical path analysis

The following shows an analysis of the time taken to carry out the different activities involved in the construction of a basic building. The shortest time for completion is 51 days, which is obtained by following the critical path. The critical path is the longest path through the schedule, which involves foundation (10 days), plus walls (20 days), plus electrical (10 days), plus electrical checks (1 day), plus paint (10 days). A delay in any of the critical events would lead to an overall delay in completion. The other activities of roofing and plumbing have some slack time. Some delay in these events would not hold up the overall completion.

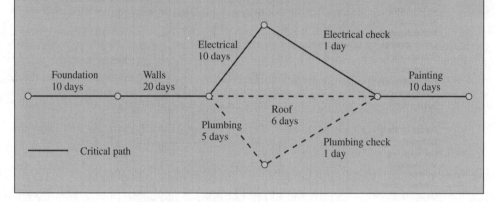

A number of points need making about the process as laid out in the flowchart shown in Fig. 12.3.

- Firstly, its iterative nature. At various points in the process it may be necessary to return to an earlier stage and amend earlier decisions. This is usually the result either of a recognition of timetabling changes, or of changes in resource (and, in particular, finance) implications. As detailed costs emerge, it may be necessary, where these exceed original estimates, to revise the objectives of the service, or the manner in which the service is to be provided.

- Secondly, the diagram emphasizes the need for a planning group, composed of planners, service managers, and hopefully user or community representatives. One of the key functions of this group is to develop the type of operational policy discussed earlier.

- A third point to note is the relationship between the physical planning activity and the service planning activity. The relationship between health planners and architects is a delicate one, which, when working well, can produce imaginative, workable, and productive results. When it works poorly, however, it can lead to buildings which constrain the function for which they were intended. The role of the architect in planning is to convert the service requirements into a workable environment. For this to be successful the architect needs to be given sufficient and accurate information on how the service is to operate. A brief to an architect which requests 'an out-patient clinic' has little chance of meeting the real, albeit unstated, requirements. At the other extreme lies the service planner who is a frustrated architect and wants to impose her/his design solution on the service requirements. What is required is a recognition on both sides of the appropriate respective roles. The planner's role is to ensure that the health service provides the architect with a clear statement of its needs. That of the architect is to provide solution(s) to this with respect to the building and in line with cost constraints. One important role for the planner in this context is ensuring that the budget is adhered to and, where necessary, that the costly desires of either the health professionals or the architect are kept in check.

- A final point relates to the last stage of the implementation prior to the actual commencement of the service itself. Too often insufficient attention is paid to orienting staff to their new positions, commissioning new equipment, and obtaining agreement on maintenance procedure. It is important that adequate time is allotted for these key startup activities.

MONITORING

One of the functions of the planner during the implementation period is the overall monitoring of activity. In this context monitoring is the process of observing whether the planned shifts in an activity or service are occurring. Monitoring needs to provide the opportunity to spot difficulties in implementation that are occurring early enough to take any remedial action. Various means of doing this have already been referred to, including the use of logframes, activity plans, and schedules. Another important method of monitoring is through financial management information systems. Financial monitoring can be used not only as a means of ensuring that budgets are adhered to, but also as an indicator of general planning activity. However, it is important that such information is not viewed as the sole indicator of progress. Unfortunately, this is the practice with some large donor agencies which are more concerned with ensuring that expenditure occurs as planned rather than that appropriate changes are accomplished.

It has become the practice of some large donors to insist on the development of specific project units to monitor the implementation of specific projects. This vertical approach to project monitoring has a number of serious drawbacks.

- Firstly, the dislocation of such implementation units from the broader planning process can be very distorting. Planning and implementation, it has been argued, should be seen as part of the same process. Planning that does not result in implementation is widely recognized to have failed. However, the converse can be equally serious, though this is not always recognized. Implementation that does not link into the broader process of planning (particularly where there is a flexible approach to planning which builds in the possibility of plan changes periodically) can result in the carrying out of activities that are no longer relevant. Large donor projects are frequently implemented several years after their conception and design. It is essential that linkages into the broader planning system are made in order to keep such projects consistent with changing needs, and to allow the possibility of change during implementation.

- Secondly, the development of project implementation units may serve the needs of donor agencies well. They help to ensure that the completion of activities and the disbursement of funds occurs as intended. However, where they are project-specific, they are unlikely to develop a more sustained institutional basis for implementation within an organization.

It is strongly suggested that donor agencies need to take a longer-term and broader perspective on the need to develop institutional capacity to implement within an organization, and to design their project-implementation arrangements accordingly.

The adoption of *Sector Wide Approaches* with donors pooling resources in support of a broad health ministry strategy which is being tried in some countries (see p. 110) is in part a recognition by donors of the unrealistic and unnecessary pressures placed by them in the formulation and monitoring of specific donor projects and may lead to an amelioration of the above difficulties.

LOCATION OF PROJECTS AND PROGRAMMES

One common cause of delay in the implementation of (particularly though not exclusively construction) projects is difficulties over their location. A specific function of the planner is to ensure that the location of the new or expanded facilities is specified. In doing so, a number of factors need to be borne in mind, including the following:

- health plans
- the nearest existing facilities of similar type (in distance and time)
- the catchment area and its population
- the nearest existing referral facilities
- political factors (community desires, community leaders' desires, politicians' desires)
- the availability and cost of suitable land or building
- accessibility and travel time and ease
  - for staff
  - for support services
  - for the community

- other agency/ministry developments
- the availability of staff accommodation.

IMPLEMENTATION OF SERVICES PROVIDED BY OTHER AGENCIES

The preceding treatment has concentrated on aspects of the implementation of developments within a health plan over which the health planner has a degree of direct control. However, we have suggested that plans should take as broad a perspective as possible, and incorporate the activities of other organizations and sectors, both health and health-related. In these cases, the health planner working from within the health ministry will have a far more limited role in implementation. This may include joining the project team to ensure co-ordination. Where the information systems allow, assistance in the monitoring role may also be possible.

SUMMARY

This chapter has looked at the stages of programming and implementation. A number of the causes of poor implementation of plans derive from poor earlier planning. However, even where activities have been well specified, implementation may be delayed or distorted by a lack of skills at the implementation stage. There are a number of techniques which can be used to assist in ensuring that activities are carried out in a comprehensive and timely fashion.

INTRODUCTORY READING

For an introduction to the problems behind implementation see Bowden (1986) and Hogwood and Gunn (1984). Goodman and Love (1980) provide management techniques for assisting in overcoming problems with the implementation rather than the design aspects of programmes. Nancholas (1998) describes the use of logframes in planning. For the physical aspects of planning, Wells (1976) is a classic example of health centre design. The four volumes by Kleczkowski and Pibouleau (1976, 1977, 1979, 1983) are also useful sources of information. Issues of the location of facilities are introduced by Massam *et al.* (1986) and Stock (1983). Unger and Criel (1995) look at health infrastructure planning and Doherty *et al.* (1996) look at locational criteria for primary health planning. Gosling and Edwards (1995) provide a useful guide and monitoring and evaluation.

EXERCISE 12

A new training programme is being designed for community health workers (CHW). It will have the following components:

Training of trainers	3 weeks
Curriculum development	6 weeks
Recruitment of community health worker trainees	3 weeks
Approval of funding	4 weeks
Training of community health workers	4 weeks
Purchase of first-aid kits for CHWs	6 weeks

Draw up a chart showing the order in which you feel these activities need to occur. From this determine the critical path. How long would the overall programme take? If the training of trainers was extended to 4 weeks, what would the overall length of the programme be?

REFERENCES AND FURTHER READING

Allen, D. E. (1979). *Hospital planning.* Pitman Medical, London.

Bowden, P. (1986). Problems of implementation. *Public Administration and Development,* 6, 612–71.

De Winter, E. (1992). Are we ignoring population density in health planning? The issues of availability and accessibility. *Health Policy and Planning,* 7(2), 191–2.

Doherty, J., Rispel, L., and Webb, N. (1996). Developing a plan for primary health care facilities in Soweto, South Africa: part II: applying locational criteria. *Health Policy and Planning,* 11(4), 394–405.

Goodman, L. J. and Love, R. N. (1980). *Project planning and management.* Pergamon, New York.

Gosling, L. and Edwards, M. (1995). *Toolkits: a practical guide to assessment, monitoring review and evaluation.* Save the Children, London.

Hogwood, B. and Gunn, B. (1984). *Policy analysis for the real world,* Chapter 11. Oxford University Press, Oxford.

Kleczkowski, B. and Pibouleau, R. (1976). *Approaches to planning and design of health care facilities in developing areas,* Vol. 1. World Health Organization, Geneva.

Kleczkowski, B. and Pibouleau, R. (1977). *Approaches to planning and design of health care facilities in developing areas,* Vol. 2. World Health Organization, Geneva.

Kleczkowski, B. and Pibouleau, R. (1979). *Approaches to planning and design of health care facilities in developing areas,* Vol. 3. World Health Organization, Geneva.

Kleczkowski, B. and Pibouleau, R. (1983). *Approaches to planning and design of health care facilities in developing areas,* Vol. 4. World Health Organization, Geneva.

Kleczkowski, B. and Wilson, N. D. (1984). *Health care facility projects in developing areas: planning, implementing and operations.* WHO, Geneva.

Llewelyn-Davies, R. (1976). Planning health facilities in developing countries: some case studies and their lessons. *World Hospitals,* 12, 159–63.

Massam, B. H., Aktar, R., and Askew, I. D. (1986). Applying operations research to health planning: locating health centres in Zambia. *Health Policy and Planning,* 1, 326–34.

Mein, P. and Jorgenson, T. (1978). *Design for medical buildings: a manual for the planning and* building of health care facilities under conditions of limited resources. Housing Research and Development Unit, University of Nairobi.

Nancholas, S. (1998). How to do or not to do a Logical Framework. *Health Policy and Planning*, 13(2), 189–93.

Palmer, C. and Innes, C. (1980). *Operational research by example*. Macmillan, London.

Phillips, D. (1981). *Contemporary issues in the geography of health care*. Geo Books, Norwich.

Ross, D. (1990). Aid co-ordination. *Public Administration and Development*, 10, 331–42.

Stock, R. (1983). Distance and the utilization of health facilities in rural Nigeria. *Social Science and Medicine*, 17, 563–70.

Unger, J. P and Criel, B. (1995). Principles of health infrastructure planning in less developed countries. *International Journal of Health Planning and Management*, 10(2), 113–28.

Wells, M. A. (1976). *A model health centre*. London Conference of Missionary Societies.

Planning human resources

Of all the inputs into the provision of health-care, human resources are the most important, constituting up to 75% of expenditure in some countries. In recognition of this, a sub-specialty of planning, *human resource planning*, has grown up. This chapter introduces human resource planning and looks at its role in, and relationship to, the broader function of health planning. Within the wider literature the term 'manpower planning' is commonly used, but it will be deliberately avoided here because of the gender bias present in the term 'manpower'.

WHAT IS HUMAN RESOURCE PLANNING?

The objective of human resource planning is to ensure that there is the right number of personnel with the appropriate skills available in the right place at the right time. This definition clearly begs a number of questions, including what is meant by 'right' and 'appropriate'. As we shall see, these questions are only to be answered by reference to the broader field of health planning, of which human resource planning is one sub-activity.

Human resource planning is a critical activity within the broader sectoral planning activity. Health services rely heavily on personnel. They are very labour intensive, with between 60% and 75% of the health-sector recurrent budget being spent on the provision of this particular resource. If human resources are poorly planned, therefore, the implications for the health sector itself can be extremely serious. Indeed, some argue that if planners concentrated solely on human resource planning then the task of planning the health sector itself would naturally follow; however, this is an extreme and unrealistic position. There are numerous examples of adequate numbers of well-trained staff frustrated and unable to operate as a result of a poor supply of other complementary resources such as, for example, drugs.

Later in the chapter we will discuss the various possible relationships between the broad activity of health sectoral planning, and the more specific activity of human resource planning. Suffice it to say at this point that a balance between overall sectoral planning and human resource planning is needed. However, this is not to deny the importance of human resource planning as a specialty in itself, as indicated by the number of specialist books on the subject which have been written.

THE RECORD ON HUMAN RESOURCE PLANNING

Despite the above, however, the record on human resource planning is still poor in many countries, as is evidenced by a variety of symptoms of malaise. Common problems include the following:

- *Too few trained and available personnel.* Most countries have shortages of certain groups of health professionals, particularly in those fields which require extensive education, such as doctors, pharmacists, laboratory technologists, and nursing specialists. Which particular cadres are in short supply will vary from country to country.

- *Too many trained and unemployable personnel.* In contrast, in some countries there has been an overproduction of certain groups of health professional, leading either to their being inefficiently employed in inappropriate situations, or their remaining unemployed. It should, of course, be noted that it is not uncommon to have both too many of one cadre, and too few of another, within the same country.

- *Distributional difficulties.* It is perfectly possible for either of the above problems to manifest itself within a particular subsector or region of a country, while overall in the country there may be a balance of personnel. For example, within a country there may be an appropriate overall number of doctors, but their concentration in urban hospital settings may lead to shortages elsewhere.

- *Inappropriate use of personnel.* Even in situations of balanced supply, staff may be inappropriately used for their levels of skill. For example, to employ highly trained nurses to carry out basic bedside nursing duties which could be performed by less trained staff may be an inefficient use of such staff, although it is possible that the other benefits gained through the contact with the patient (e.g. observation) provided by basic nursing care may make the use of more skilled staff in such situations worthwhile.The development of auxiliary cadres might be an appropriate response to such inefficiency. Elsewhere such inefficiency may be the result of an oversupply of a cadre. For example, overproduction of doctors in some countries has led to their routine employment in management positions requiring no medical skills.

- *Unproductive or demoralized staff.* A less measurable and tangible problem which can have serious implications for the delivery of health-care is that of demoralized staff, whose output is consequently lower than it should be. Low morale may arise from a variety of factors, including low pay or poor conditions of service (including, for example, poor access to housing) relative to the same cadre in the private sector or in neighbouring countries, or to comparable workers in other sectors. It may also be due to low job satisfaction, perhaps arising from a lack of adequate complementary resources such as drugs, from poor equipment, or from a poor management style.

WHY IS THE RECORD ON HUMAN RESOURCE PLANNING SO POOR?

There are various reasons why, in any particular country, the record on human resource planning is poor, resulting in one or more of the symptoms described above. Clearly human resource planning can suffer from any of the pitfalls which face planning in general, and which are discussed in earlier chapters. However, in addition to these, there are problems specific to human resource planning, including the following:

- *High supply lead-times*. In many of the health professions, training times are substantial. Medical training, for example, may require a minimum of six years. As a result, decisions to alter the supply of a cadre through changing training numbers are often slow to filter through to the service.

- *Professional attitudes*. Although planners rightly regard personnel as only one of several resource inputs, it clearly has special attributes not shared by other resources. In particular it is typically not passive in its response to proposed changes in the roles or functions of professions. The aspirations or attitudes of the health professions may run counter to those of whoever is planning the service. For example, doctors in some countries may see the introduction of medical auxiliaries as a threat to their livelihood or status, and may resist it. Similarly, attempts to redress distributional imbalances may meet strong opposition. In this sense the previously mentioned role of a planner as a political analyst with the task of anticipating resistance or indeed support from particular quarters should not be underestimated.

- *Lack of an appropriate body responsible for human resource planning*. In some countries, there is no clearly defined organization or unit responsible for health-sector human resource planning, resulting in a confusion of planning roles. In other countries a body does exist with defined human resource planning responsibilities, but with little power, or not tied into the broader planning process. Human resource planning failures may occur, for example, when health training schools fall under the education ministry, with health planners unable to influence either the curriculum or the intake of such schools. Other scenarios encountered include the responsibility for human resource planning functions being held either by a central government department or by a health ministry personnel department with poor relationships with the same ministry's planning department.

- *Lack of accurate or usable data*. Partly as a result of previous inattention to the importance of human resource planning, there is often a major lack of information on various aspects of personnel. This information gap may range from basic data on present staff numbers and deployment to more sophisticated information on retirement or attrition rates.

- *The presence of a significant private sector*. One major confounding factor in human resource planning relates to the presence in some countries of a significant private sector. The consequent drain of staff from the public sector is clearly a problem for the health ministry, and attitudes to this will reflect attitudes to the private sector as a whole. However, the more specific difficulty which faces the human resource planner is often the unpredictability of the private sector. If the private sector were to siphon off a known number of staff annually, this would, of course, have implications for the training budget, but such information could be built into a human resource planning model, alongside the public sector requirements. However, lack of such information is a frequent characteristic of the private sector.

HUMAN RESOURCE PLANNING — AN APPROACH

It would appear, then, that the record on human resource planning is often poor, for a number of reasons. Let us now turn to approaches to human resource planning. The elements of human resource planning can be most easily conceptualized as a model, the basis of which is given in Fig. 13.1.

A significant part of human resource planning is related to quantifying the factors which impinge on this model, and analysing the effect which different policies will have on these variables. It is essential, however, to recognize the dangers of reducing the process simply to that of a quantified model, looking only at inputs and outputs and ignoring the less measurable effects which the process itself will generate. Such effects may include resistance by professional groups to particular proposals which they perceive as affecting them. We will begin by examining the model, and then return to these variables.

There are essentially two components in the process of human resource planning: supply of, and demand (or requirements) for, personnel. This is complicated firstly by the fact that these variables are not static, but alter over time, so that data on projected flows over a number of years are required; and secondly by the fact that constant revision and updating is required as assumptions prove to be wrong, or change. An equilibrium situation is aimed at, in which the demand and supply are equal for each set of staff for each year.

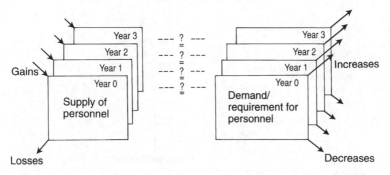

Fig. 13.1   Human resource planning — the essential components

- The *supply* of human resources describes the available (trained and willing to work) personnel. This supply will be affected by gains such as new trained staff, or losses (for example through retirement).

- The *demand* for human resources is the funded requirement (available posts) for personnel. It should be remembered that the term 'demand' is again being used here in the economic sense, to mean a recognized need for staff together with funds to pay for them.

Human resource planning involves estimating projections of each side of the supply-and-demand equation. Where an imbalance is foreseen, steps need to be taken to correct or prevent it. Human resource planning can be carried out at various levels. In particular it is important to be clear whether a comprehensive national perspective is being taken, or one relating primarily to the health ministry or the public sector. Here we will take a national perspective, thereby including the private sector on the overall demand side of the equation. If a purely public sector approach were taken instead, the private sector would still be taken account of, but as one of the drains on the supply side.

The steps involved in drawing up a human resource plan are shown in Fig. 13.2, and are considered separately. The diagram refers to a single cadre of health professionals. Overall the plan would need to repeat the process for each cadre.

The model is essentially straightforward, requiring the estimation of projections of the number of staff needed (the demand) in each cadre and the number likely to be available (the supply). Where there is a mismatch between the demand and supply of any cadre the variables which influence either the demand or supply need to be examined and where necessary policy to respond to these developed. Each of these steps is now examined.

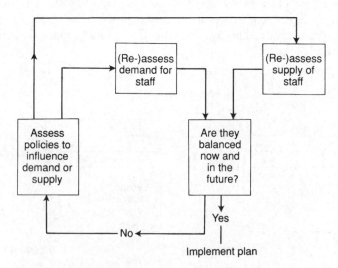

Fig. 13.2   Human resource planning for a single cadre: the major steps in the process

ASSESS DEMAND

The first step involves estimating the demand or requirements for each different professional group for each year over the plan period. Ideally a 10 year period is chosen, given the long lead-times involved in changing levels of personnel.

Four possible models for assessing demand
Four methods of calculating health personnel requirements are to be found in the relevant literature; in particular, see Hall and Mejia (1978) and Hornby *et al.* (1980). They are known as the *health-care demands*, the *health needs*, the *personnel to population ratio*, and the *service targets* methods. These methods are illustrated in Fig. 13.3, and are now briefly introduced.

• The *health-care demands approach* to estimating the demand for health staff forecasts likely future health service utilization. The forecast of this is derived from projections of future socio-economic factors which are assumed to be the major influencing variables. Forecasts of changes in the utilization then lead to forecasts of the likely demand for health staff. By viewing the main determinants of health-care provision as economic factors, such an approach derives from market-driven

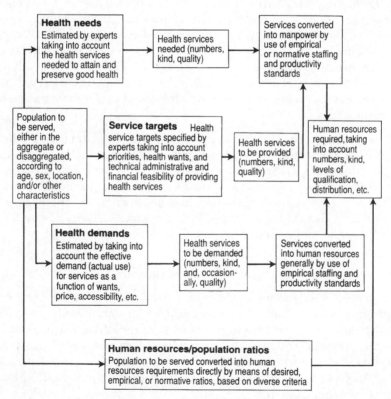

Fig. 13.3 Schematic representation of four method of estimating human resource requirements Reproduced, by permission, from Hall, T. L. and Mejia A. Health Manpower Planning: principles, methods, issues. Geneva, World Health Organization, 1978, p. 62.

approaches to health-care. It therefore unsuitable for a public sector needs-based planning approach, although it may be entirely suitable for a private sector wishing to project future demand for private health-care.

- The *health needs approach* uses assessments by health professionals, based on demographic and epidemiological forecasts, of the future health needs of a population. Although more suited to needs-based planning than the first approach, it has two deficiencies:

  - it is essentially a top-down approach, not allowing community determination of needs, and may reinforce a vertical strategy as health needs become translated into 'diseases'
  - it takes no cognizance of other resource constraints (such as technology) on service expansion. Thus personnel demand is seen to be predicated purely on health needs, and not affected by the need to have a balanced and complementary set of inputs.

- *Personnel to population ratios approach.* In many countries, human resource planning demand estimation is based on the use of set ratios between the population and health personnel. This approach relies on the setting of ratios (often known as *norms*) for health professionals as related to the population size: for example, one doctor per 10 000 population. Once norms have been established, the approach is clearly easy to apply. It is, however, either dependent on professionals' assessment of the personnel needs of a given population, or uses norms from other countries. In both approaches there is an implicit assumption of a consistency both of needs and of health service responses — either between different parts of the same country, or between different countries which is one of the fundamental weaknesses of the approach.

- *Service targets approach.* This last approach involves the setting of specific health service targets and then assesses the personnel requirements to accomplish each of these. Thus for example, the health plan may call for the provision of 10 new health centres each year, each requiring a set number of staff in different categories. As we shall see later in this chapter, when we look more closely at this approach, its major advantage is its close linkages with service plans which allows a more integrated approach to resource (including personnel) planning.

Which approach to demand estimation is most suitable?

In practice it is unlikely that any single method will be used for determining demand, and likely that elements of all of the above will be present. Indeed, it is difficult to conceptualize how either the health needs or norm-based approaches can operate without some prior conception of the services (and hence personnel) needed. Often the issue is the degree to which a method is explicit or implicit. In assessing a specific country approach to determination of the requirements for personnel, a number of questions are worth considering.

However, it is clear that certain approaches are likely to be less appropriate to a needs-based approach to planning. In particular:

- *norm-based planning* may mask issues of distribution and hence of equity

- the *health demands approach* implies a demand- rather than needs-based orientation to planning, and again therefore, for reasons discussed earlier in the book, runs counter to the principle of equity.

- the *health needs planning* may reinforce a more vertical approach to planning through its disease-based approach.

In addition there is a wider danger that human resource planning can be very top-down and centralist, particularly under the health needs and norms approaches.

As we saw in Chapter 8, need is not an absolute concept, and perceptions of it vary depending on the 'perceiver'. Three possible perceptions can be distinguished here: that of the health professional, the planner, and the community. Table 13.1 illustrates how these different perceptions are treated by each of the four models outlined.

The most appropriate approach to human resource planning demand appears to be a *service-targets approach*. Figure 13.4 illustrates this approach, which is now described in more detail..

Table 13.1 Roles under different approaches to human resource planning demand estimation

Model	Roles in human resource planning of:		
	Health professional	Planner	Community
Health demands	No role	As quantifiers	Community demand (not need) used
Health needs	Determined by health professionals	As quantifiers	No role suggested
Norms	Determined by professionals Basis unclear	As quantifiers	No role suggested
Service targets	Dependent on degree of participation in process	Personnel requirements derived from service plans	Dependent on degree of participation in process

Service-targets estimation of demand for human resources

As we have seen above, under this approach, the sectoral plan objectives are translated into services, which in turn are subdivided into a series of tasks, each requiring different skills. A publication from WHO (Shipp 1998) provides details on the methodology for estimating detailed levels of staffing requirement through Workload Indicators of Staffing Need.The skills identified then determine the number and type of personnel required to carry out the service. Breaking down services into tasks

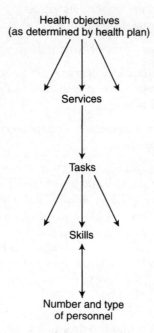

Fig. 13.4   Service targets approach to demand estimation

and then skills leads to the possibility of different staff usages. Such an approach reduces the chance of particular services being immediately identified with particular professionals. It thus allows the possibility of a more creative and efficient use of staff.

One advantage of this approach is that, where the skills identified for carrying out a new task are not all present in one type of staff, the need for training or even new cadres may be identified. Unfortunately this type of detailed task-based examination of services is rarely easy. Where it is not feasible to carry out such a bottom-up approach, the alternative of extrapolating health-personnel requirements from broad service descriptions or indeed from other equivalent services is often used. Box 13.1 provides an example of the approach for mobile immunization services.

ASSESS SUPPLY

The second step in human resource planning involves the estimation of the present and future supply of each cadre of health workers. Supply estimation is conceptually the easier part of human resource planning, although the information required is frequently not available. Some items of information may be estimatable (such as retirements or deaths over time), but others are highly sensitive to policy changes. In particular, the number of trained staff not working as health professionals depends on the style of personnel management and the remuneration policies.

The supply of personnel is essentially a function of six variables, illustrated in Fig. 13.5. The first two of these represent the current stock, and the others represent

Box 13.1   Service targets approach example: mobile immunization programme

Part A shows some of the key tasks that need to be performed to achieve the objective, together with the skills needed to carry out the tasks. Part B illustrates examples of the current cadres who have a particular skill as part of the their training and other staff who could obtain these skills through further training.

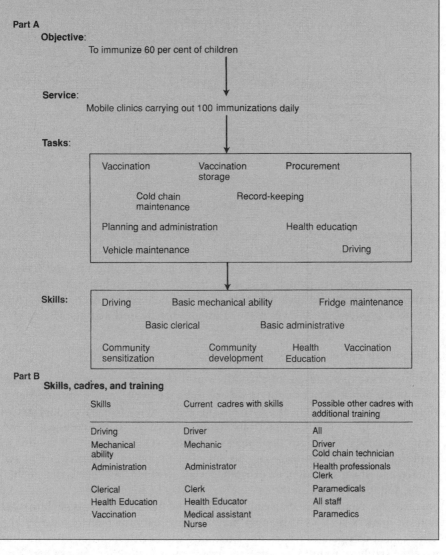

Part A

Objective:

To immunize 60 per cent of children

Service:

Mobile clinics carrying out 100 immunizations daily

Tasks:

Vaccination	Vaccination storage	Procurement
	Cold chain maintenance	Record-keeping
Planning and administration		Health education
Vehicle maintenance		Driving

Skills:

Driving	Basic mechanical ability		Fridge maintenance
	Basic clerical	Basic administrative	
Community sensitization	Community development	Health Education	Vaccination

Part B

Skills, cadres, and training

Skills	Current cadres with skills	Possible other cadres with additional training
Driving	Driver	All
Mechanical ability	Mechanic	Driver Cold chain technician
Administration	Administrator	Health professionals Clerk
Clerical	Clerk	Paramedicals
Health Education	Health Educator	All staff
Vaccination	Medical assistant Nurse	Paramedics

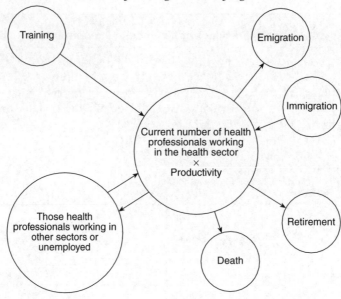

Fig. 13.5   Effective supply of health professionals

dynamic variables which will affect the future stock. In addition, there is a further variable, productivity, which will alter the effective productivity. The process of identifying current and future supply is one of quantifying each of these variables. The steps involved are shown in Fig. 13.6 and briefly outlined below.

Professionals currently working in the health sector

The largest group is those staff currently working in the health sector. Information on those in the public sector ought, in theory, to be relatively easy to obtain from records. However, the reality may be different in some countries where staff records are incomplete. In such situations, information may have to be obtained in the short term by a survey of staff. In the longer term, however, personnel information systems need to be set up. Often these can be linked to the payroll information on staff.

Information on the number of trained staff working in other parts of the health sector, and in particular in the private sector, may be much harder to obtain. In many countries the relationship between the public and private sectors is such that information on matters such as personnel may be provided either on request or regularly. Where such co-operation does not exist, and the health ministry does not currently have the statutory right to insist on information on staff, other sources may have to be used. These will include the professional registers, such as the medical register, where these exist.

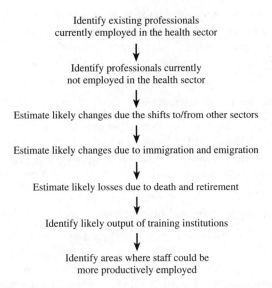

Fig. 13.6 Steps in estimating supply of personnel

Professionals currently not working in the health sector

Information is also needed on trained health professionals who are not currently working in that capacity. Some of these may be actively seeking work and yet, in situations of oversupply, unable to obtain it. Information on these may be available through the personnel office of the health ministry, in situations where such records are kept. Other professionals may, for a variety of reasons, be working in different occupations, and information on these may be far harder to obtain. Where a national picture of the human resource situation is being sought (rather than purely one for the public sector) it should be remembered that staff working in the private sector will already have been included under the first category.

Shifts in trained staff into and out of the health sector

The above information relates to the current situation, which is not static. Shifts may occur as a result of a variety of factors, including the economic situation or personnel policies. Information on losses from, or gains to, the public sector at least should be available from past personnel records.

Immigration and emigration

The stock of health professionals can also be altered by losses as a result of emigration, and by gains as a result of immigration. Although for many countries this may not be significant, elsewhere it can be a major factor. The Gulf states, for example, the health service has relied heavily on migrant labour for a number of years. More recently, migration has become an important factor in the countries of southern Africa, in part as a result of economic and political changes. Information may not always be easy to obtain, although the government department responsible for the issuing of passports or entry or work permits may be able to provide information.

Future losses from death and retirement

The penultimate factor affecting the overall supply of health personnel is the losses arising from the natural factors of retirement and death. These are unlikely to be major factors, but in large professions such as nursing they are likely to be reasonably predictable, provided information on the age-profile of the profession is available.

Future gains to the supply from training schools

The third category of information required is the number of professionals expected to enter the labour market each year from training. These are the outputs of training schools. Information on this is usually readily available from in-country training schools, and can be projected forwards on the basis of intake figures, likely annual attrition rates, and final pass rates. Where training takes place outside the country it may be harder to obtain information. However, information should be obtainable on individuals trained under State scholarships.

Changes in productivity

Lastly, the effective supply of staff will depend not only on personnel numbers but also on their levels of productivity. Where staff can be more efficiently deployed, this can effectively raise the overall supply in real terms. Productivity is affected by the relationship of staff both to other resources, such as equipment, and to other cadres. Appraisal techniques can help to analyse more efficient combinations of different types of staff and of staff with other resources. In addition, productivity is affected by the organizational framework within which staff work, and by the terms and conditions (both monetary and non-monetary) under which they are employed. These are less likely to show up under a more traditional appraisal, and yet may be a major factor in low productivity.

   The above analysis is made from the perspective of the whole health sector, and not just of the public service provision. From the perspective of the State sector a further breakdown as to the likely internal effects of these factors on the different constituent parts of the public sector supply of staff is needed.

   The information should, where possible, be broken down to give both a sub-national picture, particularly where regional imbalances are expected, and a picture of the differences between the public and private sectors. As we have seen, sources of information on the supply of personnel are often not immediately available. However, until a proper personnel information system can be set up it is usually possible to estimate the numbers in each category. Table 13.2 summarizes possible sources of information.

Table 13.2   Possible sources of personnel supply information

Data on:	Source of information
Current supply	Personnel returns, survey, professional registers
Emigration	Foreign affairs records
Immigration	Foreign affairs records
Training output	Training school records, government scholarship records, education ministry
Deaths	National age-specific mortality rates
Retirement	Personnel records
Transfers	Survey register

DETERMINE MISMATCHES BETWEEN THE ESTIMATED DEMAND AND SUPPLY OVER TIME AND LOCATION

Having estimated the demand and supply of each cadre for each year in the plan period, the next task in the development of a personnel plan involves comparison of demand and supply and subsequent analysis of where mismatches leading to either an oversupply or a shortage of a particular group are likely to occur. It might for example recognize that, with current policies, there will be a significant shortage of midwives in four years' time.

DETERMINE APPROPRIATE ACTION TO MINIMIZE MISMATCHES

Once potential mismatches have been identified, policy alternatives as to how such mismatches can be avoided or minimized need to be identified. Such alternatives can be best understood as operating on any of the variables affecting either demand or supply. The broad categories of alternative policy options are given below, and can be seen to relate back to the model variables shown in Fig. 13.1.

Demand-targeted policies

There are two possible policies:

- alter the service targets (up or down) and hence the sectoral plan and consequent personnel requirements, or
- alter the means of providing the service through using alternative personnel mixes (for example the doctor to auxiliary ratio).

Supply-targeted policies

Here there are several alternatives:

- alter the output (up or down) of training institutions
- alter the content of the training programmes to produce different skills
- identify areas where staff can be used more efficiently
- alter personnel policies to recruit health personnel currently not working in the health sector
- alter personnel policies to improve retention rates of staff
- recruit personnel from outside the country.

REGULARLY REVIEW AND UPDATE PLAN

This book argues for a dynamic approach to sectoral planning, with built-in review mechanisms which allow changes to be identified as early as possible. Regular up-dating of information through a personnel information system is desirable, in the same way as we discussed in Chapter 6 in connection with other planning information. Under such an approach personnel plans should be reviewed alongside the sectoral plan, as changes in the one have repercussions on the other. Although it has been suggested that a 10 year human resource plan is advisable because of the lead times involved, this does not prevent its being updated on a regular basis. In Chapter 14 we introduce the use of rolling sectoral plans. Such an approach is also well suited to the process of human resource planning.

HUMAN RESOURCE PLANNING IMPLEMENTATION

Once a personnel plan has been drawn up, there are three major approaches to ensure its implementation. These are control of the overall establishment, development of a training plan, and ensuring that personnel policies are consistent with the plan.

Establishment control

It is important that once one has, in the personnel plan, identified the needs for staff, these targets are adhered to as far as possible. The estimation of demand should lead naturally into the forecasting of requirements for new posts, and indeed in some cases into planning for a reduction or abolition of posts. Although the plan should not become a rigid tool, it is important that reviews of the establishment should take account of the plan, and that it should only be deviated from in exceptional circum-stances. If the plan is a rolling one, then there is an opportunity for any changes in its contents to be considered as part of the annual review process.

Training plan

The second element relates to the need to develop a training plan which follows on from the personnel plan. This would include ensuring that training institutions are following the intake requirements and that their curricula accord with the skill requirements identified. It would also set up a system for ensuring that appropriate students are selected in good time for entry to training courses either in-country or overseas. Thirdly, policies dealing with issues of scholarships and, where appropriate, bonding of students returning from training need to be set out in a clear and explicit way.

Personnel policies

The third element concerns personnel policy. It is important that this meets the needs of the personnel plan both in terms of attracting and retaining staff and in ensuring that staff morale is kept high to ensure productive working. It is also important that personnel policies are consistent with the principles of primary health-care (PHC); for example, they should allow equal opportunity to all members of a society irrespective of their sex, their age, or any disability they may have.

RELATIONSHIP TO THE PLANNING PROCESS

As suggested earlier, the relationship between human resource planning and broad health-sector planning is of key importance. If the relationship is inappropriate the problems which we saw at the beginning of this chapter can occur. A number of scenarios involving this relationship are possible, including the following:

- *Human resource and sectoral planning carried out in isolation from each other.* Such a scenario is all too commonly encountered, with health planners and human resource planners working separately and with little co-ordination. Although common, such an approach is, of course impossible to justify. It is essential that personnel should be seen as a means (albeit a very special one) to the end of providing health-care in a planned manner.

- *Minimalist sectoral planning.* Proponents of the free-market approach to health-care may argue that although sectoral planning is unnecessary, human resource planning is required to respond to the market's future needs. Such an approach sees the role of human resource planning as being one which responds and reacts to the projections of demand. Inasmuch as this book has rejected the market approach to health-care, such a scenario is unacceptable and irrelevant.

- *Human resource planning takes the lead role.* In this scenario, the view is taken that because personnel is ultimately the crucial input, attention should be focused on its planning. Sectoral planning, it is argued, will then follow the lead of human resource planning and devise plans to fit around the personnel element. Such an approach ignores the possibility of substitution between personnel and other resources. Thus, for example, there is often a variety of possible combinations of personnel and technical equipment to perform the same services. The appropriateness of any particular approach in particular circumstances is dependent on (among other factors) the relative costs of the personnel and technology and the social acceptability and feasibility of alternatives. Such an approach also ignores constraints on the provision of other inputs which could have implications for personnel plans.

- *Sectoral planning leads and determines human resource planning.* In this scenario, personnel estimation is seen as the planning of one (albeit a crucial) resource, with the services to be provided being the focal planning point. Such an approach, by recognizing the strong relationship between personnel costs and total costs, also permits the potentially heavy cost implications arising from changes in personnel to be allowed for.

This last approach fits most closely with the concept of planning argued for in this book, as a means of ensuring that limited resources are directed towards the provision of services which meet priority needs. Such an approach emphasizes *service delivery* (resulting from a combination of resources) rather than solely the presence of personnel.

HUMAN RESOURCE PLANNING AND HEALTH SECTOR REFORM

Chapters 3 and 4 discussed a number of issues concerning Health Sector Reform (HSR) policies being considered in a number of countries. Two such policies in particular have an important bearing on human resource planning: the promotion of the private sector and decentralization. The implications of these are briefly discussed below.

Private sector

One of the elements of some HSR policies involves the promotion of the private sector as a health-care provider. The discussion in this chapter has been in terms of the personnel needs of the whole health sector. Already in many countries the private sector is a major drain of professional staff from the public sector, through its ability to provide better conditions of service. This can have serious implications for the ability of the public sector to recruit and retain staff. The desire and ability of a government to deal with this drain on public services will largely depend on the political climate and ideology of the country. Countries with a clear commitment to policies of equity are likely to develop stronger policies towards the control of the private sector. Such policies were discussed in Chapter 4. It is in the area of personnel that the private sector may have the greatest (negative) impact on the plans of the public sector. It also represents a cost (in terms of the training investment) on the public sector which is rarely paid back. Furthermore, as we have seen, one of the difficulties with the private sector is the difficulty in obtaining information about its plans, as a result of both its fragmentation and its often strong reluctance to divulge information for various reasons about its plans.

An increased role for the private sector brings with it both challenges and opportunities in the area of human resource planning. On the one hand the scale of the problem of public sector staff haemorrhaging is likely to intensify, leading to increased pressure to increase public sector salaries. However, as the public/private mix becomes more recognized, then there are potential opportunities to regularize the information exchange, flow of staff, and private sector training contributions.

Decentralization

The second major HSR policy with a particular implications for human resource planning is decentralization. Genuine decentralization brings with it the power to set staffing levels in response to locally determined plans. However, in most countries, staff retain the right to move freely between areas, in response to the labour market. This can cause significant difficulties for human resource planning, particularly where local areas are empowered to set their own salary levels. It is suggested that, even with policies of decentralization, a strong central human resource planning role is required. However, such a planning function will need to respond to the demand determinants of local plans, with a greater emphasis on providing projected information to local planners and on influencing supply side factors.

SUMMARY

This chapter has introduced the principles of human resource planning. The two elements of supply and demand for staff were discussed as the basis for any plan. The chapter has described the major stages of developing a human resource plan. It has argued that demand should be based on the plans for services implicit in the broader sectoral plan. Lastly various policies for balancing the supply of and demand for personnel and the implications for two key areas of HSR policies have been outlined.

INTRODUCTORY READING

The two classic texts on health planning are Hall and Mejia (1978), which is a series of chapters on different aspects of human resource planning, and Hornby *et al.* (1980) which uses a similar approach, but in manual form. Adams and Hirschfeld (1998) look at human resource issues for the next century. The recent publication from WHO (Shipp 1998) focuses on the demand side of human resource planning by looking at indicators of staffing need. Wheeler and Ngcongo (1990) provide a good case study from Botswana, and Kan (1990) provides one from China. Butter and Mejia (1987) and Meerhoff and Lewis (1988) look at the problems of oversupply of doctors. Much human resource planning has focused on the quantitative aspects. Other qualitative and organizational aspects are examined by Cumper (1986), looking at the legal aspects; Rutabanzibwa-Ngaiza *et al.* (1985), and Jesani (1990) at aspects of equal opportunities and Simmonds (1989) at wider issues of personnel management.

EXERCISE 13

What is the record on human resource planning in your country?

- Are there trained staff unemployed?
- Are there vacancies for which there is funding but no staff?
- Are there areas where staff are not efficiently used?
- How high is morale?
- What policies could be adopted to address any of these problems?
- Which agency or department is responsible for human resource planning in your country? How does it relate to the overall planning function?

Consider the following problem.

A hospital is faced with a staffing crisis. Its budget is being squeezed, and its administrator is looking for ways of increasing its efficiency. She calls for reviews of the nurse and medical staffing pattern, and discovers:

(a) 40% of a registered nurse's time is spent making beds, bathing patients, taking temperatures and dispensing routine medicines.

(b) 30% of a medical officer's time is spent taking patient case histories, and in treating minor illnesses.

From the training curriculum of registered nurses and nurse assistants it is recognized that with some additional in-service training, registered nurses could perform the tasks set out in (b) above, and nurse assistants those in (a).

Complete the following table and answer the following questions.

1. What medium-term improvements can be made, given the present staffing pattern set out below, and the staff costs?
2. What advantages and disadvantages are there arising from the policy?
3. What obstacles would exist to carrying it out, and what policies would be needed?
4. What information would be needed to determine such information in the first place? How would it be collected?

	Current number	Annual unit cost	Staff nos.		Financial implications
			Increase	Decrease	
Doctors	10	10 000			
Reg. Nurses	40	5 000			
Nurse assts.	30	2 200			
Total	80				

REFERENCES AND FURTHER READING

Abel-Smith, B. (1987). Counting the cost. *World Health*, April, 18–19.

Adams, O.B. and Hirschfeld, M. (1998). Human resources for health — challenges for the 21st century. *World Health Statistics Quarterly*, **51**(1), 28–32.

Butter, I. and Mejia, A. (1987). Too many doctors. *World Health Forum*, 8, 494–500.

Cumper, G. (1986). Neglected legal status in health planning: nurse practitioners in Jamaica. *Health Policy and Planning*, 1, 30–6.

Fulop, T. (1986). Health personnel for 'Health for All': progress or stagnation. *WHO Chronicle*, **40**(1), 194–9; (2), 222–5.

Fulop, T. and Roemer, M. I. (1987). *Reviewing health manpower development*. Public Health Paper 83, WHO, Geneva.

Hall, T. L. and Mejia, A. (ed.) (1978). *Health manpower planning: principles, methods, issues*. WHO, Geneva.

Hornby, P., Ray, D. K., Shipp, P. J., and Hall, T. L. (1980). *Guidelines for health manpower planning*. WHO, Geneva.

Jesani, A. (1990). Limits of empowerment: women in rural health care. *Economic and Political Weekly*, 19 May, 1098–1103.

Kan, X. (1990). Village health workers in China: reappraising the current situation. *Health Policy and Planning*, 5, 40–8.

Kolchmainen-Aitken, R.-L. and Shipp, P. (1990). Indicators of staffing need: assessing health staffing and equity in Papua New Guinea. *Health Policy and Planning*, 5, 167–76.

Meerhoff, R. and Lewis, D. (1988). Oversupply of medical doctors in Uruguay: a policy dilemma. *Health Policy and Planning*, 3, 280–90.

Ojo, K. (1990). The crisis in the distribution of health personnel in Nigeria. *Health Policy and Planning*, 5, 60–6.

Rutabanzibwa-Ngaija, J., Heggenhougan, K., and Walt, G. (1985). *Women and Health in Africa* EPC Publication No 6, London School of Hygiene and Tropical Medicine, London.

Shipp, P. J. (1998). *Workload indicators of staffing need — a manual for implementation*. WHO, Geneva.

Simmonds, S. (1989). Human resource development: the management, planning and training of health personnel. *Health Policy and Planning*, 4, 187–96.

Wheeler, M. and Ngcongo, N. (1990). Health manpower planning in Botswana. *World Health Forum*, 11, 394–405.

14

The state of planning and planning for the State

Chapter 1 suggested that, for many countries, the record on health planning has not been good. The final indicator of success for planning is whether necessary and appropriate changes are both identified and achieved. Yet for many countries the health system continues to have deficiencies, and, in particular, an imbalance of resources, described in Chapter 7, which is avoidable even with the low level of overall resources available to the health and related sectors. Up to this point in the book we have focused on various components and techniques of planning on the basis that an understanding of these is a necessary condition for planning. However, such an understanding, although necessary, is insufficient in itself to improve the planning record. Two other broad conditions also need to be satisfied.

- Firstly, the application of these techniques needs to occur within a coherent and overarching *planning system*.

- The second, and possibly more important, factor is the need for the development of a *planning culture*. This culture must not be confined to the offices of specialist planners, but must permeate the health system.

Such a positive attitude to planning is not easy to cultivate, given in particular the individualism inculcated in many health professionals (and in particular the medical profession) by their training. Such individualism can be the antithesis of the collective decision-making process which underpins planning. However, if planning, as the agent of change for the future, is itself to have a future, a strengthening of the planning systems and the development of a planning culture are needed in many countries.

This final chapter brings together some of the themes that have been discussed earlier in the book, and focuses on the management of the planning process. As in the rest of the book, there are no easily generalizable and transferable blueprints that can be advocated for all situations. Each system needs to be seen as specific to the social, political, institutional and economic context of its own country. However, there are broad principles and guidelines that can be used as the basis for the development of a workable system, and to help develop a positive attitude to planning. This chapter first looks at appropriate criteria and characteristics of a planning system. It follows this with a case study of such a system, and concludes by looking at a number of myths in planning which need to be dispelled if the record of planning is to be improved in the future.

A set of criteria, in the form of questions for assessing the strengths and weaknesses of a health planning system, are summarized in Table 14.1 and briefly outlined below.

Table 14.1   Criteria for assessing a health planning system

Is the purpose and role of the health planning system[a] clear and appropriate?

Is the health planning system based on explicit values?

Are the functions of, and inter-relationships between actors in, the health-care system well defined?

Are the decision-making structures of the planning system open and transparent?

Is there an appropriate balance between central and local decision-making?

Is there consistency between planning and other decision-making processes?

Does the planning system balance technical and political analyses?

Does the system facilitate planning for health rather than solely for health-care?

Does the planning timetable balance long-term direction with short-term flexibility?

Is there an adequate information base for planning and is it used?

Is there a variety of appropriate and well-used planning processes and tools

Is planning adequately and sustainably technically resourced?

Is the aid programme well managed?

[a] It is important to distinguish between the objectives of a planning *system* and those of a *plan*; this table is concerned with the former.

ASSESSMENT CRITERIA

Is the purpose and role of the health planning system clear and appropriate?

Within any health system, it is important that there is agreement on the role and purpose of the planning system itself. The design of any system should be based on the objectives that the system is trying to achieve. For example, a health planning system may be seen to have four major objectives:

- to provide the framework to enable the setting of medium to long-term policy

- to translate policies into plans of action

- to ensure the implementation of these plans

- to co-ordinate the aid programme to the health sector.

Narrower objectives may exist, but these may not be appropriate. For example, managing the capital budget may be seen as the sole role of the health planning system but, as we have seen in Chapter 11, this is inappropriately narrow.

Is the health planning system based on explicit values?

Health planning decisions are the product of a combination of technical considerations and value judgements. It is important that the latter are as clear and well defined as possible to inform subsequent decisions and planning processes. Potential values (see Bryant *et al.* 1997) and criteria for decision-making include the following:

- equity (explicitly defined)

- participative, democratic and accountable decision-making processes

- commitment to appropriate mix of central and local decision-making

- recognition of the importance of process as well as inputs–outputs.

The importance of being clear over values can be illustrated by one value stressed in Primary Health Care (PHC) policies — equity. One important function of the planning system is the promotion of equity within the health field. There are two ways in which the planning system can do this. Firstly, the resource allocation process, discussed in Chapter 11, must be based on principles of equity. This implies not only ensuring that resources provided centrally are distributed to the local areas on the basis of need, but also taking account of their existing resource levels and ability to generate resources locally. Secondly, clear guidance is needed from the planning process, backed up by an appropriate information system, as to what is meant by equity, and how it can be monitored. This has been discussed in Chapter 3.

Are the functions of, and interrelationships between actors in, the health-care system well defined?

As we have seen, there are four main functions any health-care system has to perform:

- policy-setting, including strategic planning

- financing

- health-care provision

- regulation.

In many countries, Health Sector Reform (HSR) policies are leading to changes in the roles of different agencies. For a planning system to be effective, it is important that its relationship with the other functions of the health-care system is well defined. The relationship between policy and planning is particularly critical. It is also important that as new roles are defined, attention and resources are devoted to developing the capacity to carry out this function effectively. The roles of government in strategic planning and regulation are likely to require particular attention.

Are the decision-making structures of the planning system transparent and open?

A variety of groups may claim a right to involvement in planning decisions. Possible groups include politicians, communities, other health-related agencies, health workers including managers and professionals and a variety of technical perspectives, ensuring a multidisciplinary set of views. The means of decision-making will affect access by these groups. It is important that there is a clear recognition of who should be involved, and at what stage. This has various implications for for the planning system.

The roles of planners, managers and communities need to be clear. This book has stressed the need to view planning as an activity that is the responsibility of all managers, and not solely as a set of tasks conducted by specialist planners. For plans to be implemented, they must be seen both to be relevant to the needs of the service as perceived by health staff and by users, and to be workable. Plans must not be viewed as having been imposed extraneously on health professionals and communities. However, managers and other health staff have constraints on the amount of time that they can devote to planning. In the situation of tight resources that faces busy managers, it is easy and understandable for concerns about the future to be overshadowed by concerns about the present. In this sense, resources, in the form of specialist planners, are needed to act as guardians of the future.

Specialist planners are needed also as advocates of the needs of minorities. Involvement of communities and indeed of managers of mainstream services, unless carefully handled, can result in the neglect of minority health-care needs. In such situations, planners are potentially able to ensure the expression of these minority needs.

Broad-based ownership of the plans is essential. Planning as an activity therefore needs to be structured in a manner that encourages full participation in the process. At the same time it has to be recognized that there are specialist skills — in epidemiology and economics, for example — which need to be available to support this planning process.

It is important therefore that the means by which planning decisions are made are open and explicit and that mechanisms for input into the planning decisions by different groups are well understood. These mechanisms may, for example, include:

• planning committees or groups with clear terms of reference

• timetables for the planning system

• issuance of planning guidance and circulars

• consultative processes

• use of media and publicity

• legislation

• published documents in an accessible form.

Openness does not necessarily mean that all groups have an equal right to influencing decision-making. It is important that the system has mechanisms for controlling the input of other groups into the planning processes. In particular commercial, professional, and donor interests need to have a means to access the process without having undue influence.

The preceding treatment has argued for broad involvement of a variety of non-specialist planners in the planning process. It is important to remember that such people are not likely to be familiar with either the broad outlines of planning or the procedural details. In order to assist in making the planning system more open and transparent, three actions are therefore necessary.

- Firstly, there should be *clear procedures* for planning. It is very easy to get bogged down in bureaucratic planning procedures, so it is helpful to have clear documentation on the nature of the various planning processes, and who is involved in each of them. A simple planning manual, distributed to all the people involved directly in the planning process, can be a useful way of doing this, provided it is does not become unwieldy. It should not, for example, attempt to answer all the detailed procedural questions. However, it should set out the relations with other parts of the management process, including budgeting and human resource planning.

- Secondly, a *clear timetable* must be set for the various planning activities. This is important to ensure that key dates are adhered to, but is also necessary if involvement on the part of health professionals and communities is to be more than token. It is also important that due notice is given as to when particular activities need to be undertaken — through the issuing of official circulars, for example. Where specific information is sought on plan proposals or budgets it is also helpful to use agreed formats.

- Thirdly, it is important that documents produced in the process of planning are *comprehensible*. Like any other specialist group, planners have their own technical jargon, which can be very alienating to non-planners. This may mean that various versions of documents, including short summaries, are necessary if genuine participation is to be possible. It also means, as we saw in Chapter 6, that attention has to be paid to how information is presented. Few planners have fully recognized the real implications of community participation in terms of how specialist planning information is presented to communities. The forms of communication techniques that have been developed in the area of health education need to be harnessed to the process of planning.

Are the planning processes and tools integrated and appropriate?

Health planning is ultimately concerned with identifying and implementing necessary changes to the health sector. There are a variety of processes and tools for doing this, of which the development of written plans themselves is a key, but not the sole one. Planning involves a number of processes as set out in the planning cycle. Although this may not be formally or sequentially followed, it is important that the steps are all undertaken and consistent with each other. A number of different activities can be seen within the overall planning process, including:

- information gathering and analysis
- policy formation
- plan design
- resource allocation

• human resource planning

• plan implementation.

As we have seen in earlier chapters, some of these areas may end up marginalized and not integrated with the overall planning process, and yet all are necessary ingredients for successful planning. It is, for example, all too common to find human resource planning activities performed by a personnel department with little or no reference to the overall service planning occurring elsewhere. Although not all these activities are necessarily the prime responsibility of a planning secretariat, it is essential that some integrating process is provided.

Each of the acticities listed above requires different skills, and may occur at different stages of the planning process, but it is essential that there are clearly defined organizational and functional links between them. For example, as we have seen, it is important that information collected is relevant to the needs of planning. One area where dislocation of functions is common is between plan design and implementation. There are strong arguments in favour of having specialist planners responsible for the co-ordination of the implementation of plans, but there are equally convincing arguments to suggest that those who have been involved in the design of a programme are best placed to implement it. Whichever solution is chosen, in any particular system, will depend on a variety of other factors. However, the links between these functions must be well defined.

State planning has often focused heavily (even solely) on the services directly provided by the public sector. However, all planning processes need to take account of all the institutions and actors involved in the health system, and to consider mechanisms for influencing other sub-sectors. The State has a particular responsibility to take a broad view, and may need to use a variety of mechanisms and tools to influence the actions of other sectors outside its direct management control. There is a variety of tools available for planning. It is important that planners follow the steps in the planning cycle, and in particular that realistic and acceptable prioritization, the key element of planning, occurs. It is important that planners are aware of potential tools. It is also important that the tools are used consistently and in the same direction to send the same signals to the health system. Examples of such tools are provided in Table 14.2.

Lastly, a word of caution is needed. Although clear, well-documented processes are essential for a health planning process that is to be open and consistent, this must not be allowed to lead to inflexible bureaucratic obsession with process at the expense of the ultimate aims of health planning — changes that will improve health.

Is there an appropriate balance between central and local decision-making?

Planning, as an activity, needs to be closely tied in with the general decision-making processes of the health ministry. Furthermore, we have seen decentralization of certain parts of the decision-making process is a necessary, though not a sufficient, condition for PHC. In some countries decentralization is occurring more generally within the overall government system. Given the resultant trend towards decentralization of the

Table 14.2   Examples of tools for planning

Budgeting
● capital and recurrent
● project and programme

Resource allocation mechanisms

Health financing and funding flows

Managed markets

Contracting of services and outsourcing

Development of health-care packages

Human resource planning

Planning of other inputs (pharmaceuticals, etc.)

Organizational restructuring in the health service

Health systems research

Incentives and controls (over other sectors and actors)

Tax, pricing and subsidization policies

Legislation

Norms and standards of care

Plan statements

Policies in health-related sectors (e.g. agriculture policy, tax policy)

Privatization of public sector assets

Projects

Development of quasi public bodies

Regulation and licensing of supply of health facilities

Regulation and licensing of health professions

Advocacy

Use of the media

External aid support

---

managerial process, it is important that certain planning decisions are similarly decentralized. Furthermore, it has been argued earlier that there are good reasons, in themselves, for some elements of the planning process to be decentralized. Localized planning allows for needs assessment to reflect the differences in both epidemiological and demographic patterns between areas, and for the responses to these needs to be consistent with differences in patterns and modes of service delivery. It also allows for differences in community views to be incorporated. Decentralization may also be a more appropriate means of fostering multisectoral solutions to health problems. Since this is so, where resources permit, the development of locally-based plans would appear to be entirely consistent with the tenets and objectives of promoting PHC. It is important, however, to add a word of caution. Decentralization of planning ahead of decentralization of broader managerial functions can lead to frustration and unrealized expectations. In particular, delays in the decentralization of budgetary responsibility can provide a major obstacle to the full decentralization of planning functions.

The speed at which decentralization is possible, in practice, however, depends largely on the availability of sufficient personnel with the requisite skills. During the transitional stage, it is likely that central support will need to be provided for the peripheral planning personnel. Indeed, it is likely that certain specialized skills will always be in such short supply that they remain at the centre, providing expert advice to the peripheral units. These may include, for example, planning skills in the area of human resources. In such situations the relationship between central and peripheral planners needs careful attention. Genuine decentralization would suggest that peripherally-based planners are seen as accountable to the broader peripheral decision-making process rather than to the centre. There may, however, be a temptation to view such planners as outposts of the centre, with prime responsibility to the central planning function. If this temptation is not resisted, then there is a danger that local managers and communities will not identify with the planning process, and will see it as an imposed central process.

Even where resources do allow full decentralization, some planning functions will need to remain at the centre. Under a policy of decentralization is it is essential that there is a mix of central policy framework coupled with local decisions which reflect local needs and priorities. It is also important that all levels understand their roles and functions.

Table 14.3 sets out a possible division of responsibilities between the centre and the local level.

Where the form of decentralization is not restricted to the health ministry, but is more general, an additional role of the planning function at both national and local levels may be to ensure that adequate funds are provided to the health-sector elements of an integrated local plan.

Table 14.3   Possible roles of centre and district levels in health planning

Central functions	Joint activities	Local functions
Broad policy leadership		Local needs assessment
Resource generation and allocation		Development of local plans
Donor co-ordination		Implementation of local plans
Liaison with central ministries		
Co-ordination of local plans		
Planning of central specialist services		
Human resource planning		
Technical planning support		
Legislation		
	Monitoring and evaluation	

Is there consistency between planning and other decision-making processes?

It is essential that the planning system is developed in such a manner that it is consistent with other decision processes both within the health sector and outside.

As we have seen, there is a danger within large organizations that the functional decision-making processes develop a life of their own and fail to work in a cohesive integrated manner. In particular, human resource planning and budgeting may not be related closely with the strategic planning function. It is essential to develop mechanisms that ensure this: for example, committees with a remit for both planning and budgeting may be one method.

It is also important that relations with central government are clearly defined. To a large degree this will be determined by the requirements of the central government system, and it is important that there is consistency with the overall system. This can at times be frustrating, especially where the central systems are seen as restrictive. However, such constraints must be viewed as like any other external constraints. Health planners can try and remove them by changing the central system; however, where this is not possible in the short term, the constraints must be worked within. This does not however remove the possibility of creativity within them!

Does the planning system balance technical and political analyses?

As we have seen, planning may not result in change if it fails to take account of different groups and their views. Techniques such as stakeholder analysis, political mapping, consultation, and broad membership of planning bodies will assist in achieving this. Planning systems which focus narrowly on technical skills are likely to be unsuccessful.

Does the system facilitate planning for health rather than solely for health-care?

Health-care is only one aspect of the overall health system. The health planning process needs to reflect this and promote a recognition of the inputs made by other sectors in the promotion of or constraints on health. This includes developing tools to influence other non-health-care factors.

Where government has a cross-agency form of integrated decentralization, led by a local government authority, this can provide a strong basis for a multisectoral approach to health. The health planning response in such an organizational frame-work is likely to be very different to that where health is defined within narrow boundaries.

Does the planning timetable allow a combination of long-term direction and short-term flexibility?

Plans are a statement of planning intention. There is a variety of different time-scales for planning including:

- long-term (perspective plans)
- medium-term (strategic plans)
- short-term (operational plans).

It is important that a variety of such statements of intention exist and are consistent with each other. It is also important that they combine long-term vision with short-term flexibility. The use of rolling plans may assist in this.

The planning process needs to combine a long-term perspective which provides policy continuity with the flexibility to respond to changes in the short term. In particular, they need to be able to respond to changes in the external environment, such as resource availability or political change. Chapter 2 introduced the concept of the planning spiral as a series of conceptual stages that need to be gone through in sequence. Part of the process of managing a planning system involves ensuring that a realistic timetable which allows this to occur is set and adhered to.

One major decision that any planning body needs to make in the development of a planning system is the life cycle of a plan. Twenty years ago most plans were based on five year cycles, often as part of a wider development plan. One advantage of such a long-term planning process, in addition to the obvious longer-term perspective possible, is that it allows for incorporation and adequate lead-time for larger projects (such as hospitals). Recently, however, there has been an increasing recognition that such a cycle is unduly rigid, and may not provide sufficient information on the degree

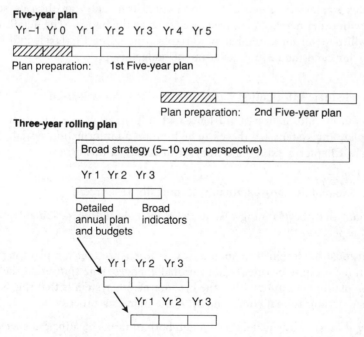

Fig. 14.1   Five year and three year rolling plan cycles

of detail in plans that is needed for their operationalization. Such five year plans also have the drawback of quickly becoming out of date and out of touch with changing needs. Figure 14.1 illustrates this. At the other extreme, annual plans done in isolation have no broad framework within which to fit.

One process increasingly being adopted, which allows the benefits of a long-term perspective as well as satisfying the need for detailed operational information, is the rolling plan cycle illustrated in Fig. 14.1. At any time within the three year rolling plan there is a medium-term perspective (provided by the overall three year framework).

- Year 3 of the plan is provided in broad outline (giving, for example, information on the overall number of health centres to be constructed).

- Year 2 provides information in more detail — for example a breakdown of the number of such facilities by region or district.

- Year 1 is the most detailed, and provides an operational plan with information on the precise location of such facilities, and start and finish dates for construction.

The plan is often set against a broader strategy which sets longer-term aims and objectives, and may be updated every three years or so. Every year the plan is rolled forward in such a way as to put more flesh on what were previously Years 2 and 3, and to bring in a new Year 3. The rolling-forward process allows therefore for changes in emphasis due to changing needs or resources, but not for major deviations from the broad strategy or momentum already set.

Within this framework, a more detailed annual timetable can then be set that is consonant with other management processes such as the budget. The details of such a timetable will depend on a number of variables, including the levels and degree of decentralization, and the central government budgetary process.

Is there an adequate information base for planning, and is it used?

Planning requires information (both hard and soft, quantitative and qualitative). A successful planning system will therefore be built on an information system and use it appropriately. Chapter 6 explored a number of issues in this area.

Is planning adequately and sustainably technically resourced?

It is important that the planning system developed should be sustainable. There are two related aspects to this.

- Firstly, it must be designed in such a way as to ensure that the planning function will continue, despite broader organizational changes. One spin-off of the development of a planning culture within the broader health system is that this is likely to strengthen organizational commitment to the planning process.

- Secondly, it must be adequately resourced, both in terms of sufficient specialist staff and associated other costs. The exact requirements for resources for the planning function will of course vary, as will the means of supplying those resources. In some cases many of the specialist planning skills may be available outside a specific planning secretariat. Elsewhere, certain skills will have to be provided internally within the planning secretariat.

Support to the planning function has been a favourite target for external donor aid; it is important that such aid is provided in a way that is institution-building rather than institution-weakening. Unfortunately, such planning is frequently linked into specific projects, often through separate parallel implementation units. Such units are not only time-limited to the length of the project, but frequently also fail to link into the broader health planning system. This may be understandable from the point of the view of the donor, concerned to ensure the proper and prompt disbursement of donor funds, but the long-term price for this may be a weakening of the internal planning capacity.

One question frequently asked is 'What is the ideal make-up of a planning unit or department?' Unfortunately, there is no easy or uniform answer to such a question. There are certain skills that are required in the planning process. However, the broad approach to planning which has been advocated here suggests that not all of these need necessarily be located within the planning secretariat. The disciplines required in planning are wide-ranging, and include:

- economics

- social epidemiology

- sociology

- law

- community development

- quantitative techniques

- political science

- organization theory

- health systems research

- operations research

- physical planning.

Amongst these, there has been a shift in a number of countries from an epidemiologically dominated process to one in which economics is seen as the key discipline; see the readings at the end of the chapter for examples of views on the role of economics in planning. Interestingly. at one level this mirrors a shift in international dominance of the health policy scene from WHO to the World Bank.

The two disciplines of epidemiology and economics clearly do have a particular role in health planning. However, neither on its own is adequate or desirable. An epidemiologically driven planning process may fail to take sufficient account of the resource implications of strategies, and an economically driven process may result in too narrow a focus on efficiency. In addition, a number of other skills are required for a successful planning system, as the above list suggests.

Although specialist planners certainly do not need detailed knowledge of all the above skills, they do need to have an understanding of what is offered by each of these disciplines, and how their expertise can be accessed. For example, health planners do not need to be experts in economic appraisal techniques; they do, however, need to know how to set the terms of reference for one to be carried out on their behalf, and how to interpret the results. In addition to a broad base of general knowledge in these areas, specialist planners need to have large doses of common sense, imagination, and flexibility! It is also important that technical resources are continuously updated. Career structures and staff development programmes for planners are an important ingredient in this.

Governments need to recognize the importance of ensuring that the policy and planning process is adequately resourced. Unfortunately, the emphasis on HSR, and downsizing the role of public sector provision, has often led to a neglect of the central planning capacity at precisely the time when it needs to be strong.

Is the aid programme well managed?

One of the functions of a planning system must be to ensure that the aid programme supports the health planning system, and is consistent with it. Otherwise it is possible for the aid programme to dominate the planning system, with negative consequences in terms of a balanced and owned strategic direction. A strong internal strategic capacity whereby a government is clear as to the direction in which it wishes to move is a necessary (though not necessarily sufficient) condition to ensure a locally acceptable health strategy. Too often the policy-making vacuum that exists in the health sector of some countries leads to a (sometimes understandable) filling of this vaccuum by externally 'imposed' policies.

One of the key tasks of the planning function is liaison with external donor agencies. Although there is often considerable reluctance on the part of other departments to lose their contacts with aid agencies, it is essential for the coherent and consistent implementation of plans that a single department should have the overall responsibility for seeking and agreeing the terms of donor assistance. As with all other aspects of planning, this does not obviate the need for, or the appropriateness of, direct discussions between service delivery managers and aid agencies. However, this must be seen as occurring within the context of the overall plan. Without such a framework it is very easy for plans to lose their sense of purpose, as each donor agency has its own agenda and favoured areas for assistance — a situation which, if not managed properly, can easily lead to distortions of the overall plan.

Some health ministries have found donor conferences a useful way of both providing information in a cost-effective way to potential donors about their plans and soliciting support for specific parts of the plans. Such conferences can of course also rebound on ministries, when donors use the opportunity to exert concerted joint pressure about particular areas that are of concern to them. Recent developments in the area of Sector Wide Approaches, as discussed earlier (see p. 110), may also be a valuable way forward.

AN ILLUSTRATIVE CASE STUDY OF A PLANNING SYSTEM

The preceding part of this chapter has discussed a number of criteria for a planning system that will facilitate the achievement of planning objectives. How these are translated into practice in different countries will depend on a variety of country-specific factors. However, in order to illustrate aspects of the above criteria, we now describe elements of a possible planning system, designed for a small country with a deconcentrated health organization with one level of organization (districts) below the central level, and with various centrally provided services. It should be stressed that this is not intended to be seen as a blueprint for planning, but rather to illustrate the application of the above criteria within a system.

Overview of the system

The system is based on a three-year rolling plan cycle. This involves each year a review process of the previous year leading to specific plans for the following three years. Each year the previous plan is reviewed and updated to extend it.

The planning system has the following elements:

- A *central planning and budgeting committee*, chaired by the chief officer (such as a principal or permanent secretary (PS)) of the health ministry, with core membership consisting of designated senior staff in the ministry. In addition, the membership is supplemented at key points — such as at the development of policy — by representatives of other levels of the health sector and of other health-related agencies and the community. This body is ultimately responsible for advising the minister on all policy in the ministry, and for reviewing, reconciling, and monitoring the plans of districts and central services (known hereafter as 'units'). The committee is serviced by a planning unit, and meets on a fortnightly basis. The committee in addition sets up working groups, as necessary, to examine particular policy areas.

- A *directorate of planning and information* responsible to the PS, with a *planning unit* responsible for servicing the planning and budgeting committee and working groups, preparing policy papers, co-ordination of the implementation of plans, and co-ordination of donor activity; and an *information unit*.

- An *annual statement of policy guidelines* from the planning committee. This indicates the areas that the planning and budgeting committee view as important to emphasize in the development of unit plans, together with any budgetary guidelines and constraints.

- *District, specialist services, and headquarter (including support service) plans (unit plans)* based on the overall policy guidelines, but taking account of local variations, and reconciled by the ministry planning and budgeting committee into an overall rolling national health plan. These provide not only the means to assess the proposals of different units, but also the basis for the monitoring of implementation. The plans set out the requirements for development (capital) expenditure (from both government funds and donors). They also form the basis of the annual recurrent budget estimates exercise. The national document is also key in negotiations with donors for assistance.

- An annual rolling *human resources plan*, based on the national health plan. This provides the basis not only for any adjustments in the supply of human resources, but also, where necessary, adjustments to service proposals.

- An *information system*, to provide, amongst others catchment-based utilization information, infrastructural information, economic information such as costs, and information on the demand for and the supply of staff.

Planning cycle timetable
Table 14.4 sets out the timetable for the planning cycle based on the above for a country with a financial year beginning in April.

Table 14.4   Planning and budgeting timetable

Month	Activity
March	Budget for following year approved
	Units provided with information on budget allocations
April	Financial year begins
May–July	Health ministry planning committee reviews previous year and develops policy guidance
August	Circular sent, together with policy guidance and information on likely resources, requesting development of plans to districts, specialist hospitals, and central units
September–November	Local and service plans developed and submitted to planning unit
November–December	Planning unit analyses local plans for feasibility (including budgetary and personnel constraints), and for consistency with national policies. Planning committee meets units, where necessary, to discuss proposals
January	Revisions of plans made as necessary; national plan drawn up
February–March	Discussion with central agencies
March	Approval of budgets and plans

Decentralization and planning
The role of the centre in this system is largely one of setting broad policy and technical guidelines, broad resource allocation, co-ordination, support, and monitoring. The implementing units — the districts, specialist hospitals, and central programmes — have the major responsibility for developing their own plans within the framework set by the centre. Where the resources in terms of trained personnel do not exist within

these decentralized implementing units to perform this task, the ministry planning unit provides support to these units in the development of the plans.

Relationship between planning and budgetary and personnel systems
The planning system described combines these closely related functions into a single system. The budget (both for development and recurrent expenditure) for each year is determined from the information provided in the planning process. Similarly the information sets out the personnel requirements for the following three years.

Roles of the planning and budgeting committee and the planning unit
A clear distinction is made between the role of the planning and budgeting committee and that of the planning unit. The planning and budgeting committee has a core membership of senior officers. In addition it can co-opt, as necessary, others for relevant meetings. The planning and budgeting committee may also set up working parties to examine particular policy issues or implementation problems. The working groups report to the planning and budgeting committee.

The terms of reference for the planning and budgeting committee are set out in Table 14.5.

The planning and budgeting committee is the ultimate decision-making body in planning under the minister, and it requires a secretariat. This function is provided by the planning unit, whose terms of reference are given in Table 14.6.

Table 14.5 Terms of reference for planning and budgeting committee

To set overall policy guidelines for the health sector

To ensure the development of annual plans consistent with these policies, and within existing resource constraints

To allocate resources to, and approve budgets for, the various implementing units consistent with these policies and resources

To approve the human resource plan

To co-ordinate the implementation of plans

To oversee the evaluation of programmes

Planning and information
The information unit forms the other section of the planning and information directorate, and is therefore closely linked to the planning unit. However, it is organizationally parallel to the planning unit, as it provides an information service wider than that required for the planning function alone.

Implementation
The major responsibility for implementation lies with the operational units responsible for a particular development or project. The role of the planning unit is one of co-ordination and monitoring. This is achieved by the production of plans of

Table 14.6 Terms of reference for a planning unit

To provide technical support to the planning and budgeting committee, and to act as its secretariat

To draw up draft policy papers for the planning and budgeting committee's consideration

To liaise with central government ministries over planning and budgeting matters

To provide the first point of contact with donor agencies and to liaise with them over aid funding

To develop, or ensure the development of, human resource plans

To provide the contact point with technical services over construction projects

To monitor the implementation of plans and projects, and provide a monthly report to the planning and budgeting committee on implementation

To assist units in the development of plans and budgets

To advise the planning and budgeting committee on the feasibility of such plans and their consistency with the national health policy guidelines set by the planning committee

In co-ordination with the information unit, to commission, and where appropriate, to carry out evaluation studies and operations research studies

---

action each year linked to the budgets, based on the overall three-year agreed plan. Monitoring is achieved by the requirement for monthly progress reports on each new project, together with financial monitoring of spending.

Procedures — forward planning

There are a number of different activities that relate to the development of the three-year plans. Each of these stages is described in turn.

National situational analysis
The planning cycle starts in June each year with the presentation of a broad situational analysis to the planning and budgeting committee by the planning unit. This situational analysis reviews the previous year, and the current state of the health sector. The analysis includes the following:

• health status changes from previous years

• the structure of the health services; and major changes from previous year, including what has occurred in other, non-government sectors

• the resources situation — finance, personnel, buildings, equipment, and transport

• technical changes (for example, in the immunization schedule)

• major health and health service issues.

Though the review concentrates on the public sector, it includes information on the state of the private and NGO sectors, and other health-related activities. Every three years a full analysis is conducted. In intervening years, the review only notes major changes from the previous year, rather than attempting to be exhaustive.

Policy statement
Following approval of the (amended if necessary) situational analysis, the planning unit presents a draft policy statement based on the situational analysis to the planning and budgeting committee for discussion. This document is short, and sets out the broad policy that the ministry intends operational units to follow in the development of their plans. It also gives guidance on the resource levels likely to be available to units in the development of their plans and budgets. The planning policy statement is agreed by the end of July.

Planning circular
In August, the planning unit issues a circular to all units requesting them to prepare their plans and budgets for the following financial year. This circular:

- sets out key dates
- includes the national situational analysis and policy statement
- provides pro formas for the completion of the budgets and plans.

Preparation of unit plans and budgets
Following the issuing of the circular, units develop plans and budgets. Planning activity at this level is of course not confined to this period of the year. Planning groups involving other sectors and the local communities should be active throughout the year, carrying out at the local level similar functions to the national planning committee. As an illustration a district plan might have the following sections:

- district situational analysis: the health situation specific to the area, and its present health services
- objectives and targets of the district
- gaps or deficiencies in health services and resources
- service proposals for meeting targets, including resource implications
- recurrent budget requirements
- capital requirements
- personnel requirements.

The plan covers a three-year period. However, detailed budgets are only required for the first year of the plan, with indications of any further recurrent and personnel implications for Years 2 and 3. The provision of these plans and budgets is the responsibility of the units. Assistance is provided by the planning unit, as necessary.

Assessment and reconciliation of plans
The plans from the units are returned to the planning unit by the end of November. The next stage of the process is the analysis of the plans for:

- consistency with overall national policies

- consistency with other unit plans

- internal consistency

- feasibility in terms of resources — both financial and staff.

The results of the preliminary analysis by the planning unit on the above criteria are presented to the planning committee, who, where necessary, meet with the units to discuss these. These meetings take place in December.

Draft national health plan
Following discussions with the units, the planning unit prepares, for presentation to the planning committee, a draft national health plan bringing together the various plans and budgets in a format consistent with the requirements of the central government. However, it also includes information on objectives and projections. Following approval by the planning committee, this is the document used in discussions with central government ministries. The document provides information on:

- health policy

- objectives

- service changes proposed

- other necessary changes, such as legislative or organizational changes

- recurrent budget implications

- changes in posts (new or redundant posts, or those with changed job descriptions)

- development budget requirements.

Human resource plan
One criterion against which the unit plans are assessed is feasibility in terms of human resources. In order to assess the implications, and where possible to take remedial actions, a human resource plan is drawn up as follows:

- *Supply analysis.* By the end of September each year the planning unit, with the assistance of the personnel office in the ministry, analyses the current supply and future projections of health staff under present assumptions — taking account of the output of training schools and the effect of attrition.

- *Demand analysis.* In parallel with the above the planning unit analyses the present and known future demands for health professionals, based on current and known planned post expansions.

- *Supply and demand matching.* The above information provides information on likely shortfalls or surpluses by cadres under existing plans. This information is compared with the unit plans and their future requirements for staff, to provide a picture as to the feasibility of these plans. Where necessary and possible this leads to changes in the staff parameters, for example changing the number of training places for different cadres. This leads to the production of a human resource plan as part of the overall national health plan.

Central government approval
Following the production of the draft national plan and budgets the ministry holds discussions with the central ministries. During such discussions the plans and budgets may need further revision, after which the agreed national health plan is produced.

National health plan and unit budgets
The last stage in the forward planning and budgeting process is feedback to units. Information is provided on the agreed budgets and plans of each unit in a form that allows implementation and easy monitoring.

Procedures — implementation

Annual plan of action and budgets
The above paragraph described the final stages in the forward planning activity as the production of a national health plan and of unit budgets for distribution to the units. This plan forms the basis of the implementation activity. Each unit is required to develop a simple action plan setting out the key dates for each activity (for example for the purchase of equipment, or for the completion of buildings), which then forms their management tool for monitoring. The responsibility for implementation rests with the units, though in the case of major construction projects it may be handled by the planning unit in conjunction with the local unit.

Monitoring and progress reports
On the basis of the action plans the units are required each month to complete a progress report for internal monitoring indicating whether their plan is being achieved and where problems are being encountered. Where necessary this is followed up by the planning unit. Regular reports providing an overview of the implementation of plans are provided to the planning and budgeting committee by the planning unit. These reports are accompanied by budget statements for each unit, for analysis by the accounts staff.

Training plan
On the basis of the broad human resource plan, a training plan for the ministry is produced covering both in- and pre-service training needs. The responsibility for this lies in the personnel office, which is also responsible for arranging for the selection of students and for logistical arrangements.

Donor co-ordination

There are two ways in which donor co-ordination can be handled:

- The production of a plan itself forms the focus for an annual donor conference

- The requirement is placed on donors that all initial co-ordination of aid should be effected through the planning unit.

Co-ordination of donors by the planning unit ensures that donor policies are consistent with those of government, and that any conditions placed by donors are acceptable and adhered to. However, such co-ordination is primarily aimed at the initial contact. Technical discussions take place within the implementing units.

The preceding has been a case study of a planning system to illustrate the components. The different contexts facing each health system will inevitably, and rightly, lead to different systems.

A PLANNING CULTURE

The second broad precondition for successful planning is the development of a *planning culture*. It is not uncommon for a country to have a highly skilled and well-resourced planning unit, but for plans developed by the unit to fail to be implemented. Various attitudes are still dominant in some countries which run counter to the success of planning, and which need to change. These misperceptions are now outlined.

Misperceptions about planning

- *Planning is about the production of plans*. There is a common view that planning is about the production of plan documents. Much planning activity is concentrated on ensuring that plans are produced. Although plan documents are an important part of the planning process, they must not be allowed to take over. They must remain a means to the planning end, rather than an end in themselves. Planning must be seen to be concerned with action, not with documentation.

- *Planning is about capital or development budgets*. Involvement in such budgets is an important part of planning, but overconcentration on this aspect to the exclusion of other tools, including the recurrent budget and legislative and organizational change, severely limits the potential of planning to achieve the necessary changes.

- *Planning is primarily concerned with projects*. The concentration on projects bedevils a number of planning systems. Projects can be important agents of change, although they can also be counterproductive. Concentration on projects to the exclusion of broader service changes can be very restrictive. Donor agencies have to shoulder the blame for pushing the adoption of project-based changes, and for much of the resultant fragmentation of planning activities and service delivery.

- *Planning is a highly technical and specialist activity.* There are a number of techniques that planners can usefully employ, and indeed the earlier parts of this book have explored some of these. However, much planning activity involves the application of common sense, and attempts to mystify this in professional jargon should be resisted. Indeed, one of the functions of specialist planners is to demystify such jargon and to empower service providers and users by turning these techniques over to them.

- *Planning should be carried out solely by specialist planners.* Where planning is seen to be the sole responsibility of officers working behind the doors marked 'Planning Office' it is a sure sign that such planning is unlikely to be successful. Although we have argued earlier in this chapter that specialist planners are needed, it is essential that they are seen as supports to a much wider system, rather than as the system itself.

- *Planning is an objective and neutral activity.* We have throughout this book stressed the fact that planning cannot be neutral. By being concerned with the promotion and implementation of policies that reflect the principles of PHC, it is based on a set of values. Such values are undoubtedly threatening to some groups in society. Indeed PHC, with its emphasis on equity and social justice, can be seen as a revolutionary creed for many countries. It is naive to pretend, therefore, that planning is a neutral activity.

- *Planning should result in a correct plan.* There is, of course, no such thing as a 'correct plan'. Not only are plans, as we have seen, the product of a series of values, which can alter; but there are many different ways to achieve a particular end.

THE FUTURE OF STATE PLANNING

Planning, as a means of achieving change, has a long way to go. The above misperceptions have to be challenged and changed. However, of possibly greater significance is the rise in recent years of the New Right and its market ideology. The desire to reduce the role of the State (a central feature of the New Right neo-liberal ideology) has significant implications for the field of health and health-care delivery. We have argued in this book that if equity is to remain as a central objective of the health-care system, then the market cannot function as a means of allocating. Unfortunately the failures of State planning in the past have fuelled the arguments of those opposed to a significant interventionist role for the State.

The planning system has a responsibility to show that it can provide better answers to the dilemma of the scarcity of resources and unlimited health needs than that provided by a market solution. In order to do this it must dispel the myths of planning that have been outlined above. Only if these can be dispelled and positive attitudes inculcated can planning, as a means to bettering the future, itself have any real future. It is an important function of planners, policy-makers, and training institutions, and indeed of donor agencies, to look for means of dispelling these misperceptions about planning, and to seek to replace them instead with positive and broad-based attitudes. If this book has assisted at all in this process then it will have achieved its purpose.

INTRODUCTORY READING

There are various articles that deal with the general issue of the changing role and capacity of health planning in the light of HSR, including Bossert *et al.* (1998), Cassells (1994), and Green (1995). Cassells and Janovsky (1992), Green *et al.* (1997), and Jeffery (1986a) include case-studies of specific planning systems.

There is a growing body of literature on the role of economists. Some examples include Andreano (1993), Donaldson (1992), Green (1990), Hanson (1992), Hsiao (1995), Lee (1983), and Normand (1991).

Articles on the role of aid and aid agencies include Buse and Walt (1996 and 1997), Hiscock (1995), Lob-Levyt (1990), Stefanini and Ruck (1992).

EXERCISE 14

Using the criteria set out in Table 14.1, assess the planning system of a country known to you. How could it be strengthened?

REFERENCES AND FURTHER READING

Andreano, R. (1993). Reflections on the economist and health economics in an international setting. *Social Science and Medicine*, 36(2), 137–41.
Bossert, T. *et al.* (1998). Transformation of ministries of health in the era of health reform: the case of Colombia. *Health Policy and Planning*, 13(1), 59–77.
Bryant, J. H. *et al.* (1997). Ethics, equity and renewal of WHO's health for all strategy. *World Health Forum*, 18, 107–15.
Buse, K. and Walt, G. (1996). Aid coordination for health sector reform: a. conceptual framework for analysis and assessment. *Health Policy*, 38(3), 173–87.
Buse, K. and Walt, G. (1997). An unruly melange? Co-ordinating external resources to the health sector: a review. *Social Science and Medicine*, 45(3), 449–64.
Cassells, A. (1994). Health sector reform: key issues in less developed countries. *Journal of International Development*, 7(3), 329–47.
Cassells, A. and Janovsky, K. (1992). A time of change: health policy planning and organization in Ghana. *Health Policy and Planning*, 7(2), 144–54.
Creese, A. *et al.* (1998). Health systems for the 21st century. *World Health Statistics Quarterly*, 51(1), 21–8.
Dievler, A. (1997). Fighting tuberculosis in the 1990s: how effective is planning in policy making? *Journal of Public Health Policy*, 18(2),167–87.
Donaldson, C. (1992). Agenda for health: an economic view. *British Medical Journal*, 304, 770–1.
Gish, O. (1977). *Guidelines for health planners*. Tri-Med, London.
Green, A. (1990). Health economics: are we being realistic about its value? *Health Policy and Planning*, 5, 274–9.

Green, A. (1995). The state of health planning in the 90s. *Health Policy and Planning*, 10(1), 22–28.

Green, A., Rana, M., Ross, D. *et al.* (1997). Health planning in Pakistan: a case study. *International Journal of Health Planning and Management*, 12(3), 187–205.

Hanson, K. (1992). AIDS: what does economics have to offer? *Health Policy and Planning*, 7(4), 315–28.

Hilleboe, H. E., Barkhuus, A. and Thomas, W. C. (1972). *Approaches to national health planning*. Public Health Paper No. 46, WHO, Geneva.

Hiscock, J. (1995). Looking a gift horse in the mouth: the shifting power balance between the Ministry of Health and donors in Ghana. *Health Policy and Planning*, 10, Suppl. 28–39.

Honadle, G. H. and Rosengard, J. K. (1983). Putting 'projectised' development in perspective. *Public Administration and Development*, 3, 299–305.

Hsiao, W. (1995). Abnormal economics in the health sector. *Health Policy*, 32, 125–39.

Jeffery, R. (1986a). Health planning in India 1951–1984: The role of the planning commission. *Health Policy and Planning*, 1, 127–37.

Jeffery, R. (1986b). New patterns in health sector aid to India. *International Journal of Health Services*, 16, 121–39.

Lee, K. (1983). Health care in the developing world: the role of economists and economics. *Social Science and Medicine*, 17(24), 2007–2015.

Lob-Levyt, J. (1990). Compassion, economics, politics. What are the motives behind health-sector aid?. *Health Policy and Planning*, 5, 82–7.

Mooney, G. (1994). *Key issues in health economics*. Harvester Wheatsheaf, Hemel Hempstead.

NHS Confederation Briefing (1997). *Planning and priorities: guidance for 1998/99*. No. 4; September, 1–4.

Normand, C. (1991). Economics, health and the economics of health. *British Medical Journal*, 303, 1572–7.

Okuonzi, S. A. and Macrae, J. (1995). Whose policy is it anyway? International and national influences on health policy development in Uganda. *Health Policy and Planning*, 10(2), 122–32.

Rispel, L., Doherty, J., Makiwane, F. *et al.* (1996). Developing a plan for primary health care facilities in Soweto, South Africa: part I: guiding principles and methods. *Health Policy and Planning*, 111(4), 385–93.

Ross, D. J. (1990). Aid co-ordination. *Public Administration and Development*, 10, 331–42.

Sorkin, A. (1984). *Health economics: an introduction*, 2nd edn. Lexington, London.

Stanton, B. and Wouters, A. (1992). Guidelines for pragmatic assessment for health planning in developing countries. *Health Policy*, 21, 187–209.

Stefanini, A. and Ruck, N. F. (1992). Managing externally assisted health projects for sustainability. *International Journal of Health Planning and Management*, 7, 199–210.

Unger, J.-P and Criel, B. (1995). Principles of health infrastructure planning in less developed countries. *International Journal of Health Planning and Management*, 10, 113–28.

Vaughan, P., Walt, G., and Mills, A. (1985). Can ministries of health support primary health care? Some suggestions for structural reorganisation and planning. *Public Administration and Development*, 5, 1–12.

Zaidi, S. A. (1994). Planning in the health sector: for whom, by whom? *Social Science and Medicine*, 39(9), 1385–93.

Index

Note: page numbers in *italics* refer to figures,
tables and boxes

Abel-Smith B 66, 95, 145
access to health-care 51, 53
accountability 56
accounting 229–30, *231*, 232–4
activity planning 244, 247
administrative costs 109
administrative feasibility 204
advocacy
  minorities 283
  planning for health 92
Africa 12, 108, 111
  see also specific countries
age groups, unit costs 96
aid
  external donor 291
  programme 292
  projects 238
  see also donors
AIDS
  disease-pattern change 98
  programmes 66
Akehurst R 193
alcohol, government-related organization
  interests 89, *90*
allocative efficiency 99–100
allopathic private practitioners 75, 79
Alma-Ata Declaration x, 43–4, 49–50
  community participation 55
  interventions 49, 50
analysis, paralysis by 118, 142
Anand S 65, 157, 162
anti-poverty measures 7
appraisal xi
  see also economic appraisal
area characteristics 139–41
Arhin DC 108
Asia 12
  see also specific countries
autonomy, clinical 16

Bamako Initiative (UNICEF) 55, 109
Bangladesh 4, 122
barefoot doctor scheme 48
Barker C 65, 157, 162
basket funding 110
benefit to cost ratio (BCR) 201, 202
Bennett S 79, 88, 93, 97
Blades CA 204
blocking device *118*
Bryant JH 281
budgeting 33, 215, 226–9
  annual 226
  capital-led allocation 225
  cash-limited 219
  central government 227, 228
  decentralization 227
  historical incrementalist 224–5
  negotiation 228
  policy 227
  programme 217, *218*
  resource allocation 219–20, *221*, 222–6
  review 227
  service objectives 227
  volume 219
  zero-based 226
budgets
  capital 217–19
  cash-limited 219
  cycle 229, *230*
  decentralization 216, 220
  draft 229
  equity 220
  final 229
  information 179
  institutional 216–17
  management 229–7
  managers 216–17
  national health plan 299
  planning system 295, 297, 300
  programme 216–17, 217, *218*
  recurrent 217–19
Burden of Disease (BoD) 65, 124, 157, 162
business planning 39

Buxton MJ 193

capital
    allocation 223
    costs 177–8
    expenditure 218
    funding 237–8
    planning 39
    social opportunity costs 199
card scheme, Thailand 108
CARE 78
Carrin G 122
cash-flow analysis 186–7
Cassels A 110
censuses 129
Chambers R 129
change ix
    planning 6, 19, 27, 238
    resistance 62–3, 242
charitable organizations 76
child health 157
Child to Child teaching 58
Child to Child Trust 58
China, barefoot doctor scheme 48
choices 3–7
    planning 5, 6
    public health sector 5
clinical autonomy 16
clinicians, management involvement 99
clinics, child 49
Cochrane A 49
Coleman G 247
collaboration, efficiency 84
Collins C 60, 61, 63
colonies
    exploitation 48
    independence 2
    public health recognition 45
    underdevelopment 48
communicable disease programmes 66
community
    decision-making 161
    development initiatives 48
    empowerment 7
    finance mechanisms 95, 96
    financing 56–7, 66, 105, 109
    health needs perception 142
    health workers 48, 56
    need perception 153–4
    option appraisal of effects 205
    participation 55–7
    planning input 17
    priority setting in PHC 166
    real costs 191

    self-help schemes 56–7
    situational analysis 148
Community Health Councils 47
competition 61
    efficiency 84
    long-term efficiency 65
    NGOs 86
    objectives shift 65
    perfect 11
comprehensive rationalism 24, 25–6, 27
consultation 288
consumerism 46–7
consumers, knowledge 10
consumption good 8
    health 155–6
contestability 65
contingencies, costing 177, 179
contracting out 99
corporate planning 39
Corrigan P 8, 44
cost-benefit analysis (CBA) 191, 192, 195,
        196, 197
appraisal 201–2, 203
cost-effectiveness analysis (CEA) 162, 191,
        192, 195, 196
    appraisal 99
    cost per outcome 202
    discounting 200
    efficiency 33
    outcome measurement 197–8
cost-effectiveness ratio 192, 201
costing xi, 170
    accuracy 180–1
    activity identification 176, 177
    checklist 178
    contingencies 177, 179
    inflation 177, 179–80
    information 179, 180–1
    methods 176–80
    public sector 173
    resources 192, 195
        identification 177–9
    step-down techniques 184, 186
    steps 176
costs 170–1, 172, 173
    age groups 96
    apportionment of joint 184, 186
    capital 177–9
    coefficients 182
    comparison with benefits 192, 201
    economies of scale 182, 185
    escalation 98
    fixed 183, 184
    information 170–1

marginal 183–4
market prices 174, *175*, 176
options 170–1
priority setting 158–9
public sector planning 171
real prices 174, *175*, 176
recurrent 177, 178–9, 182
relationships 182–4, *185*, *186*
shunting 224
social *172*, 176
social opportunity 199
transaction 65
UK health care 4
unit 181–2
variable 183, 184
cost-utility analysis (CUA) 191, *192*, 195, 196
    cost per outcome 202, 203
    outcome measurement 197–8
Council for Health Research for Development
    130
Craft N 120
Cranshaw R 165
critical path analysis 253, *254*
cultural characteristics 139
Curry S 174

data
    aggregation 122
    collection 132
decentralization 59–61
    budgeting/budgets 216, 220, 227
    decision-making 162, 285–7
    feedback systems 132
    HSR 65, 66, 219–20, 277
    human resources planning 277
    inequity 61
    PHC 68
    planning system 285–7, 294
    public sector 84
    resource allocation 162, 220
decision-making
    central 285–7
    community 161
        participation 56
    consistency 287–8
    consumer involvement 47
    criteria 281–2
    decentralization 60, 162, 285–7
    local 285–7
    openness 283
    participation 103
    planning 5, 6, 18
    process 165
    structures 282–4

De Koning K 120
delegation of powers 59
Delphi technique 165
demand-side, finance system 101–2
demographic shifts
    resource reallocation 100
    social insurance 108
demography
    information 139
    situational analysis 31
dependency theory 48
dependents, economic 96–7
depreciation 178
developing countries v, ix
development
    funding 47
    planning 38
    priorities 156
development policy
    shifts 47–9
    social ends 47–8
    village level 48
devolution 59
    State to NGOs 87
diagnosis 119–20
Disability Adjusted Life Year (DALY) 65, 124,
    157, 159, 198
discounted cash flow analysis 191
discounting *192*, 198–9, *200*
disease
    burden 124
    classification 120
    health measure 124
    notifiable 129
    pattern changes 97–8
    ranking 163, *164*
    see also communicable disease programmes
distributional effects of project 205
Dixon J 165
donor agencies
    conferences 292
    priority setting 161
    project-based changes 300
donors 34
    co-ordination 300
    funding 238–9
    see also aid
Doyal L 120

early discharge policy *186*
Eastern Europe ix
ecological effects of project 206
economic appraisal 190
    activity objectives 192–3

alternative options *192*, 193
analysis *192*, 195–6
benefit valuing 196–7
CBA 201–2, 203
CEA 202, 203
checklist *204*
cost comparison with benefits *192*, 201
cost-effectiveness ratio *192*, 201
criteria for exclusion 193–4
CUA 202, 203
discounting *192*, 198–9, *200*
exclusion of unfeasible options *192*, 193–4
health sector benefits 195
making *192*, 193
option appraisal 203–6
perspectives 194–5
resource costing *192*, 195
resource identification *192*, 194–5
sensitivity analysis *192*, 199, *200*, 201
steps *192*
techniques 65, 162, 191–9, *200*, 201–3
see also option appraisal
economic demand, need 153
economic planning 38
economic producers 96–7
economics 291
  theories 10–11
economic shifts, social insurance 108
economies of scale 182, *185*
economy growth 155–6
educational characteristics 139
effectiveness of intervention
  priority setting 158–9
  situational analysis 147
efficiency 232, 233–4
  situational analysis 147
elasticity, economic *105*
employment
  insurance schemes 107
  see also occupational health-care providers
empowerment 7
enterprise culture 47
environmental effects of project 206
epidemiology 291
equity 50–3, *54*, 55
  budget-setting 220
  definitions 50–1, 52
  economic pressures 97
  exemption schemes 106
  finance system 101–2
  horizontal 53
  occupational health-care providers 80
  option appraisal 205
  planning 52–3

  for health 92
    systems 282, 301
  resource allocation 161–2
  situational analysis 147
  tax-based systems 109
  vertical 53
  see also inequality
Estonia 4
Etzioni A 26
Europe, State intervention 2
evaluation xi, 33, *128*, 190–1, 207–8
  implementing 211
  indicators 210
  information 210
  inputs 208–9
  methodology 210–11
  outcome effects 209–10
  outputs 209–10
  planning for health 92
  political purpose 208
  questions 208–11
  situational analysis 211
  summative 207–8
evidence-based medicine 65
exemption schemes, fee for service 106
Expanded Programme of Immunization (EPI)
    192–3
expectations of medical care 97
externalities 191

Fanshell S 44
fee for service 103, 105–7
  exemption schemes 106
feldshers 48
feminist analytical perspective 120
finanacial appraisal 191
finance/finance system x, 95
  alternative approaches 103, *104*, 105–10
  availability 205
  capital 110
  collective 103
  criteria for choosing 100–3
  deficit 110
  demand-side effects 101–2
  demographic changes 96–7
  equity 101–2
  health-care supply 101
  ideologies 95–6
  planning 110–11
  redistributive *104*
  resources 145
  revenue-generating ability 101
  sources 126
  State 12, *13*, 14

user-charge 95, 96
viability 100–1
financial control
  central government function 227
  donations 239
financial management 229–30, *231*, 232–4
  corrective actions 232–4
  implementation systems 255
  monitoring 229–30, *231*, 232
flexibility of planning system 6, 288–90
flowcharts 247, 251, *252*, 254–5
forecasting, econometric 121, 122
foreign exchange 174, *175*
funding
  development 47
  donors 238–9
  shifts for HSR 66
  supplementary 232, 233

Gantt chart 251, *253*
gastroenteritis 58
gender
  health planning 53
  information on issues 120
  option appraisal 206
geographical area 140
Ghana 122
Gilson L 145
Gish O 145
goals 32
GOBIFF programme 62
government
  policies and NGOs 81–8
  service 84
  see also State
grants 105, 110
Green A 61, 65, 76, 93, 157, 162, 184
Griffiths A 111, 145
gross national product (GNP) 9, 47, 98
  development 155

Hall TL 265
Hanson K 65, 157, 162
health
  agencies x
    impacting on 74–5, 89
  concept 44–9
  consumption good 8, 155–6
  definition 44
  education 55, 58
  gain indicators 158
  holistic notion 45–6
  investment 8–9, 155–6
  multisectoral approach 57–8
  objectives 240
  perceptions 154–9, 160
  planning 74–5, 91–2
    rationale 2–3
    system 288
  policy x
  rights 8
  state 7
  strategy 89
  systems research 130
  see also disease; ill health; need
Health for All goal 43, 49
Health by the People 48
health care
  access 8
  demands approach to human resource
    planning 265–6
  needs 124
  planning system 288
  rights 8
  sector planning 75–6, 77, 78–80
  state of health 7
  supply side 139
health centres, development 49
Health Maintenance Organization (HMO) 107
health professionals
  need perception 153–4
  planning 17
  priority setting in PHC 166
  situational analysis 148
health promotion 35
  activities impacting on 89
  change creation 90
  multisectoral approach 89, 90
  PHC 59
  planning 88–91
  public health initiatives 45
  regulatory approach 91
  suasive action 91
health-related agencies x
health sector
  funding 100
  planning 15
health sector benefits
  economic appraisal 195
  valuing 196–7
Health Sector Reform (HSR) v, 35, 63–6
  decentralization 65, 66, 219–20, 277
  funding shifts 66
  human resources planning 276–7
  market approaches 64–5
  organizational framework 245
  PHC 66–8
  planning 66–8

policies vi, 43, 193
private sector 276
separation of functions 64
user orientation 66
vertical programmes 66
health services
facilities 143–4
gaps 144
organizational arrangements 144
political control 160
situational analysis 143–4
utilization 144
health status
changes 9
improvement aim 19
indicators of change 197–8
insuree 106
need indicator 124
utilization of health-care 52
herd immunity 11
Hilleboe HE 26
holistic notion of health 45–6
Honigsbaum G 165
Hornby P 265
hospitals
city-based 224
quasi-governmental 76
household surveys 129
human capital 196
human resources xi
data 262
diversion 88
personnel supply/demand 263–4
plan 298
private sector impact 262–3
problems 261
professional attitudes 262
responsibility for planning 262
supply lead-times 262
see also personnel
human resources planning 39, 260, 263–8,
    269, 270–6
components 263
decentralization 277
demand 265–6
    estimation 266–7
demand-targeted policies 273
emigration 271–2
health demands 267
health needs 267
HSR 276–7
immigration 271–2
implementation 274–5
mismatch in demand/supply 273–4

norm-based 267
personnel to population ratio 266
private sector 276
productivity changes 272
relationship to planning process 275–6
review 274
roles 267
service targets 266, 267–8, *269–70*
supply-demand equation 264
supply estimation 268, 270, *271*
supply-targeted policies 274
trained staff 271
training schools 272

ideologies, finance mechanisms 95–6
ill health 155
    pattern developing countries 45, *46*
Illich I 49
immunity 10–11
immunization 45, *46*, 192–3
    expanded programme (EPI) 66
    mobile programme *269–70*
implementation *128*, 239–40
    bar chart 251, *253*
    critical path analysis 253, *254*
    documentation 245–7, *248*
    flowcharts 247, 251, *252*, 254–5
    improving 243–7
    Logical Framework 247, *249–51*
    monitoring 255–6
    operational policy 247, *251*
    planner role 245
    planning system 92, 295–6, 299–300
    plans 33
    poor 240–3
    services provided by other agencies 257
    timetabling 247, 251, *252*, 253–5
income
    distribution 122
    health links 158
incrementalism 24, 27–30
India, health planning 2, 15
indicators
    inequality 52, 53, *54*
    information 119
individuals
    empowerment 7
    responsibility for health care 9
    role in health/health-care 46–7
industrialized countries ix
inequality
    decentralization 61
    indicators 52, 53, *54*
inflation, costing *177*, 179–80

information 116–18
  accuracy 118–21
  aggregation 122
  analysis 131
  baseline 210
  blocking device *118*
  budgets 179
  collection 119, 127–30
  control 132
  costing 179, 180–1
  cost of obtaining 121
  data collector feedback 132
  demographic 139
  dissemination 99
  evaluation 210
  forms 117–18
  gender issues 120
  hard 117
  health systems research 130
  immeasurability 117
  indicators 119
    need 123–5
  input 210
  interpretation 119
  mortality/morbidity 120
  outcome 210
  planning system 295
  policy 127
  political context 127
  power 117
  presentation 131
  process 210
  provision for priority setting 159
  requirements *128*
  research 133
  resources 125–6
  selection 116–27
  services 125, 126–7
  skills 132–3
  soft 117
  systems x–xi, 127–32, 224
    management 132–3
  types 123–7
  underlying trend projection 121
information technology (IT) 117–18, 133
infrastructure 139–41
inputs, evaluation 208–9
input–output equation 83
insurance schemes
  comprehensiveness 108
  health status 106
  private 103, 105–7
  see also social insurance
internal rate of return (IRR) 201

International Classification of Diseases 120
International Health Policy Program 130
International Journal of Epidemiology 129
International Labour Organization (ILO) 48
    social insurance 96
International Monetary Fund (IMF) 15, 97
interventions 7
    effectiveness measurement 65
investment 8–9
    child health 157
    health 155–6

justice, planning systems 301

Kielmann AA 129
Killingsworth J 62
King M 49
knowledge, consumers 10
Koblisky M 120

labour, migrant 272
Latin America 2
    rational planning 26, 30
    social insurance 156
legal feasibility 204
legislative framework 245
Leighton C 111
Leslie J 53, 120
levels of planning 36
life expectancy of children 157
Lindblom CE 27
line item control 234
loans 105, 110
Loewenson R 51
Logical Framework 247, *249–51*
Loomes G 159
Lysack CL 55

Mach EP 145
McKenzie L 159
McKeown T 45
malaria 142
management 37
    by objectives 244
    centralized 63
    clinician involvement 99
    market approaches 64–5
    reports/returns 129
    skill lack 243
    structure lack 243
management information systems (MIS) 132
Managerial Process for National Health
    Development (WHO) 30, 40, 217, 238
managers, budgets 216–17

market
  ability to pay 11
  demand-based 151
  health care allocations 9–10
  internal 65, 99
  prices 174, *175*, 176
  private 10
  theory 84
Martin M 120
Marxist economic theory 10
maternal health 157
Matthias A 76, 93
Médecins sans Frontières 85
medical assistants 48
Meija A 265
milk, formula 58
Mills A 186
Mills M 111, 145
minority groups, advocacy 283
missionary-provided care 76
models of planning 24–31
  comprehensive rationalism 24, 25–6, 27
  incrementalism 27–30
  mixed scanning 26–7
money 125–6
monitoring plans 33
Mooney GH 196
moral hazard 107
morbidity
  health need 152–3
  information 120
  measures 159
  priority setting 158–9
Morley D 49
mortality
  health need 152–3
  information 120
  rate 155
  risk reduction value 196
  standarized ratio (SMR) 220, 222
Moser CON 53
mother-and-child health (MCH) programme
    217
multiagency collaboration 61
multisectoralism 103
multivariable decision matrices 163, *164*
Murray CJL 157, 159, 162

Nancholas S 247
national health plan
  draft 298
  unit budgets 299
National Health Service (UK) 2, 14, 151
Navarro V 48

need 124
  approach to human resource planning 266
  assessment 220, *221*
  community perception 142
  economic demand 153
  gradations 152
  health-care 124
  human resources planning 266
  indicators 123–5
  medical concepts 153
  medical perception 142
  meeting 4
  morbidity/mortality 152–3
  perceptions 152, 153–4, 160
  priority setting 151–3
  regional 222
  service split 220, 222
  situational analysis 141–2
need-focused policies 15
needs-based planning 11, 151
net present value (NPV) 201, 202
network analysis 247
New Deal (US) 1
Newell K 48
New Right 9
  competition 61
  ideology 156
  market approaches 64–5
non-governmental organizations (NGOs) 35
  advantages 82–5
  competition 86
  contracted services 85
  efficiency 83–4
  experience diversity 86
  fields of work 85
  fragmentation 86
  government policies 81–8
  grass-roots organizations 85
  health-care involvement 75, 76, 77, 78
  indigenous 78
  information availability 82
  international links 83, 84
  managerial inefficiency 86
  motives 86
  multisectoral approach 85
  organizational inefficiency 86
  personnel syphoning 86
  planning levels 36–7
  politically sensitive services 84–5
  religious 77–8
  resources 83
    generation 84
  secular 78
  size 83

volunteers 84
see also private-for-profit organizations
non-health sector inputs to situational
    analysis 143
non-profit organizations 64
Nordberg E 129
nutrition, promotion 57

objectives 32
    setting 91–2
objectivity in planning 28
occupational health-care providers 75, 77, 79–
    80
operating costs 177–9
opinion, informed 129–30
opportunity cost xi, 170
opposition to plans 34
option appraisal 32–3, 36, *128*, 190–1, 203–6
    acceptability of programme 205
    administrative feasibility 204
    checklists 206
    distributional effects 205
    ecological effects 206
    economic effects 205
    environmental effects 206
    equity 205
    evaluation 207
    finance availability 205
    forms 206
    gender 206
    knock-on effects 205
    legal feasibility 204
    long-term sustainability 205
    pilot activity expansion 206
    planning for health 92
    political effects 205
    programming 206–7
    resource allocation 207
    resource availability 205
    social effects 205
    technical feasibility 204
options, costs 170–1
oral rehydration solutions 58
Oregon, priority-setting process 165
organizational framework 245
outputs evaluation 209–10
Oxfam 78

PAHO-CENDES 26, 30, 40
paper rights 108
paralysis by analysis 118, 142
paramedical staff 48
participative planning systems 132
pay, performance-related 65

payment ability 11, 102
peri-urban community 158
personnel xi, 39
    central government function 227
    demand 263
    health service 139
    labour market entry 272
    losses 272
    plan 274–5
    planning system 295
    policies 275
    population ratio 266
    records 271
    resources 145
    supply 263
        estimation 268, 270, *271*
        information sources 273
    syphoning 86
    trained staff 271–2
    training 275
    see also human resources
perspective planning 39
Peru 122
perverse incentives 224
physical planning 39
Physical Quality of Life Indicator (PQLI) 159,
    198
planners, specialist 301
planning body membership 288
planning/planning system vii–x, 1, 280
    activity 3, 24, 37–40, 244, 247
    aid programme 292
    aims 19
    allocative 3, 24, 27, 244
    assessment criteria 281–92
    attitudes 15–18
    budgets 295, 297, 300
    business 39
    capital 39
    change 6, 19, 27
    choices 5, 6
    circular 297
    consistency 287–8
    corporate 39
    culture 300–1
    culture development 280
    cycles 289–90
    decentralization 285–7, 294
    decision-making 5, 6, 18
        criteria 281–2
        structures 282–4
    development 38
    direction 288–90
    documentation 284, 285

donor co-ordination 300
economic 38
equity 282, 301
external donor aid 291
failures 16–18, 19
finance 110–11
flexibility 6, 288–90
formalized 1–2
functions 282
health 288
health-care 288
health professionals 17
health sector 15
human resources 39
implementation 295–6, 299–300
information 295
  base 290
  systems x–xi
infrastructure 63
intention 288–9
interrelationships 282
isolation of process 17
justice 301
levels 36–7
misperceptions 300–1
monitoring 299
needs-based 11, 151
open process 18
participative 132
perception of health 7
personnel 295
perspective 39
physical 39
planning circular 297
policy statement 297
political activity 18–19
political process 33–4
priority setting xi
private health sector 6
procedures 284, 296–9
processes 284–5
programme 39
progress reports 299
projects 39, 300
public sector 171
purpose 281
range of alternatives 6
regulatory 39
resources 292
role 281
rolling cycles *289*, 290, 293–4
service 39
spiral x, xi, 31–3
  conceptual stages 289

implementation 239–40
State 1, 15, 285
strategic 38
technical resources 290–2
techniques 301
technocratic activity 18–19
terms 37–40
timetable 284
tools 284–5, *286*
training plan 299
unit plans 297
values 281–2, 301
Planning Programme Budgeting Systems
  (PPBS) 217
plans 3
  assessment 298
  capital 39
  operational 40
  production 300
  reconciliation 298
  rolling 39
  work 40
policy
  aid programme 292
  alternatives 87–8
  changes 241–2
  development 33–4
  formation by State 11
  guideline priority setting in PHC 166
  information 127
  outcome 33–4
  personnel 275
  setting 37
  situational analysis 32, 141
  statement on planning system 297
Politi C 122
political activity 18–19
political environment 141
political mapping 27, 127, 288
political process 33–4
population
  age structure 96
  characteristics 138–9
  growth 96
pressure groups 55–6
prevention, PHC 59
preventive services
  funding 109
  personal 105
prices 174, *175*, 176
pricing 11
Primary Health Care (PHC) v–vi, 7
  Alma-Ata Declaration 49–50
  appropriate technology 58–9

centralized management 63
community participation 55–7
decentralization 59–61, 68
equity 50–3, *54*, 55
health/health need perceptions 160
health promotion 59
implementation obstacles 61–3
misinterpretation 62
multiagency collaboration 61
multisectoral approach 57–8
need determination 153
origins 43–4
planning 52
  infrastructure 63
  systems ix, x
policy 282
  delivery 67–8
political resistance 62–3
preventive approach 59
priority setting 153, 165–6
resistance to change 62–3
resource allocation 161–2
selective strategies 62
service mix 58–9
priorities, changes 241–2
prioritizing 5
priority setting xi, 32, *128*, 151
activity objectives 193
costs of intervention 158–9
decision-making process 165
donor agencies 161
economic appraisal 162
effectiveness of intervention 158–9
health need 151–3
health perceptions 160
ill health effects 155
information provision 159
judgements 159
multivariable decision matrices 163, *164*
need perceptions 160
PHC 165–6
resource allocation 161–2
target groups 157–8
within planning framework 161–3, *164*, 165
private allopathic practitioners 75, 79
Private Finance Initiatives 110
private-for-profit organizations 64, 77
advantages 82, 83
allopathic sector 75, 79
resource generation 84
see also non-governmental organizations
  (NGOs)
private insurance 103, 105–7
private sector

aims 35
appraisal 191
HSR 276
human resources planning 276
impact on human resources 262–3
planning 6, 34–6
  levels 36–7
promotion 15
structure 140–1
private voluntary organizations (PVOs) 76
producers, economic 96–7
programme
  budgeting 217, *218*
  location 256–7
  planning 39
  specificity lack 243
programming 33, *128*
  planner role 245
  planning for health 92
projects 237–9
  implementation units 255–6
  location 256–7
  monitoring 255–6
  planning 39
    systems 300
public behavioural valuation 196
public health
  colonial country recognition 45
  funding 109
  initiatives 45
public sector ix
  aims 35
  appraisal 191
  choices 5
  costing 173
  decentralization 84
  large-scale projects 174
  planning 34–6, 171
    levels 36–7
  role 75
  structure 140–1
purchaser–provider split 64, 76
purchasing 84

Quality Adjusted Life Years (QALYs) 159, 198
quality of life 125, 155
  health status indicators 197
  improvement 197
quantophrenia 204

Rainhorn JD 165
rapid appraisals 129
rationalism, comprehensive 24, 25–6, 27
rational planning, realistic 31–3

rationing of resources 5
recession
    economic 97
    world 156
Red Crescent 78
Red Cross 78, 85
reform *see* Health Sector Reform
regulation, State 12–13
regulatory planning 39
Reich MR 27, 127
religious characteristics 139
Rensburg HCJ 53
reproduction 53
resource allocation xi, 151, 215
    budgeting 219–20, *221*, 222–6
    capital-led 225
    central government guidance 228
    decentralization 162, 220
    decisions 18
    equity 161–2
    health indicators 158
    model *221*
    option appraisal 207
    PHC 161–2
    priority setting 161–2, 166
    specific criteria 223–4
    weighting 220, 222, 223
Resource Allocation Working Party (UK;
        1976) 222–3
resources x
    availability 205
    costing *192*, 195
    donor pooling 110
    effective 98–100
    estimation 179
    evaluation 208–9
    financial 145
    flows *146*
    gap 242–3
    generation
        NGOs 84
        private-for-profit organizations 84
    identification for costing 177–9
    imbalance 16
    indicators 4
    information 125–6
    lack 242–3
    misallocation 16
    money terms expression *177*, 179
    NGOs 83
    personnel 145
    rationing 5
    reallocation 99–100, 219
    scarcity 4

situational analysis 32, 144–5, *146*
    transformation to services 209
revenue-earning ability, net 101
revenue generation, local 224
Revolving Drug Funds 95, 109
Rifkin S 55, 62
rights to health/health-care 8
Roemer MI 156
rolling plans 219
rural areas
    health-care 158, 224
    populations 53
Russell S 102

sanitation 58
Save the Children Fund 78
scanning, mixed 24
scarcity 3–7, 170
    resources 4
sectoral planning 275–6
Sector Wide Approach 110, 239, 256
    donors 292
Segall M 51, *53*, 224
self-help schemes 48, 56–7
sensitivity analysis *192*, 199, *200*, 201
sentinel reporting 129
service managers, situational analysis 148
services
    activity levels 234
    evaluation 209
    information 125, 126–7
    management planning 243–5
    planning 39
    provision
        by other agencies 257
        health ministry role 35
        State 12, *13*, 14
    quality
        reduction 234
        situational analysis 147
    resource transformation 209
    situational analysis 32
    targets 266
        estimation of human resources demand
            267–8, *269–70*
    user participation 56
shadow pricing 174, *175*, 176
shared assumptions 28
Shipp PJ 267
Simmonds S 211
situational analysis 31–2, 36, *128*, 137–8
    area characteristics 139–41
    commentary 147–8
    cultural characteristics 139

documentation 137
educational characteristics 139
effectiveness 147
efficiency 147
equity 147
evaluation 211
health needs 141–2
health services 143–4
infrastructure 139–41
issues *148*
national 296–7
non-health sector 143
option appraisal 206–7
performing 148
planning for health 91
policy 141
political environment 141
population characteristics 138–9
priority setting in PHC 166
religious characteristics 139
resources 144–5, *146*
service quality 147
smallpox campaign 45, 99
Smith R 89, *90*
social costs *172*, 176
social insurance 95, 96, 102, 103, 108–9
  demographic/economic shifts 108
  Latin America 156
  systems 66
social opportunity costs 199
social security institutions 14
social time-preference 199
social welfare
  responsibility 2
  shift from 156
socio-economic characteristics 31
socio-economic situation 140
South Africa 51–2
stakeholder analysis 27, 127, 288
stakeholders 18
standard of living 45
standarized mortality ratio (SMR) 220, *222*
State
  attitudes to health-care types 14–15
  devolution to NGOs 87
  duties 80
  health care
    financing 12, *13*, 14
    investment 9
    involvement 75
    provision *77*
    quality 80
  ideology 80
  intervention 2

laissez-faire towards NGOs 87
planning 1, 2, 7, 15, 285, 301–2
policy
  alternatives 87
  formation 11
  implementation towards NGOs 88
  tools 88
regulation 12–13
regulatory controls on NGOs 87
role vi, ix
service provision 12, *13*, 14
support for NGOs 87
transfer of NGO services to government
  87–8
see also government
strategic planning vi, 38
Structural Adjustment Programmes 63, 64
surveys, information collecting 127–9
sustainability, long-term 205

Tangcharoensathien V 79, 97
Tanzania 76
targets 32
taxation 102
  trade-based 109
tax-based systems 108–9
tax revenue 103, 108–9
technical efficiency 99
technical feasibility 204
technocratic activity 18–19
technology, appropriate 58–9
Thailand 97
  card scheme 108
time-preference, social 199
topography 140
Townsend P 51
traditional practitioners 75, 77, 80
training plan 299
treatment records 129
tuberculosis control 66
Turshen M 45

UK
  health care costs 4
  Second World War 2
underemployment 97
underfunding 99
unemployment 97
Unger J-P 62
UNICEF *54*, 62, 66, 95–6
  Bamako Initiative 55, 109
unit costs 181–2
United States, New Deal 1
unit plans 297

user charges 103, 105
　administration 101
users, health sector orientation 66
USSR 1
　community health workers 48
　health planning 15
utilization of health-care 51–2, 53

Vaughan JP 49
virement 232, 233
vital registration 129
voluntary organizations 76
volunteers, NGOs 84

waiting lists 151
Walsh JA 62
Walt G 33, 49, 62
Warren KS 62
water supplies 58
wealth distribution 48
web sites 21–3
Welsch HG 165
West P 52
WHO

gender issues 120
Health for All goal 43, 49
health definition 8, 44, 89
Managerial Process for National Health
　Development 30, 40, 217, 238
smallpox campaign 45
women, health plans 53
women's movement 56
World Bank 15
　Burden of Disease 65, 124, 157, 162
　DALY 124
　finance mechanisms 95, 96
　health policy 291
　loans 110
　packages of care 62
　user charges 66, 105
　World Development Report (1993) 63, 65,
　　122, 159, 198
World War II 1, 2
World Wide Web 130

Zachus JD 55
Zimbabwe 51–2